# Praise for *The Green Beauty Guide*

"All hail to the lipstick revolution! Today, our world can't afford beauty without a conscience. Even daily shopping habits that seem as mundane as our cosmetic and personal care product choices now have an enormous influence on our future. When shoppers read *The Green Beauty Guide* and put Julie Gabriel's insightful green beauty tips into practice, they are also being Green Patriot environmentalists, helping to build a safe and secure future for the world and for our children—not to mention improving their personal health and their appearance."

*David Steinman, founder of the Green Patriot movement,*
*author of* Safe Trip to Eden *and creator of* 50 Simple Steps
to Save the Earth from Global Warming

"Once we read *The Green Beauty Guide*, we recycled all of our other organic beauty tomes. Julie is the definitive source, and we never hit a beauty counter without her short list of product recommendations and ingredient red flags. Julie educates and inspires us to simply be more beautiful. We could spend hours making all of her fabulous DIY green beauty recipes. Read this book—your skin will thank you, and so will your health!"

*Lisa Blau and Amanda Freeman, cofounders,*
*Vital Juice Daily (www.vitaljuice.com)*

"I am often asked for a resource on cosmetics and ingredients. Julie Gabriel's *The Green Beauty Guide* is an easy-to-read, informative introduction to many facets of the cosmetic world and how it connects to our well-being—from green to synthetic, do-it-yourself to superexpensive. If you are new to this world or even think you know 'green,' step in and discover or rediscover this world and its underbelly."

*Suki Kramer, Suki Pure Skin Care*

"Julie Gabriel has done a stellar job of creating an excellent resource that is powerful, thought-provoking, and incredibly bold. She challenges the system and encourages us to be diligent and informed about what we put on our bodies. Too often, as consumers, we complain to friends and ourselves, but rarely do we take action. I think this book is an incredible show of force, and for the right reasons. Thank you, Julie, for this important tool. I cannot wait to give it to my family and friends."

*Anne Doulbeau, Inara*

"If you care about the health of the planet and your own well-being, Julie Gabriel's *The Green Beauty Guide* will send you running to clean out your medicine cabinet and your cosmetic bag. This book is exceptionally well-researched and a compelling read!"

*Anne Dimon, TravelToWellness.com*

"Powerful and beautifully written! *The Green Beauty Guide* asks all the right questions about the beauty products we use daily on our bodies and offers many helpful suggestions for finding safer alternatives. Tell your friends about this important book. And let's give the beauty industry a makeover!"

*Stacy Malkan, author of* Not Just a Pretty Face:
The Ugly Side of the Beauty Industry *and cofounder of*
*Campaign for Safe Cosmetics, www.SafeCosmetics.org*

"This is the book that I lie awake at night and write in my head. It's the message that we talk about every day on the phone with mamas who are concerned about toxins in mama and baby products. This is the information that pregnant women desperately need. Julie Gabriel has done a fabulous job of organizing the information in an understandable format, and mothers everywhere should start here for more information on toxic chemicals and how to decipher ingredient labels. *The Green Beauty Guide* is a must-read for all women, especially those who are carrying and nursing a baby. Our angel babies are worth it!"

*Melinda Olson, Angel Mama Earth Baby*

# the green beauty guide

## Your Essential Resource to Organic and Natural Skin Care, Hair Care, Makeup, and Fragrances

## Julie Gabriel

Health Communications, Inc.
Deerfield Beach, Florida

*www.hcibooks.com*

The information contained in this book is based upon the research and personal and professional experiences of the author and reflects the author's professional opinion. The publisher does not advocate the use of any particular healthcare protocol but believes in presenting this information to the public. Should the reader have any questions concerning the appropriateness of any procedures or preparation mentioned herein, the reader should consult a professional healthcare advisor.

**Library of Congress Cataloging-in-Publication Data**

Gabriel, Julie.

    The green beauty guide : your essential resource to organic and natural skin care, hair care, makeup, and fragrances / Julie Gabriel.

       p.   cm.

    Includes bibliographical references and index.

    ISBN-13: 978-0-7573-0747-8 (trade pbk.)

    ISBN-10: 0-7573-0747-7 (trade pbk.)

    1. Cosmetics—Environmental aspects. 2. Hygiene products—Environmental aspects. 3. Beauty, Personal. I. Title.

TP983.G26 2008

646.7'2—dc22

2008033951

Publisher: Health Communications, Inc.
        3201 S.W. 15th Street
        Deerfield Beach, FL 33442-8190

R-10-09

*Cover design by Justin Rotkowitz*
*Illustrations by Andrea Perrine Brower*
*Interior design by Larissa Hise Henoch*
*Interior formatting by Lawna Patterson Oldfield*

# contents

To my sweet little Masha

*Beauty is eternity gazing at itself in a mirror.*
*But you are eternity, and you are the mirror.*

Kahlil Gibran
Lebanese-born American philosophical essayist,
novelist, and poet (1883–1931)

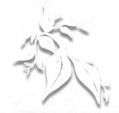

# foreword

**f**inally, some sane and accurate advice about cosmetics and beauty products! Julie Gabriel pulls no punches in this frank, honest, and totally unbiased masterpiece about the good, the bad, and the ugly sides of the cosmetic industry. First and foremost, she helps you understand that when you buy a product that makes various beauty claims, you are dealing with a business that wants to sell you something that may not necessarily be good for your health. In many cases, quite the opposite is true. How do you know? Reading this book will make you very well-versed in the numerous chemicals that come packaged in facial creams, shampoos, and cleansers. You will know what's safe and what could be harmful. Want to know what a xenoestrogen is? This book will tell you. Read this book because it could save your life.

You aren't manipulated into buying any one philosophy or specific "green" product brand. Not only does this very well-researched book tell you what to look for and avoid in buying and using various lotions, potions, and beauty creams, but it gives you a very practical approach to shopping for what's healthiest and best for your body. Additionally, you will learn how to make green beauty products yourself from raw ingredients and the recipes provided in this book. Since prepackaged green beauty products can be expensive, knowing how to make your own could save you tons of money.

Do not underestimate the advice in this book in regard to your general health. I have been in the practice of natural healing for more than thirty years, and I have had to help my patients undo damage caused by the toxins we find in our food, water, air, prescription drugs, and a long list of cosmetic or beauty products. The ingredients in most of these creams, lotions, shampoos, conditioners, cleansers, and moisturizers are loaded with cancer-causing agents. When you read this book, you will know what they are and how to find better natural alternatives that will actually enhance, not worsen, your general health.

Some of you may ask, "Shouldn't we be getting this type of advice from a board-certified dermatologist?" The answer to this is a most definite no! If you want advice on how to suppress a skin disease like acne or psoriasis with toxic chemicals, see a dermatologist. If you are interested in prevention and health promotion, read this book instead and learn how to effectively deal with cosmetic issues.

Unfortunately, acne, psoriasis, and other skin conditions are often treated with cancer-causing and liver-damaging pills and creams. Also, for seborrhea and psoriasis, coal tar shampoos—known cancer-causing agents—are commonly prescribed. Steroid creams and sunscreens are known to contain cancer-causing ingredients. Sure, such prescriptions will obliterate acne, psoriasis, eczema, and a long list of diseases, but at what price?

Another issue dealt with in-depth by Julie Gabriel is organic versus synthetic beauty products. If it's organic, is it really any better? Here, the author helps the reader sort out fact from fiction in this wildly controversial area. Sometimes what's labeled as organic may actually be a major problem for health.

While you are reading this book, keep in mind that the things you put on your scalp and on your skin can absorb into your system and cause health effects in your internal organs. Once you finish this book, you may be convinced that if it's not safe to eat, it's not safe to use on your skin or scalp. Julie should be congratulated for showing us how to be beautiful and healthy at the same time.

Dr. Zoltan P. Rona, M.D., M.Sc.
Medical Editor of the Benjamin Franklin
Award-winning *Encyclopedia of Natural Healing*

 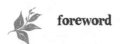

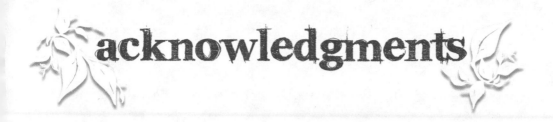

# acknowledgments

**t**his book was unknowingly inspired by Harriet Hubbard Ayer, the nineteenth-century author of *Bath and Body Splash*. It was her idea to use apple cider vinegar for bathing, bay rum for conditioning hair, and oatmeal for washing hands. Her collection of age-old beauty wisdom is the time-tested foundation of homemade, edible beauty recipes in this book. This probably explains why many beauty recipes in this book are good enough to eat. After all, your skin is what you feed it.

I must thank the people who believed that my sincere passion can become a reality. My deepest thanks go to Adina Kahn of Dystel & Goderich for her faith in me and her nonstop support. Deepest thanks to Andrea Gold of HCI Books for her stellar professionalism, warm encouragements, and kind patience. I am grateful to Stacy Malkan of the Campaign for Safe Cosmetics, Dr. Zoltan Rona, M.D., Bianca Presto of Modus Dowal Walker, Melissa Amerian, Lisa Blau, Amanda Freeman, Susie Fairgrieve, Nikki Gersten, Morgan Dub, Richard Isbel, and Katheline St. Fort. Thank you so much. Without you, this book wouldn't have happened.

I am extremely grateful to my husband and daughter for their suffering without a normally functioning mom and wife all these months. Masha, thank you so much for being such a self-contained, happy baby. You are the most beautiful girl in the world. And Mama, maybe now you'll listen and let go of your awful synthetic face creams. I care because I love you.

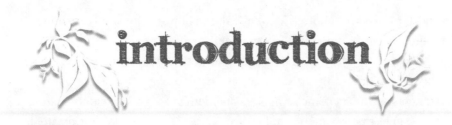

# introduction

**f**or nearly fifteen years, I have been writing about fashion and beauty. I helped women and men make sense of the latest products while declaring some shimmery nail polish an absolute must-have. I witnessed exciting moments when fashion and beauty trends were born as they crystallized in the electric air backstage of fashion shows, during glitzy, glamorous, celebrity-studded events, or in the hectic rush of a fashion shoot. And I am guilty of heralding fashion fads that were forgotten the week after the magazine hit the newsstands. I have interviewed, reviewed, analyzed, and criticized.

My true love is homemade "edible" beauty. Dieting and the subtle, yet powerful ways it shapes our looks fascinates me and makes me search for delicious cures to wrinkles and pimples. As a nutritionist, I have fallen in love with natural ways to improve the skin's clarity, tone, and vitality. When it was time to write this book, I could not resist sharing everything I have learned in those years about skin care and offering you dozens of yummy recipes that bear a very close resemblance to those you cook for dinner. In addition, there is a hefty dose of science. You will learn many things that will never be published in glossy magazines, but this essential knowledge will form the foundation that allows you to become your own beauty expert and organic lifestyle guru.

As you read this book, you will learn how your skin absorbs nutritive and toxic substances, what certain chemicals can do to your body, where to look for them, and how to avoid the most obnoxious ones. You will learn about the dangers of synthetic fragrances and paraben preservatives, and you will understand why they cause allergies and increase your risk of cancer and other devastating diseases. I strongly believe that when you know what is going on in your skin, you will understand why certain ingredients work and others do not. You will be able to follow my recipes for organic, homemade skin care more consciously and will shop for ready-made beauty products with more insight. Cosmetic products are food for our skin, and each chemical ends up in thousands of hungry mouths covering our skin—pores, that is.

Whenever we buy the latest lotion or potion, we assume that people who make it have only good intentions in mind. We assume that our governments regulate cosmetic makers and demand vigorous safety testing. We assume that cosmetic makers consciously avoid making products that contain ingredients with questionable safety records. Perhaps it is time to stop assuming anything. The chemical industry works nonstop. The amount of synthetic chemicals in use all over the world has increased twofold over the last ten years. Today, we have more than 100,000 chemicals in use in different areas of our lives, and less than 5 percent of these chemicals have been thoroughly tested for their long-term impact on human health. Even proven toxins, such as lead and mercury, were presumed innocent for years—until dozens of well-documented cases of serious adverse health effects piled up, thus prohibiting the use of these chemicals in paints, household items, and cosmetics. Which chemical will be next to get the boot? Phthalates? Or maybe parabens?

Every day we learn about recalls of toys contaminated with lead, yet no one has ever recalled toxic cosmetics. Cosmetics, unlike drugs, are not regulated by governmental agencies. The safety of skin care, hair care, and makeup are determined by the cosmetic manufacturers themselves. No one is questioning their practices or watching over their shoulders, so they make their own rules about what to use in products we rub onto (and put into) our bodies.

At the same time, no one has ever disputed the safety of a product containing coconut oil, aloe vera extract, chamomile infusion, or green tea. As of today, none of these ingredients has ever been linked to the elevated risk of cancer, Alzheimer's disease, allergies, or asthma. Plant extracts, juices, and essential oils have been a part of human lifestyles for ages, and their safety has been vetted by millions of users down through the centuries.

We have all ingested our share of carcinogenic substances, such as parabens, formaldehyde, resorcinol, and paraffin, during our lifetimes. Chronic diseases develop over decades of toxic living. Cancer researcher and avid promoter of holistic approach to woman's health, Dr. Tamara Vishnievskaya, Ph.D., told me in an interview for *Fashion Monitor* in 2004 that most women have minuscule lumps in their breasts since their

 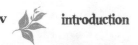

teens, and nearly all women in their eighties and nineties have cancerous formations in their breasts. However, these lumps may not become malignant for many years until the toxic load in the body tips the scale toward illness.

Environment, consumer habits, lifestyle, and diet all matter when it comes to chronic diseases that may or may not become acute. It's plain stupid to start smoking, drinking, and gorging on junk food just because there is a high chance for us to develop cancer, heart disease, or Alzheimer's disease at some point in our lives.

The human body is an amazing, complex system with incredible powers of self-regeneration. All it needs is a little helping hand. Medical science has remarkable examples how lifestyle changes helped reverse diabetes, heart disease, and even cancer. Many naturally derived powerful antioxidants can prevent and reverse sun damage and even halt the progression of skin tumors. Organic eating habits and diligent use of nontoxic cosmetic and household products will greatly diminish the toxic burden that jeopardizes our health.

Instead of continuing the old, toxic ways of treating our skin and other vital body parts, let's try to do our best to *reduce our chances of developing devastating diseases*. It's never too late, and every little bit helps.

# chapter **1**

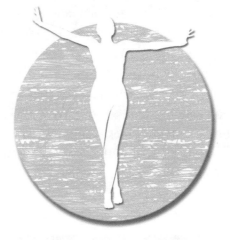

## the
## nature
## of skin

**m**ost people unconsciously treat their skin as a high-tech fabric—silky yet waterproof, glowing yet warm, silky and sexy yet resilient. The fabric benefits from regular laundering in the shower, occasional dry cleaning in a salon, and some ironing before special occasions. Many people believe that the luxurious fabric we are born in should always be spotless and fresh, no matter what it takes. We would rather bake in a tanning booth and add a glazing of shimmery lotion to hide imperfections than scrub our assets with sea salt and self-massage with virgin olive oil. We use "mattifying" lotions when our skin gets oily, hydrating creams when our skin feels dry, and battle blemishes when they become red, swollen, and very visible. When it comes to skin care, we tend to be reactive rather than proactive. Whenever possible, we opt for quick results and convenience. We are so busy fighting the consequences of the skin's imbalance that no one remembers how it feels to have normal skin.

## Anything but Normal

Normal skin does not exist anymore. Cosmetic companies invented "combination oily," "combination dry," and "dehydrated oily" skin types that require complex regimens and dozens of bottles to make skin look healthy and normal. However, a slight dryness and shiny T-zone are perfectly normal, no matter how hard the industry tries to convince us that we need to address these issues.

We are so obsessed with all the new lotions and potions that promise to make our skin appear healthy that we don't try to make it truly healthy. We are so eager to make these magic concoctions work that we do not ask ourselves whether this chemical cocktail is actually making our skin younger or any healthier. "Healthy skin isn't a quick fix," says Susan West Kurz, a holistic skin care expert and the president of Dr. Hauschka Skin Care. "If you apply a cortisone cream, the blemish will go away, but the problem still exists within the system." To support the normal functioning of your skin and naturally maintain its youthful looks, you need to first know how skin works.

Our skin is an incredibly large and complex organ. The average square inch of skin holds 650 sweat glands, 20 blood vessels, 60,000 melanocytes (pigment skin cells), and more than a thousand nerve endings. Being only 2 millimeters thick, skin does a great job protecting us from the outside world, keeping a constant body temperature, absorbing the sun's energy and converting it into vitamins while shielding us from UV radiation, storing fats and water, getting rid of waste, and sending sensations.

Skin is made up of three main layers: an epidermis, with the important top layer, stratum corneum ("horny layer"), and a dermis. Every layer of the skin works in harmony with the others. The skin is constantly renewing itself, and anything that throws its functions off balance affects all skin layers at the same time.

## Keeping Skin Moist

For most people, proper skin care starts with adequate hydration. But as shocking as it sounds, healthy skin doesn't really need any additional moisture. Our skin is perfectly able to keep itself hydrated. Its surface is kept soft and moist by sebum and a natural moisturizing factor (NMF).

Sebum, a clear waxy substance made of lipids, acts as a natural emollient and barrier. It helps protect and waterproof hair and skin and keep them from becoming dry and cracked. It can also inhibit the growth of microorganisms on the skin. Sebum, which in Latin means "fat" or "tallow," is made of wax esters, triglycerides, fatty acids, and squalene. The amount of sebum we produce varies from season to season and can be predetermined genetically, but in fact, the amount of sebum needed to keep skin moist and healthy is very small. People who are "blessed" with oily skin think their skin is dripping oil, but they produce only 2 grams of sebum a year!

For some reason, sebum became public enemy number one in the fight for clearer skin. It is just as absurd as saying that tears should be blamed for smudged mascara! Skin experts claim that sebum combines with dead skin cells and bacteria to form small plugs in the skin's pores. The only way to keep skin clean, they insist, is to completely stop the production of sebum. Instead of promoting good skin care habits that would eliminate dead skin cells and bacteria buildup, these "experts" recommend stripping skin of its vital fluid with the drug isotretinoin or "deep" cleansers that wreak havoc on the skin's nature-given abilities to cleanse and revitalize itself through cellular turnover and natural moisturizing.

Sometimes your skin may feel tight and scaly. This is when your skin's oil barrier loses its effectiveness, most often due to a cold and dry environment during the winter. Instead of letting skin readjust itself by producing more sebum, we cover it with a synthetic, oily film that physically blocks water loss. On top of this film, we may put an additional layer of waxes, petrochemicals, talc, and dyes in the form of makeup. To remove this airtight layer cake, we treat our skin with ionic surfactants and detergents that destroy the natural moisturizing factor, leaving the skin more vulnerable than before. Squeaky-clean is good for kitchen sinks, but not for human skin!

While sebum locks moisture in skin, the natural moisturizing factor (NMF) keeps skin hydrated. NMF is a mixture of water, free amino acids, lactic acid, and urea, as well as sodium, potassium, chloride, phosphate, calcium, and magnesium salts that keep the skin moist and supple by attracting and holding water. The water content of the skin's outer layer is normally about 30 percent; it rises after the skin has been treated with certain humectants, such as hyaluronic acid, that boost the skin's ability to retain moisture. To help preserve water, skin cells contain fats and fatty acids, which trap water molecules and provide a waterproof barrier that prevents transepidermal water loss (TEWL).

*It is important to feed aging skin with substances that resemble the skin's own oils.*

TEWL is the constant movement of water through the epidermis. Water evaporates through the epidermis to the surrounding atmosphere. Environmental factors such as humidity, temperature, season, and the moisture content of the skin can all affect TEWL.

Our skin gets drier as we get older because it loses some of its intercellular lipids after age forty. It is important to feed aging skin with substances that resemble the skin's own oils. These moisturizers should become oilier, but not necessarily heavier, as our skin ages. Essential fatty acids can greatly help skin retain moisture, and since they are natural, our skin accepts them more happily, which means less irritation.

  **the green beauty guide**

# Skin Eats, Too!

Advocates of synthetic skin care insist that our skin is virtually water-tight. Many say skin can be scrubbed, steamed, and washed, and nothing penetrates it deep enough to cause any damage. At the same time, many conventional cosmetics claim they deliver collagen, vitamins, and minerals to feed our skin. So do cosmetics really "get under our skin"?

In fact, beauty is skin deep. Human skin is a powerful absorption organ that seems to be constantly hungry for anything that touches its surface. Just like a curious toddler, our skin grabs every available molecule, every single drop of water, every lick of makeup, and every whiff of fragrance and takes it to its cellular "mouth" to taste, chew on, and, most likely, ingest.

Oxygen, nitrogen, and carbon dioxide, as well as toxic pollutants, enter our skin via three doors: sweat ducts, hair follicles and sebaceous glands, or directly across the stratum corneum. This ability of skin to absorb chemical substances so they can be spread throughout the body is widely used in medicine. Transdermal delivery drugs for motion sickness, cardiovascular disease, chronic pain, smoking cessation, and birth control are already widely used.

According to new estimates, our skin can absorb up to 60 percent of substances applied to its surface. Unfortunately, along with water, vitamins, minerals, and oxygen, skin soaks up potentially carcinogenic ingredients that increase our risk of having cancer at some point in our lives—as if breathing polluted air and eating chemicals was not enough!

To perform their magic, many cosmetic products need to push active ingredients deeper beyond the stratum corneum, the uppermost layer of skin comprised of dead skin cells. Traditionally, it was thought that hydrophilic (water bonding, or dissolvable in water rather than oil) chemicals do not penetrate deep into skin, while lipophilic chemicals (oils or oil-in-water emulsions) diffuse deeper inside the dermis.

Today, scientists know that the process is much more complicated. Various substances can penetrate the skin using different vehicles, sometimes as simple as water. This is when penetration enhancers, also called sorption promoters or accelerants, come into play. To deliver active ingredients, they decrease the resistance of skin's barrier. Some dissolve intercellular matrix, some change the skin's metabolism, and some damage or alter the physical and chemical nature of the top skin layer.

Most common penetration enhancers include alcohols (ethanol), glycols (propylene glycol), and surfactants. Liposomes, biomolecular spheres that encapsulate various chemicals from drugs to active components of cosmetic products, also serve as penetration enhancers. The most common liposome is phosphatidylcholine from soybean or egg yolk, sometimes with added cholesterol. Nanoparticles, currently used to deliver sunscreens and vitamins A and E, can boost the skin's permeability by up to 30 percent. Some penetration enhancers, such as transferomes, which are made of surfactants and ethanol, are able to deliver up to 100 percent of the drug applied topically! The greater its alcohol content, the deeper the solution is able to penetrate. Many essential oils have been reported to be gentle yet effective penetration enhancers.

What happens when a potentially toxic substance passes the skin's barriers? It ends up in blood vessels and lymph ducts located in the epidermis and dermis layers. Skin cells get their nutrients and excrete toxins thanks to an endless circulation of blood and lymph. Lymph, a colorless fluid made of plasma, performs a vitally important drainage function since it provides white blood cells that produce antibodies to fight infection.

As chemicals are absorbed, they enter the bloodstream and travel with lymph across the body, to be eventually filtered out by the liver and flushed away by the kidneys. However, some substances remain inside the body, adding to the systemic load that can accumulate for decades. Since the skin is the largest organ in our body, it soaks up contaminants in much larger amounts than the intestines or lungs.

Most skin care products on the market contain hundreds of synthetic additives whose safety is based on animal, not human, studies. These studies usually analyze the action of separate ingredients applied on an animal's skin in enormous doses for short periods of time. Granted, humans are unlikely to encounter such doses. But many of us are loyal to cosmetic products. As a result, we are exposed to small doses of the same toxic chemicals for decades. No one can tell how daily applications of SPF50 sunscreen may impact our health ten years from now—apart from pale skin and possibly a lower risk of skin cancer—simply because these sunscreens have been introduced quite recently, and clinical studies do not cover long periods of time.

Chemical industry insiders say that only small amounts of potentially toxic ingredients are used in cosmetics, from 1 to 10 percent, or just a few micrograms. Medical researchers today are concerned about the long-term, snowballing effect of small doses of questionable chemicals that people absorb from products used consistently over long periods of time.

Let's say you have been using a fruit-smelling shampoo that contains 1 percent of potentially carcinogenic diethanolamine (DEA), a surfactant that helps to stabilize foams, every day for five years. That is 2 ml of DEA per 200 ml bottle of shampoo. You may have switched from brand to brand, picking a "volumizing" or "energizing" shampoo variety, but core ingredients remained the same (emollients, penetration enhancers, and shine-boosting silicones). With daily shampooing, you end up using nearly an ounce of pure, industrial-strength DEA in a year. Now imagine that you pour a glass of this transparent, gooey substance over your head and start massaging it vigorously into your skin. Then you wash it off with a stream of hot water so this goo spreads over your freshly scrubbed, warm, and unprotected body. Does it make you feel healthy or more beautiful?

*Skin can absorb up to 60 percent of substances applied to its surface.*

Part of the problem is that no laboratory has ever found a human volunteer to participate in a study that would involve voluntarily rubbing your head with undiluted diethanolamine—whether derived from coconut or petroleum. Only rats can handle this tough job. A recent study by a team of researchers from the University of North Carolina at Chapel Hill found that fetuses of pregnant mice that were exposed to DEA showed slower cell growth and increased cell death in parts of the brain responsible for memory. Simply put, they were smaller and less smart. This happened because DEA has a similar structure to choline, a molecule that is needed in large quantities for normal brain development (Niculescu et al. 2007).

When potential cancer-causing poisonous chemicals are absorbed by the skin and carried with the blood all over the body, the offending chemical can interact with other chemicals in our system. Sometimes these reactions produce substances that provoke cells to evolve in the wrong way, resulting in cancer. Diethanolamine can combine with amines present in cosmetic formulations to form nitrosamines, among them N-nitrosodiethanolamine, which is known to be highly carcinogenic. Toxic ingredients may lead to many other serious diseases, including allergies, fertility problems, diabetes, and Alzheimer's disease. In the best-case scenario, they may worsen existing acne or cause an allergic reaction that resembles acne. If you do not understand that toxic chemicals in cosmetics make us sick and age prematurely, you will remain a victim of the chemical industry, and it is not good for your skin or the health of the planet.

## PREDICTING HOW WELL YOUR SKIN WILL SOAK UP
## THE GOOD AND BAD IN COSMETICS

*How strong is the solution?* If the concentration of a certain ingredient is high, then it has a better chance of sneaking though the skin's protective barriers. For example, the skin will be exposed to more retinoic acid from a potent prescription-only cream than from an over-the-counter lotion that contains the same ingredient.

*How long will it remain on the skin?* The longer the product sits on the skin's surface, the more of its ingredients will be absorbed. Our skin will soak up more paraben preservatives from a moisturizer that remains on the skin for hours than from a cleanser that is quickly washed off, but if you rub the cleanser vigorously, the absorption rate will increase.

*How much water does it contain?* It was once thought that oil-based skin care products penetrate the skin more readily than those that contain water. Today, we know that well-hydrated skin absorbs chemicals at a much higher rate. Besides, hydration can be increased by paraffin, oils, and waxes. Paraffin, oils, and waxes as components of skin creams, ointments, and water-in-oil emulsions—basically anything that prevents transepidermal water loss—can improve the amount of chemicals soaked up by skin. Water acts as an excellent natural penetration enhancer. That's why your skin can absorb more chemicals when you soak in synthetic bath foam for long time.

*How healthy is the skin?* Undamaged, strong skin can shield us from many toxic substances and germs, but even a slight scratch or cut becomes a welcome sign for anything we do not want inside our bodies. Even something as innocuous as the removal of outer layers of skin with a facial scrub or a peeling mask can dramatically increase dermal absorption. Inflamed, swollen acne pimples absorb more benzoyl peroxide than the healthy skin just a millimeter away.

*Where do we apply the product?* Skin on different areas of the body varies in thickness. For example, facial skin will absorb ingredients twenty times faster than the thicker skin on the palms of the hands.

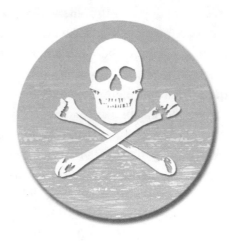

# beauty
## and the toxic
# beast

**W**hat is in your morning bathroom routine? Most likely, you take a shower with a zesty, invigorating shower gel; you shampoo and condition your hair; you wash and maybe scrub your face with a foaming fresh-smelling cleanser; if you are a man, you also shave. You splash your skin with a toner or an astringent, top it with a moisturizer with (hopefully) some sunscreen in it, followed by makeup (again, optional), rub some antiperspirant under your arms, and add a spritz of a fragrance to seal the deal. Within fifteen minutes, you have exposed yourself to a whopping amount of chemicals—and you haven't even left home yet!

After a quick count of ingredients contained in a typical cleanser, toner, moisturizer, eye cream, facial scrub, body wash, body lotion, and sunscreen, I came up with more than two hundred different chemicals that we diligently apply to our skin daily. This is not counting hundreds of synthetic fragrance ingredients in your favorite eau de toilette! Soon you will inhale car emissions, pesticides, radon, volatile organic compounds, persistent organic pollutants, tobacco smoke, dust, and microscopic droplets of grease. You will eat food that contains artificial preservatives, flavors, and colors, and you will drink water that has subpar purity standards, adding to the already brewing cocktail of chemicals that enter your system nonstop.

In 2006, a consumer advocacy group, Environmental Working Group, with the support of the Breast Cancer Fund, Breast Cancer Action, and the National Environmental Trust, released a study of the listed ingredients for 7,500 bestselling beauty products. Here are some of the findings:

About 90 percent of cosmetic ingredients have never been analyzed for health impacts by the Cosmetic Ingredient Review Board, a panel that oversees cosmetic safety. More than seventy popular hair dye products contain ingredients derived from coal tar, a known carcinogen. Nearly 55 percent of products contain "penetration enhancers" that increase the ability of chemicals to enter the bloodstream.

> About 90 percent of cosmetic ingredients have never been analyzed for health impacts.

# Too Good to Be True?

How many times have you stumbled upon the phrases "our studies show" and "dermatologist tested"? These marketing clichés are so common, you hardly pay attention. The cosmetic industry, one of the largest and most profitable of all industries, spends more on advertising than any other trade. Each advertisement claim should be validated, and there's a well-established claim validation business that serves the beauty industry.

A cream delivers 300 percent more moisture? The shampoo makes hair five times shinier? Show us the proof, officials say. "The Cosmetics Directive does require that when a claim for efficacy is made for a cosmetic product, full substantiation for the claim should be available," says the European Union's Cosmetics Directive 76/768/EEC. Most often, such claims are validated by consumer testing, surveys, and clinical studies. Women slather creams on freshly washed, dry faces, and miracles happen—skin looks moisturized, and wrinkles are less visible. Women wash their greasy, limp locks with a new fruity shampoo and, what do you know, their hair looks shiny and clean. What a breakthrough!

Rarely do we learn if the dermatologist involved in the study was on the payroll of the cosmetic company, or if the study was peer-reviewed, double-blind, or carried out by an independent laboratory. No one bothers to tell us whether a sufficient number of participants was involved. (Most studies are done in vitro, in a glass tube.) If people were involved, how many participants were there? Most studies involve thirty to eighty volunteers, of whom "67 percent reported firmer skin" after a few applications. Did they apply the cream to clean skin? Did they sleep well? Did they drink lots of water? We will never learn, but these factors are important. We never know who conducted the study—the company itself or a laboratory, or whether this laboratory was founded by the company to substantiate this and many other marvelous claims, such as "makes you look ten years younger." What would happen if an eighteen-year-old started using it? Will she suddenly look like a preschooler? Such claims look impressive in press releases and ads, but they are never published in scientific journals and validated by the scientific community.

Pseudoscientific blabber and impressive sales pitches aside, none of these so-called tests gives any information that is helpful for your skin and for a good reason: no one tests the skin care product to find out if it is making skin truly healthy—or at least not hurting it. All that matters is instant cosmetic effect. Beauty products are evaluated for safety *after* they are released to the marketplace.

Beauty products are evaluated for safety *after* they are released to the marketplace.

In most countries, it's up to the manufacturers to ensure that their personal care products are safe. In the United States, the cosmetic industry-funded Cosmetic Ingredient Review (CIR) evaluates the safety of cosmetic ingredients and products. It is very unlikely that a group of cosmetic manufacturers would voluntarily question the safety of the ingredient they buy in hundreds of tons and use in thousands of products. Neither cosmetic products nor cosmetic ingredients are reviewed or approved by the government health agencies before they are sold in stores.

The U.S. Food and Drug Administration (FDA) employs a hands-off approach to cosmetics: there is no harm until harm is proven. Instead of testing beauty products before they appear on the market, the FDA regulates products only after they are sold, investigating health complaints when and if complaints are filed. At the same time, the FDA estimates that only 3 percent of the 4,000 to 5,000 cosmetic distributors have ever filed reports on injuries to consumers with the government agencies.

If there is a safety problem with a cosmetic product—for example, a number of allergic reactions arising in many people—the FDA can take action to obtain the manufacturer's safety data on the product and ask for detailed safety testing results. Most of the tests are performed to ensure that the product is effective in delivering the promise. Human studies conducted by manufacturers often focus on overall appeal—such as a pleasant smell, silky feel, or a light texture—or short-term results, such as an "instant lifting effect." The U.S. Department of Agriculture reminds us that label claims of a product being "dermatologist tested," "sensitivity tested," "allergy tested," or "nonirritating" carry no guarantee that it will not cause those reactions. Such tests only prove that the product is effective against wrinkles, dandruff, or sunburns, and the results can be visible in a matter of minutes, days, or at least a few weeks.

All safety-related tests are performed on animals. Since there is not yet enough information on alternatives to animal testing ensuring human safety to validate the use of certain chemicals, the FDA at this point will only accept animal safety data. While the European Union (EU) has banned animal testing of cosmetic products since 2000, elsewhere beauty products are most often tested on genetically modified mice or rabbits whose lifespan is much shorter compared to that of a human being.

Even if a complaint is filed, sometimes it takes decades to come up with a sizable body of complaints to invoke an investigation. Then it may take another decade to convince legislators that they should ban the substance from cosmetic products. The FDA has the authority to declare a product misbranded, adulterated for reasons such as improper labeling, or dangerous to health. Generally, the FDA must prove these allegations in court. For this reason, the FDA will often accept the industry's action of voluntarily withdrawing a substance from use. Many manufacturers prefer to voluntarily recall the questionable product or quickly reformulate it to remove the dubious ingredient. In June 2008, when California filed a lawsuit against the manufacturers of shampoos, body washes, and dishwashing liquids contaminated with 1,4-Dioxane, only one manufacturer, Beaumont, quickly reformulated its products, removing the ethoxylated compounds from the ingredients. This proves that cosmetic manufacturers are well aware of the potential harm caused by some of their ingredients but will do nothing until they face a lawsuit.

And in most cases, even lawsuits are powerless. The investigation can take years, and during all this time no one can prohibit the manufacturers and stores from selling potentially cancer-causing beauty products. No one will voluntarily slap a sticker saying "Warning: Can Cause Cancer" on their so-called organic products. You see, such stickers won't help sales.

In sixty-seven years, the FDA has banned or restricted only nine personal care ingredients. It took the FDA twenty years to ban the use of lead in paint on toys and furniture. However, a recent wave of recalls of millions of children's toys that were contaminated with excessive amounts of lead in paint shows that such bans mean very little when it comes to the millions of items sold in thousands of stores. Testing of toys, as well as of the rest of consumer products, is voluntary, sporadic, time-consuming, and money-consuming— and, therefore, rare.

> In sixty-seven years, the FDA has banned or restricted only nine personal care ingredients.

Medical research has already proven that synthetic fragrances trigger asthma (Curtis 2004), that the detergents in shampoos can damage eye tissue (Scaife 1985; Neppelberg 2007), and that hair-dye chemicals can cause bladder cancer and lymphoma (Zhang et al. 2008). Absorbed into the body, toxic chemicals can be stored in fatty tissue or organs such as the liver, kidneys, breasts, ovaries, and brain. Cosmetic companies accuse the media of alarmism, but scientists are finding plastic components called phthalates in urine (Adibi et al. 2008), parabens and antibacterial agents such as Triclosan in breast-tumor tissue (Darbre 2006), as well as the hormone-disrupting fragrant component xylene in human breast milk (Reiner et al. 2007).

Still think that blue metallic eye shadow is your cosmetic bag's worst secret?

## 1,4-Dioxane: Silent Killer

This hidden cancer-causing petrochemical has been found at high levels in dozens of babies' and adults' personal care products, including baby baths and hair dyes. In July 2007, laboratory tests revealed the presence of this petroleum-derived contaminant in popular baby products, including bestselling baby baths and baby washes sold worldwide. The tests also found the carcinogen in some of the most popular shampoos, body washes, and many other personal care products used daily by millions of women worldwide.

1,4-Dioxane is considered a probable human carcinogen by the U.S. Environmental Protection Agency (EPA). Animal tests have indisputably proven its tumor-promoting activity (Stickney et al. 2003). 1,4-Dioxane is also on California's Safe Drinking Water and Toxic Enforcement Act (Proposition 65) list of chemicals known or suspected by the state to cause cancer or birth defects. U.S. federal regulators, particularly the Integrated Risk Information System, consider 1,4-Dioxane's potency to be equivalent or greater than many pesticides (EPA 1992, 2000).

This carcinogen forms during a procedure called ethoxylation, a cheap shortcut that companies use to provide mildness to harsh ingredients. This process requires the use of the cancer-causing petrochemical ethylene oxide, which generates 1,4-Dioxane as a byproduct.

This is why you will never find 1,4-Dioxane in ingredient lists. No warnings are given either. Because this contaminant is produced during manufacturing, the U.S. Department of Agriculture does not require 1,4-Dioxane to be listed as an ingredient on product labels, and the practice of assessing risk one chemical at a time does not account for the combined effects of very low levels of hidden contaminants in personal care products and from other sources.

The FDA has been measuring 1,4-Dioxane levels since 1979, but because the agency has little authority over the cosmetic industry, it has no power to make the manufacturers reduce levels of 1,4-Dioxane. All you can do at this point is carefully scan the ingredient label. Check product labels for ingredients that contain "eth" in their name, such as sodium laur*eth* sulphate, (PEG) poly*eth*ylene glycol, ol*eth*, myr*eth*, cetear*eth*—basically, any ingredient that has an *eth* in its name most likely tests positive for 1,4-Dioxane. Unfortunately, many so-called "natural" and "organic" beauty products contain ethoxylated synthetic ingredients, and many well-known shampoos, baby products, and even dish detergents bearing words "organic" and "eco-friendly" on their labels revealed whopping amounts of toxin during tests carried out by the Organic Consumers Association. For more information, check www.the greenbeautyguide.com.

## Some Greenwashed Products Are Contaminated, Too

The shocking results of the recent study by the Organic Consumers Association revealed that many personal care and household cleaning products claiming to be "natural" or "organic" are contaminated with traces of 1,4-Dioxane. Astonishing amounts of 1,4-Dioxane were found in "natural" dishwashing liquids and other so-called earth-friendly products.

In June 2008, the attorney general of California filed a major lawsuit against Avalon Natural Products (manufacturer of the Alba brand), Whole Foods Market California (manufacturer of the Whole Foods 365 brand), Beaumont Products (manufacturer of the Citrus Magic brand), and Nutribiotic, the manufacturer of well-known shampoos and conditioners, whose products tested highest for 1,4-Dioxane. The lawsuit alleges that these companies should have put warning labels on products con-

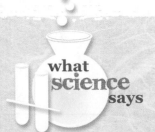

## what science says

When laboratory animals were tested with 1,4-Dioxane at the lowest parts per billion level—over the animal's lifetime—they developed cancer. However, the levels of 1,4-Dioxane found in many personal care products are often thousands of times higher than those found to cause cancer in laboratory animals. We need to remember the synergistic effects of chemicals; toxins add up and even multiply to create greater risk. Cosmetics contaminated with 1,4-Dioxane might also have traces of formaldehyde, nitrosamines, phthalates, and other contaminants.

The risk is even greater when you are using body products contaminated with 1,4-Dioxane. According to a California state health official's memorandum, 1,4-Dioxane is readily absorbed through the lungs, skin, and gastrointestinal tract. Bath products contaminated with 1,4-Dioxane are particularly dangerous. Warm water is an effective penetration enhancer. When our pores are opened, 1,4-Dioxane enters the bloodstream more easily. 1,4-Dioxane is also released as a gas and is inhaled more intensely in the warm and humid area of the bathroom or a shower stall. When studying the risks of 1,4-Dioxane under California's Safe Drinking Water and Toxic Enforcement Act (Proposition 65), researchers found that a single product containing 1,4-Dioxane could lead to 970 excess cancers in one million. "Even if this were off by a factor of ten, the risk would still be 97 excess cancers, and this remains noteworthy—especially for a cosmetic product," noted Campaign for Safe Cosmetics on their website (full article: http://www.safecosmetics.org/faqs/mvf_dioxane.cfm).

taining high levels of 1,4-Dioxane, stating that they may cause cancer. As the investigation continues, check www.thegreenbeautyguide.com for more information.

## The Solution

It's no secret we are ready to pay more for beauty products that claim to be clean from contaminants. However, a visit to any health food store unfortunately reveals the majority of products in the personal care section with "organic" brand-claims contain only cheap water extracts of organic herbs and maybe a few other token organic ingredients to justify the "organic" claim on the label. The core of such products is composed of conventional synthetic cleansers and conditioning ingredients usually made in part with petrochemicals, often containing toxic contaminants like 1,4-Dioxane.

The general rule of thumb is to avoid products with unpronounceable ingredients. To avoid 1,4-Dioxane, the Organic Consumers Association urges consumers to search ingredient lists for indications of ethoxylation including: myreth, oleth, laureth, ceteareth, and any other "eth," PEG, poly-ethylene, polyethylene glycol, polyoxyethylene, or oxynol in ingredient names. Watch out for "eths" and PEGS, and your health will thank you.

When I was writing this book, I suffered a lot of sleepless nights because I couldn't stop thinking about all the damage I have possibly done to my baby by using a breast pump made of plastic with bisphenol-A or treating her bottom to PEG-containing baby wipes. The new research on 1,4-Dioxane came out when the book was almost ready, and I developed a sort of mental immunity to these sort of shocks. Without much surprise, I discovered that I was washing my baby's cutlery and bottles with a fruity-smelling dishwashing liquid that claimed to be "pure, earth-friendly, and all-natural." It had the name "Masha" scribbled on it to let all fellow dishwashers know that this supernatural and super clean detergent must only be used on baby cutlery, cups, and bottles. Down the drain it went in an instant. From now on, we wash our dishes with unscented organic liquid soap, and for baby cups and bottles, it's baking soda and a chunk of plain old-fashioned olive soap. I'd rather not take any chances.

### Green Fact

Most products tested positive for 1,4-Dioxane are foaming cleansers with sodium laureth sulfate, ammonium laureth sulfate, or both, as the main ingredients.

It may be good to remember, though, that the recent laboratory studies show 1,4-Dioxane is nonexistent in the variety of products produced and certified under the USDA National Organic Program, because the regulations disallow ethoxylation and any other synthetic petrochemical modification, as currently outlined in the National List of Allowed and Prohibited Substances of the United States National Organic Program. For your peace of mind, look out for this label—but only if it refers to the whole product, not one of its ingredients. We will discuss organic labeling more in Chapter 4.

## Phthalates: Hormonal Disharmony

A study by the Women's Environmental Network, Swedish Society for Nature Conservation, and Health Care Without Harm found phthalates in almost 80 percent of the popular cosmetic products tested, none of which listed these chemicals on the labels.

About 1 billion pounds of phthalates per year are produced and sold worldwide. Phthalates are widely used industrial compounds known technically as dialkyl or alkyl aryl esters of 1,2-benzenedicarboxylic acid. Phthalates are all around us: in shower curtains, rubber ducks, PVC furniture and clothes, sex toys, fragrances, MP3 players (including earphones and cords), perfumes, hair sprays, and nail polishes. Some of the bestselling fragrances contain phthalates, a group of dangerous toxic chemicals that is linked to reproductive birth defects and other illnesses, according to the FDA, National Toxicology Program, and other governmental agencies. The majority of Americans tested by the Centers for Disease Control and Prevention have metabolites of multiple phthalates in their urine at any given time. Phthalates are so ubiquitous it is impossible to completely avoid them, but you can distance yourself from a great deal of them.

Phthalates are known reproductive toxins, and while these chemicals may be safe in extremely low levels, women are exposed to phthalates from many sources that join forces to create dangerously high levels of phthalates in the body. That new car smell, which becomes especially noticeable after the car has been standing in the sun for a few hours, is mainly the toxic brew of phthalates emitting from a hot plastic dashboard and seats. This is why some doctors recommend that pregnant women do not buy new cars or even ride in them, especially during the first crucial weeks of pregnancy.

"All synthetically scented products, such as shampoos [and] deodorants, contain phthalates, but perfumes contain the highest levels of phthalates," says Stacy Malkan, cofounder of the Campaign for Safe Cosmetics.

The chemicals in question include di-n-butyl phthalate (DBP, commonly found in nail polish) and di(2-ehtylhexyl) phthalate (DEHP, found in perfumes). Most often, they are hiding under the word "fragrance" in the ingredient list. Even though the amounts of these toxic chemicals in beauty products are minuscule, scientists warn that their combined effect could pose health problems. While cosmetic manufacturers insist that phthalates are "safe as currently used," and phthalate manufacturers produce websites praising phthalates for making our lives better and safer, recent medical data contradict this notion. There is nothing good or safe about phthalates.

## what science says

In all living creatures, phthalates tip hormonal scales, making males and females more feminine. Solid research links phthalates to the rising incidence of hormone-related medical conditions, including polycystic ovarian syndrome, infertility, and breast cancer. Young women, who use a lot more cosmetics and fragrances than men, are at particular risk.

A 2000 study at the University of Puerto Rico in San Juan linked the use of phthalates in beauty products to early puberty in girls (Colón et al. 2000). A study by the Atlanta-based Centers for Disease Control and Prevention found that phthalate levels in young women may be twenty times higher than average (CDC 2001).

Unborn baby boys are in particular danger since phthalates have been shown to damage developing testes in males. This could result in many systemic disorders such as low sperm count, sexual dysfunction, and hormonal imbalance. Men who come in contact with phthalates from plastics, fragrances, hair care products, and even MP3 player earphones risk even more than their sexual identity. A 2007 study done by scientists from the University of Rochester School of Medicine and Dentistry in Rochester, New York, found that phthalates, already connected to reproductive problems in women, are linked to abdominal obesity (think Homer Simpson's body shape) and insulin resistance in men (Stahlhut et al. 2007). The study found that men with the highest levels of phthalates in their urine had more belly fat and insulin resistance. Studies conducted at Harvard University in Cambridge linked phthalates to decreased sperm counts and testicular cancer in men (Hauser 2006). "This doesn't mean that women are safe. Women are exposed to phthalates when they are pregnant, and boys actually come from women," reminds Stacy Malkan, "and the damage to baby boys is done when they are most vulnerable. Most of the research was done to check the effects of phthalates on males, but hopefully there will be more studies researching the effects of phthalates on females. There are some links to breast and uterine cancer, and these findings date to quite some time ago" (Singh et al. 1975, Harris et al. 1997, Högberg et al. 2008).

The newest research reluctantly admits that babies are exposed to phthalates at a much higher rate than adults. Many baby care products contain high levels of phthalates hiding in baby lotions, powder, and shampoo, and leaking from PVC-containing toys, spoons, and pacifiers. Scientists "observed that reported use of infant lotion, infant powder, and infant shampoo were associated with increased infant urine concentrations of [phthalate metabolites], and this association is strongest in younger infants. These findings suggest that dermal exposures may contribute significantly to phthalate body burden in this population. Young infants are more vulnerable to the potential adverse effects of phthalates given their increased dosage per unit body surface area, metabolic capabilities, and developing endocrine and reproductive systems" (Sathyanarayana, Karr 2008).

Cancer, diabetes, allergies, infertility . . . are phthalates worth the risk? Scientists answer in unison: no, they are not, especially when there are so many alternatives available.

## Double Standards

The European Union has banned some phthalates from many cosmetics and toys, while in the United States, the state of California banned phthalates from use in children's toys starting in 2009. The bill prohibits the manufacture, sale, and distribution of toys and childcare products used by children under the age of three that contain phthalates. But these measures do not lull consumer activists.

"Sometimes the stuff they find is just the tip of the iceberg," says Stacy Malkan. "In Europe, they banned just two types of phthalates, but cosmetic companies continue using the rest of them. There's evidence that those other types are even more toxic, especially when used in combination."

Some cosmetic brands, including Body Shop and Aveda, both segments of the Estée Lauder beauty empire, and Urban Decay, part of Moet-Hennessy Louis Vuitton (LVMH), have already volunteered to remove phthalates from all their products. But the majority of United States–based cosmetic companies are balking at the proposed ban. The U.S. Cosmetic, Toiletry, and Fragrance Association (CTFA) calls the European regulation "unnecessary" and dismisses research on phthalates.

"We are facing increased regulatory clout from the European Union, which is affecting our industry on a global basis, notably in China," noted Marc Pritchard, chairman of the CTFA board of directors and president of global cosmetics and retail hair color at Procter & Gamble, in the annual report in 2005.

Phthalates have many high-profile defenders. "Health-related allegations about cosmetic ingredients are generally based on the results of high-dose laboratory testing in animals and have little relevance for humans," wrote Dr. Gilbert Ross, the medical and executive director of the American Council on Science and Health, in his 2006 paper, "A Perspective on the Safety of Cosmetic Products." The paper goes on to say that "The health-related allegations involving specific chemicals (e.g., phthalates, parabens, and 1,3-butadiene) fail to consider important scientific studies and recent regulatory conclusions about these chemicals, which have found that they are not hazardous."

While the National Toxicology Program listed many phthalates as carcinogens in 2003 (NTP-CERHR Monograph 2003), medical studies directly link phthalates to a higher risk of cancer in humans. Dibutylphthalate (DBP) was found genotoxic when German scientists investigated the development of squamous cell cancer (Kleinsasser et al. 2000). Di-n-butylphthalate altered breast cells, particularly genes involved in fertility, immune response, and antioxidant status in a study conducted by the Molecular Epidemiology Team at the U.S. National Institute for Occupational Safety and Health (Gwinn et al. 2007). Both di(n-butyl) phthalate (DBP) and di(2-ethylhexyl) phthalate (DEHP) appeared to promote drug resistance to tamoxifen in breast cancer, South Korean scientists found in 2004 (Kim et al. 2004).

While American cosmetic manufacturers refused to reformulate their products and remove phthalates from products sold on American soil, in 2004 they agreed to use substitutes for phthalates in beauty products shipped to Europe.

Today, nail polishes made by Revlon, Procter and Gamble's Max Factor and Cover Girl, and Estée Lauder's Clinique and MAC are phthalate-free. That is pretty much it. United States' cosmetic companies are not required by law to mention phthalates or many other chemical compounds on their labels. Hundreds of bestselling beauty products, including foundations, blushers, hair sprays, leave-on hair conditioners, fragrances, baby shampoos, and lotions, as well as bestselling MP3 gear, are still loaded with gender-bending phthalates.

## Aluminum: No Sweat About It

Going around with wet and smelly underarms for most of us is just as unthinkable as rinsing freshly brushed teeth with water from the toilet basin. Clearly, there is nothing less attractive and socially unacceptable than sweaty underarms. But rubbing your freshly shaven underarm skin with a zesty-scented stick of antiperspirant may cause you more problems than you think. In fact, you may lose the ability to think at all.

All antiperspirants rely on aluminum in the form of aluminum chloride, aluminum zirconium, aluminum chlorohydrate, and aluminum hydroxybromide. These aluminum salts dry out sweat by injecting aluminum ions into the cells that line the sweat ducts. When the aluminum ions are drawn into the cells, water flows in; the cells begin to swell, squeezing the ducts closed so sweat cannot get out.

Aluminum is a known potent neurotoxin, and it is loaded in our systems in generous doses. An average over-the-counter antiperspirant might have a concentration of aluminum anywhere from 10 to 25 percent. The FDA also requires that all antiperspirants must decrease the average person's sweat by at least 20 percent. This means that antiperspirants should work hard to keep us dry!

Aluminum does much more than mess up the natural process of toxin elimination. When it enters the bloodstream, it alters the function of the blood brain barrier. Granted, aluminum is not considered as toxic as heavy metals, but there is evidence that aluminum from hygiene products and antacids does contribute to two serious diseases: breast cancer and Alzheimer's disease.

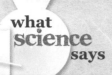
Aluminum is suspected to increase the risk of developing Alzheimer's disease (AD), a neurodegenerative disorder and the most common cause of dementia, affecting millions of men and women worldwide. Scientists have found that plaques in the brain of AD sufferers contain aluminum. While AD origins are still a mystery to many doctors, evidence is accumulating to show that aluminum may be involved in the formation of the plaques in the human brain (Shcherbatykh, Carpenter 2007) and is therefore a prime and, most importantly, avoidable risk factor for this devastating disease.

Every day we rub aluminum-loaded antiperspirant in underarm areas where many lymph nodes are located close to the surface of the skin. Recent evidence has linked breast cancer with aluminum-based antiperspirants. In research published in the *Journal of Applied Toxicology*, Dr. Philippa D. Darbre of the University of Reading in England has shown that aluminum salts increase estrogen-related gene expression in human breast cancer cells grown in vitro, which makes aluminum a powerful metalloestrogen (Exley et al. 2007). The new 2008 study found that aluminum content of breast tissue in the outer regions (closer to the underarms) was significantly higher than the inner regions of the breast (Gee et al. 2008). This happens because aluminum works as a strong genotoxin, capable of causing both DNA alterations and gene mutations, according to numerous studies that link breast cancer to various common chemicals, from aluminum to Triclosan and parabens (Gee et al. 2008).

"Lifetime exposure to estrogen is the risk factor which is tied most strongly to breast cancer," Dr. Darbre told WebMD in 2006. "If the aluminum salts in antiperspirants enter the body and mimic estrogen, it stands to reason that constant exposure over many years may pose a risk" (full article: http://www.medscape.com/view article/524555).

Opponents of the use of aluminum in personal care products agree that this metal is not the sole cause of breast cancer and Alzheimer's disease, but that it may play a role. Both diseases are caused by multiple factors, and aluminum is just one of them. Still, this factor is easily avoided. All it takes is a small change in consumer habits.

# Propylene Glycol: Beauty Dissolved

Do you know what baby wipes and aircraft deicing fluid have in common? Both have glycols as a main ingredient. Members of this family of multitasking chemicals are used in many cosmetic products, including baby washes, bubble baths, deodorants, shampoos, hair dyes, and personal lubricants (where propylene glycol works to deice the passion, most likely). All members of the glycol family are easily biodegradable and do not accumulate in soil or water, which is the only good thing about them.

There has been a lot of confusion between propylene glycol (PG), diethylene glycol, ethylene glycol, and polyethylene glycol (PEG). While all of them have similar-sounding names, these chemicals have different safety ratings. Propylene glycol is a popular humectant (an ingredient that helps draw moisture from the air to the skin) and a penetration enhancer used in many cosmetic products. It helps products such as stick deodorants retain their solid form and prevents melting. The FDA considers propylene glycol to be "generally recognized as safe" for use in food, cosmetics, and medicines. However, it banned this chemical from cat food in 2001.

Ethylene glycol is considered less safe. Apart from its use in antifreezes and deicing fluids, ethylene glycol is found in photographic developing solutions, hydraulic brake fluids, and in inks used in stamp pads, ballpoint pens, and print shops. There is a higher dose of ethylene glycols in children's shampoos and baby washes, to make them "less irritating" to a baby's whisper-thin skin.

Diethylene glycol is toxic to humans and animals. It is not allowed for food and drug use but can be found in polyethylene glycol in very low concentrations.

Polyethylene glycol (PEG) is another popular cosmetic ingredient. It's frequently used in "natural" cosmetics as well as in laxatives and other medications that have to be delivered in a slippery, syrupy form. PEG, just as propylene glycol, is also used as a food preservative. It is considered generally safe to use by cosmetic manufacturers "with a maximum concentration of use of 20 percent," with a warning: "On damaged skin, cases of systemic toxicity and contact dermatitis in burn patients were attributed to a PEG-based topical ointment" (CIR Expert Panel 2006).

  **the green beauty guide**

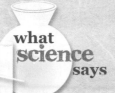
When it comes to short-term effects from daily use, contact allergic dermatitis is the most common side effect of using products containing propylene glycol and various PEGs. These chemicals are known to aggravate acne and eczema by rupturing skin cell membranes (Gonzalo et al. 1999). Propylene glycol, used as a penetration enhancer and humectant, has been found to provoke skin irritation and sensitization in humans in concentrations as low as 2 percent, while the industry review panel recommends that cosmetics can contain up to 50 percent of the substance (Johnson 2001).

Current studies have not shown that propylene or the other glycols can cause cancer when used in cosmetics. Female animals that ate large amounts of ethylene glycol had babies with birth defects, while male animals had reduced sperm counts (Anderson et al. 1987). Ethylene glycol and propylene glycol affect the body's chemistry by increasing the amount of acid, resulting in metabolic problems. However, these effects were seen when animals were fed very high concentrations of these chemicals. It is very unlikely that you will gulp PEG-containing toothpaste by the tube. However, your two-year-old toddler might happily do that, given the chance.

Then there is another potential danger. Impurities found in various PEG compounds include ethylene oxide, 1,4-Dioxane, polycyclic aromatic compounds, and heavy metals such as lead, iron, cobalt, nickel, cadmium, and arsenic. The toxicity of PEG compounds increases when products are applied to damaged skin. These contaminants could be easily and economically removed by vacuum stripping during manufacture. Still, there is no guarantee that the PEG in your baby wash has been treated to remove any possible toxins. In spite of these concerns, PEG compounds remain commonly used in "natural" cosmetics and personal care products, often disguised by giving plant names to them.

Simply because propylene glycol has many different applications does not make all PEG-containing beauty products equally toxic. Industrial-strength solutions are very concentrated and require caution in handling them. The cosmetic industry uses only very small amounts of propylene and polyethylene glycols. Chances are you've been using products containing various PEGs and PGs for years, and there's little use in being paranoid about it. But if you would like to reduce your current personal toxic load, it may make sense to avoid using products containing glycols, especially now when many alternatives are available.

# The Big Preservative Debate

All personal care products have a shelf life. You can usually find out how long the product will remain fresh by locating a "best before" date stamped on the sealed end of a tube or directly on the bottle's label. Have you ever noticed a sketch of an opened jar on a box of a beauty product? Sometimes there is a symbol of a jar along with a number preceding the letter M: 6M means six months while 12M means twelve months. If these numbers accompany a jar with a closed lid, it means that a product will remain fresh for six months from the manufacture date (as long as it remains closed and sealed), while a jar with an open lid indicates that once opened, with normal use the product will remain fresh for six, twelve, or more months.

Preservatives contained in beauty products ward off bacteria, fungi, microbes, and oxidation. Such preservatives halt enzyme activity in the formulation, stop the oxidation process, or kill bacteria and any living creatures that wandered inside the bottle. The more preservatives that are loaded into the product, the longer it can remain "pure" and uncontaminated. This way, beauty products can be manufactured in mass quantities and be warehoused for a longer period.

Of all cosmetic ingredients, preservatives are the most frequently targeted by open-minded research doctors, consumer groups, and non-governmental organizations. Preservatives keep products clean and fresh, which is a good thing because we often store our beauty products in bathrooms, which tend to be warm and moist. Also, family members may share cosmetic products, which often come in wide-neck jars—think body balm used as an aftershave lotion and hand salves doubling as creaking door menders. Under such conditions, even the most stable formulation can grow some fussy colonies.

Microorganisms can do much more than make the cream smell weird. While using out-of-date products may not please your senses, decaying ingredients can actually affect your health. The bacteria growing in outdated products can cause rashes and breakouts when applied to skin that is irritated or scratched, or to the fragile, thin skin around the eyes. *Staphylococcus aureus,* a pathogenic bacteria, can be fatal when applied to broken skin (Nguema et al. 2000), and incidences of blindness caused by contaminated mascara have been reported (Reid, Wood 1979).

the green beauty guide

No wonder many cosmetic companies are now searching for preservatives that are paraben- and formaldehyde-free yet are effective against the effects of air, light, bacteria, yeast, and fungi even at low concentrations.

In addition to eliminating parabens from their formulations, marketers are also removing phenoxyethanol. Fenilight and Feniol have the same full bactericidal activity but are much safer than phenoxyethanol. Tinosan is a natural, silver-based preservative.

Chemists are also working on creating cosmetic compounds that would not require preservatives at all. Ritative AN is a blend of emulsifiers and humectants that has built-in, broad-spectrum microbiological activity. Despite its militaristic name, the B52 preservative (based on benzyl PCA) doubles as a gentle, nonirritating moisturizer and emollient. It can be used in moisturizers, lotions, and bath products.

All of these preservatives are synthetic. They are safer than conventional preservatives, but they are hardly green. Are there any completely natural preservatives out there?

Suprapein (created by Bio-Botanica) is a totally natural preservative made of oregano and thyme oils, as well as cinnamon, lavender, lemon peel, goldenseal, and rosemary extract. Lemon peel oil, grapefruit seed extract, vitamin C (ascorbic acid), and vitamin E (tocopherols) are also used to prevent oxidation. The chemical benzanthracene, found in lemon and lime oils, has potent microbial properties. Potassium sorbate and sodium benzoate are considered safe and have a lower likelihood of causing cosmetic-related allergies and sensitivities. Many cosmetic companies are switching to aseptic manufacturing and airtight packaging, which minimizes the exposure to air and bacteria.

You can do your own share to prevent contamination of your paraben-free products, which have a much shorter life span than their synthetic counterparts do. Handle all cosmetics in a way that prevents bacterial contamination. Do not leave product containers uncapped. Do not share them. Do not use your fingers instead of applicators. Some products, such as lip and body balms, body and hair butters, oil-based serums, perfumes with or without alcohol, oil-based salt and sugar scrubs, bath and body oils, and liquid soap have a shelf life of several months to a year. Nevertheless, most organic creams and lotions that contain water must be used within six months.

While keeping bacteria away, preservatives themselves often act as contaminants and powerful skin allergens. It was once believed that parabens, known as esters of para-hydroxybenzoic acid, were not stored in human tissue. However, recent findings prove the contrary. When rubbed into the skin, parabens are rapidly absorbed and metabolized, but they also accumulate in the human body. In 2002, parabens, due to their estrogenic activity, were found to cause increased uterine growth in animals. The same study first linked parabens to the proliferation of two estrogen-dependent human breast cancer cells (Darbre et al. 2002). Two years later, parabens were found in breast milk and breast cancer tumors. In a 2004 study, tests found parabens in breast cancer tumors in nineteen out of twenty women with breast cancer (Darbre et al. 2004). This study, while small and statistically insignificant, proves the ability of paraben preservatives to penetrate skin and accumulate in living tissue, such as breasts. In the body, parabens mimic our own hormones and can have an endocrine-disrupting action. The hypothalamus, the ovaries, the thyroid—parabens affect virtually every system, even though their action is much milder than that of natural estrogens and other xenoestrogens (synthetic estrogens that mimic natural hormones).

Granted, science currently has no direct evidence that any cosmetics containing parabens result in a higher risk of cancer, and the American Cancer Society insists that parabens are perfectly safe from an oncologist's point of view. The cosmetic industry's panel, the Cosmetic Ingredient Review (CIR), reviewed the safety of methylparaben, propylparaben, and butylparaben in 1984 and concluded they were safe for use in cosmetic products at levels of up to 25 percent of the finished product. However, not a single study has yet focused on chronic, decades-long, direct exposure to parabens that act synergistically with other xenoestrogens and the body's own estrogens.

While the jury is still out, the use of parabens, often disguised by tongue-twisting names such as benzoic acid, isobutyl p-hydroxybenzoate, or p-methoxycarbonylphenol, has been strictly regulated in European-made cosmetics, and current European Union legislation allows their use only in extremely weak concentrations. It is unlikely that parabens will be removed from cosmetics sold in the United States anytime soon. There is strong support of paraben use coming from the chemical industry, especially preservative suppliers, which is very understandable.

## PRESERVATIVES TO AVOID

Other preservatives to avoid include imidazolidinyl urea and diazolidinyl urea. Often disguised as Germall 115 and Germall II, they are a mixture of allantoin, urea, and formaldehyde. Both preservatives are known skin irritants (de Groot et al. 1988; Bosetti et al. 2007). During use, they can release formaldehyde, whose ability to increase the risk of cancer is well-documented (Blackwell et al. 1981). In liquid form, formaldehyde is contained in other widely used preservatives as DMDM-hydantoin and quaternium-15. Beginning in September 2007, the European Union has banned the use of formaldehyde for embalming purposes. Bronopol, often listed as 2-bromo-2-nitropropane-1,3-diol, can contribute to the formation of cancer-causing nitrosamines, according to the FDA. It can also break down to produce formaldehyde. European regulators have also questioned the safety of iodopropynyl butylcarbamate (IPBC), a common wood preservative used in cosmetics, and may restrict its use in moisturizing body lotions. Many agencies are concerned about the levels of iodine found in IPBC, and regulators claim that iodine may be absorbed into the bloodstream, travel to the thyroid gland, and affect its functioning.

"Artificial preservatives are only necessary if your product formulation is weak or unstable," says Roger Barsby of Weleda. "If you dilute your ingredients [with water] to make the product cheaply, then you will need artificial preservatives. Also if your formulation is not balanced and carefully created, you will need stabilizers and preservatives to hold it together." To keep their lotions, shower gels, and baby products safe, Weleda uses essential oils, which provide a natural preservative action.

While writing this book I tested and studied ingredients in hundreds of cosmetic products. Too often, when thoroughly reading the ingredients in a 72 percent "organic" hand cream, I discovered that methylparaben was shyly hiding at the end of the list of ingredients, almost blending in the luscious floral design. The ingredients list further revealed triethanolamine and fragrance (unlikely to be naturally derived), both printed in very small, all-capitalized letters, making it very difficult to read. There was plenty of blank space on the label permitting a larger type, but the company usually chose not to attract attention to synthetic bulk in their "organic" creations.

Our skin eats anything that we put on its surface. I bet you already know that junk food, with all its flavor enhancers, preservatives, synthetic fillers, and highly processed ingredients, is not good for our bodies. When you use beauty products loaded with chemical ingredients, you are feeding your skin highly processed, artificial junk food. If you try eating healthfully, why use junk beauty products?

## Allergies: When Pink Is Not Pretty

Although experts say that only one in ten people has ever developed an allergy to a cosmetic product, I have yet to meet a woman whose skin would happily accept anything applied to it. Most of us have experienced a pink spot or an itch after using a new foundation or a facial treatment. For most of us, something as minor as itching is not a reason to panic.

Contact dermatitis is the most common skin disorder. It can be an irritant reaction (most commonly caused by irritating substances) or allergic reaction (caused by allergens, less common but more severe). Irritant contact dermatitis happens when harsh chemicals directly injure the outer layer of epidermis and irritate the skin. Allergic contact dermatitis occurs when the immune system reacts against a specific chemical that it considers foreign and harmful. While irritant dermatitis flares up almost immediately, an allergic reaction can develop even after you have used a cosmetic product for some time. Lips, eyes, ears, neck, and hands are the most common sites for cosmetic allergies. Symptoms of cosmetic allergy include itchiness, redness, swelling, mild fever, and blistering—definitely not pretty!

**Green Fact**

Pimples, redness, itchiness, and rashes are all signals that our body rejects certain ingredients in cosmetic products.

It may take a while to figure out what causes the allergy. You use about a dozen products on a daily basis, among them makeup, moisturizers, cleanser, toner, sunscreen, and antiaging serum. How do you go about finding the cause of the problem? While strong irritants such as fragrances cause a reaction within seconds, weaker irritants such as preservatives may take up to ten days to trigger an allergic response.

Some cosmetics are labeled "allergy-tested" or "hypoallergenic," but do not let this fool you. "Hypoallergenic" means that the manufacturer thinks the product is less likely to cause an allergic reaction. To justify this claim, some companies simply do not include fragrances or pack the lotion with fewer preservatives. The claim "dermatologist-tested" on cosmetic products only means that a skin doctor has checked the ingredient list to see if the product will generally cause allergenic problems. Other label claims that are meaningless include "sensitivity-tested" and "nonirritating." Still, you have a slightly less chance of developing an irritation when you use these products than those with a full-strength fragrance and preservatives occupying the whole ingredients list.

Sometimes you may develop a reaction to a specific ingredient that haunts you even if you stop using a suspected product and buy a similar one from another brand. You may even show symptoms of skin allergy to a product you have used for years. This happens because of a well-known synergism effect: two chemicals are working together to produce a stronger effect than they normally would when used separately. In addition, the chemical balance of the human body constantly changes. Our skin starts to produce more oil or loses water; our blood becomes more or less acidic; we develop invisible skin conditions that make our skin react in a different way to a chemical that was once safe and gentle.

"I am not allergic to synthetic chemicals because I am unhealthy," said Aubrey Hampton, creator of Aubrey Organics, in his book *Natural Organic Skin and Hair Care*. "I am allergic to synthetic chemicals because I am healthy. Your body is natural, and if your immune system is doing a good job, it will attempt to reject chemical allergens" (Organica Press, 1987).

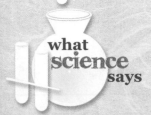

Fragrances, formaldehyde, and other preservatives used in cosmetics are among the most common allergens causing contact allergic dermatitis (Diepgen, Weisshaar 2007). And new allergens are uncovered daily. One such emerging cosmetic allergen is dicaprylyl maleate, an inexpensive synthetic emollient that has been rarely reported as a cause of allergic contact dermatitis. Now scientists have confirmed that this common cosmetic ingredient causes skin irritation in most of the participants of a recent European study (Lotery et al. 2007).

Natural beauty products are not a panacea for allergy sufferers. Many people are allergic to essential oils, especially those of peppermint, orange, and lemon. Tea tree oil, when it oxidizes in a cosmetic product, is capable of causing an irritation, which is especially annoying since tea tree oil is often used to treat acne. Lanolin, derived from sheep's wool, is a known allergen. Trace amounts of honey and propolis can cause a reaction in those allergic to pollen, and a newly found allergen, hyaluronic acid, once thought to be completely safe, is known to consistently cause an inflammatory reaction based on recent studies (Bisaccia et al. 2007; Alijotas-Reig, Garcia-Gimenez 2008).

Advocates of synthetic skin care rejoice at such news. "Citrus often shows up in skin-care products, but most of us have gotten lemon or lime juice on a slight cut while cooking and know it burns like crazy because it's irritating to the skin," Paula Begoun wrote in her book *The Beauty Bible* (2002), which is filled to the brim with praise for mineral oil, isotretinoin, dishwasher liquids-cum-facial-cleansers, and laser surgeries when everything else fails. Well, I cannot imagine that a sane person would think of applying undiluted lemon juice to the skin or rubbing the open wound with poison ivy. It is simply stupid! To please her supporters in the chemical industry, Begoun continues, "Hanging on the notion that 'natural' equals good skin care or better makeup products will waste your money and probably hurt your skin. . . . For many women, it's hard to resist the pressure to believe the lie about natural products being good for skin. . . . The notion that natural ingredients are better than synthetic ingredients is even more distressing because it just isn't true."

Criticizing natural cosmetics because poison ivy stings is the same as criticizing the use of water because a certain number of people drown while swimming or sailing each year. There are many wonderful synthetic ingredients (such as coenzyme

Q10 or palmitoyl pentapeptide), and there are some noxious plant extracts. I hope this book will empower you with the knowledge of how to combine the best of both worlds to create your own green, ecoconscious beauty routine. Let "chemophiles" defend the chemical beauty giant with feet of clay.

So what can you do if you end up with an array of itchy, scratchy spots while trying to hide a blemish? Apart from ditching makeup for a little while, it may be wise to discard all old cosmetics. Preservative agents break down over time, creating new irritating compounds, and other ingredients in cosmetics may oxidize, causing additional problems. For the time being, limit yourself to one cleanser (organic baby soap or baby wash), one toner (rose hydrosol or witch hazel), and only one moisturizer containing no preservatives and only natural, soothing ingredients such as green tea, feverfew, brown algae, and mugwort. While chamomile and marigold are traditionally used to soothe irritated skin, they may cause allergic dermatitis in some people, so use them with caution. For sunscreen, choose a mineral-based version containing zinc or titanium oxide. Whenever possible, use mineral makeup and avoid any foundation or blusher in gel or lotion form. Stay clear of deeply colored eye makeup. Stick to basic black, nonwaterproof mascara and pencil (not liquid!) eyeliners. Keep eye shadows earth-toned—no deep purples, greens, and bright metallics! Avoid looking for an offending product by patch testing with old cosmetics, because oxidation byproducts are strong allergens. Instead, make it a rule to discard all skin care products after three months of use.

## Synthetic Fragrances: I Smell Danger

What is the first thing you do when you try a new moisturizer or lipstick? You smear it on the top of your hand and then you smell it. At this moment, you are not much different from a glue sniffer: substances that make cosmetics smell attractive are very similar to those that send addicts on their chemical trips.

It seems to be vitally important for us to use cosmetic products that smell nice, and this is quite understandable: beauty products make us look and feel better. Even people who admit to having sensitive skin would choose a lotion that had a barely noticeable scent over a completely unscented formulation that smelled like beeswax, green tea, and sunflower oil combined, no matter how beneficial these substances were for human skin.

When we smell an odor, a complex process begins in the brain. The Roman philosopher Lucretius said that different odors are created by molecules of various shapes and sizes. As we inhale fragrance molecules, they trigger a complex chain of reactions. There are many theories about how our nose decodes scents, and there is no theory that explains olfactory perception completely. While the human tongue can distinguish only five distinct tastes, the nose can recognize hundreds of substances, even in microscopic quantities.

So what is fragrance, and why is it so important to us? Odorant (fragrant) molecules dissolved in the air cause a certain sensation. This is a complex process: First, the molecule triggers receptors in the nose. After that, the limbic system, a part of the brain that governs emotional responses, decodes the information. That is why messages sent by odor molecules are powerful mood enhancers. It is no secret that certain odors can evoke distant memories, raise spirits, soothe jagged nerves, and even boost self-confidence.

For most people, the process of smelling gives little information about the ingredients of a particular scent. Most of us think, *What the heck, one spray won't hurt!* The same with food: we may diligently cook organic vegetable meals at home, but sometimes we need to "recharge the batteries" with a chocolate milkshake or a burger. In one meal, we consume a hefty dose of FD&C colors and preservatives. One slip, and a week's worth of pure and clean eating goes down the drain!

It is now possible to dissect any natural scent and recreate it using synthetic fragrances.

This is when technology comes into play. While perfume makers hire famous "noses" to create perfume compositions, mass production of artificial fragrances relies heavily on smelling machines, or "electronic noses" that use chemical sensors to produce a fingerprint of any scent. It is now possible to dissect any natural scent and recreate it using synthetic fragrances. While advocates of synthetic skin care insist that everything comes from nature and nothing is created via alchemy, in the case of serious fragrance synthesizing, it's simply not true. Today, the chemical industry can recreate any scent known to man, including dirt, earth, leather, snow, or freshly cut grass—and all of them can be surprisingly beautiful when mixed in the right proportions with floral and wood notes.

Every year, fragrance compositions are becoming more and more complicated. More and more products become heavily scented: laundry detergents, dryer sheets, cosmetics, stationery, candles, and pet products come in a variety of "naturally inspired scents." Even baby toys are now infused with lavender and vanilla. To meet these needs, hundreds of new fragrant chemicals are being developed. Of the more than 5,000 materials currently available for use in fragrances, only 1,300 or so were tested for safety. Many of them are known fragrance sensitizers that have to be used in microscopic doses, if at all. Bear in mind, these synthetic fragrance molecules are programmed to turn on switches in our brains! Scientists believe that the ubiquitous nature of synthetic fragrance in modern society, coupled with the growing number of fragrance products for children and men, likely contributes to the sharp increase in allergies and respiratory illnesses.

Smart manufacturers rarely disclose the full list of ingredients that go into a fragrant composition. Fragrance formulas are considered trade secrets, and manufacturers do not have to tell anyone, including health authorities, what is in those formulas. However, many manufacturers attempt to list at least some ingredients. For example, a full list of ingredients of the average musk body mist reads as a huge list of synthetic and organic fragrance ingredients plus a "secret" fragrance, which most likely contains synthetic musk that has strong potential for triggering adverse effects in sensitive people.

There are plenty of organically derived fragrance ingredients used to enhance and enrich existing trademark compositions. All of the following naturally occurring fragrance ingredients are capable of causing allergic dermatitis and rhinitis: citronellol (found in citronella essential oil), linalool (a floral, slightly spicy odor chemical found in many plants, including mint, scented herbs, and even birch), geraniol (a fragrant component occurring in geranium, lemon, and many other essential oils), farnesol (found in citronella, neroli, cyclamen, lemongrass, tuberose, rose, balsam, and tolu), cinnamal (a flavor component in the essential oil of cinnamon), and eugenol (extracted from spices such as clove oil, nutmeg, cinnamon, and bay leaf).

A typical perfume contains a mixture of fragrance chemicals (often between 50 and 100) produced from coal tar and petroleum distillates or plants and herbs. In terms of "greenness," the fragrance industry is unique: scented, natural, and synthetic ingredients can be equally harmful. But while organically derived aromatic alcohols can irritate skin, make you sneeze, or trigger existing eczema or asthma, benzene derivatives, aldehydes, phenols, phthalates, and many other fragrant toxins are capable of causing cancer, birth defects, and central nervous system disorders. These substances can get into the body by being absorbed through the skin and when inhaled.

Studies constantly reveal new irritating fragrance ingredients. Some of the oldest known toxic synthetic fragrances are nitromusks, such as musk ambrette, musk xylene, and musk ketone. In clinical studies dating back to the 1980s, musk ambrette has caused eczema, jawline dermatitis, acute contact dermatitis, and chronic actinic dermatitis (Wojnarowska, Calnan 1986). The use of nitromusks in cosmetics has been banned, but synthetic musks are still found in musk-scented incense candles and may be lurking under the vague name "fragrance" in popular scented products.

Hydroxyisohexyl 3-cyclohexene carboxaldehyde (also known as Lyral) is the most allergic fragrance chemical currently used. It caused contact dermatitis and eczema in 79 percent of participants in a recent study. Lyral irritated the skin of even healthy people who were not prone to allergies (Baxter et al. 2003). Lyral is currently listed as an allergen but is contained in many of the popular fragrances as well as every other deodorant on the drugstore shelf.

Benzyl alcohol, an aromatic substance naturally found in essential oils including jasmine, hyacinth, and ylang-ylang, may cause various toxic effects, such as respiratory failure, very low blood pressure, convulsions, and paralysis. However, to cause real damage, it has to be used in high concentrations. Benzyl alcohol was used up to 0.9 percent as a preservative in neonatal medications, but after sixteen newborns died of acute toxic poisoning in 1982, benzyl alcohol was banned for use as a preservative. In spite of this, as a fragrance ingredient, and possibly a preservative, it is currently used in popular moisturizers, facial cleansers, aftershaves, and baby wipes and lotions. For more information, check www.thegreenbeauty guide.com.

As I was writing this chapter, I could not help but feel a tiny bit smug. *Perhaps I am not a very bad mom*, I thought. *I do not use fragrances at home. I am feeding my baby organic food and homemade purees; she drinks her organic formula from glass bottles and sleeps on organic cotton sheets. Her mattress is pure wool. There is no chance she would be exposed to such a horrible substance as benzyl alcohol.* Yeah, right. Just as I finished writing this chapter, something clicked inside my head. I went to our nursery and picked up the pack of baby wipes. These award-winning wipes contained benzyl alcohol as the third ingredient, right after water and glycerin. I sent a letter to the manufacturer of these wipes giving them specific research on how dangerous these baby wipes can be. The manufacturer responded with a canned letter that defended their use of benzyl alcohol as a disinfectant but promised they would revise the formula someday soon. Needless to say, we abandoned all wipes made by this brand, and instead I brew a cupful of organic chamomile tea, pour it in a spray bottle, and use it with a plain cotton face towel to gently cleanse my daughter's bum. Please note that some babies (and adults, too) are allergic to chamomile, so if you have a family history of allergies, always perform a patch test before using any herbal infusions, flower distillates, or essential oils.

Lesson learned: never assume anything. Just because a company makes chlorine-free, plastic-free, disposable diapers and packs them in smart bags with handwritten letters and cute baby faces, it does not mean that all of their products are safe for your baby. Do not assume that if a company makes a great moisturizer, you should buy the rest of their products.

Also, do not assume that people succeed in the cosmetic business while being led by only one aim: to make you healthier and help you live longer. Every enterprise is started with a business plan that involves some sort of profit gained at the end of the year. The manufacturer can save millions by replacing just one costly natural extract with some synthetic brew. So always check the ingredients; be vigilant and skeptical, even if it comes to organic beauty.

Back to synthetic aromatics. Benzyl acetate, a jasmine-flavored relative of benzyl alcohol, was generally recognized as safe by the Flavor and Extract Manufacturers Association (FEMA) expert panel. However, a 2002 study conducted at the University of Louisville, Kentucky, suggested that this synthetic fragrance compound may be carcinogenic in rodent studies, causing liver and bladder cancer (Waddell 2002). This study caused quite a stir in the scientific community, but so far benzyl acetate sits happily in drugstore aisles, listed among ingredients in many bestselling products, including award-winning moisturizers, mascaras, and antiaging products.

Butylphenyl methylpropional (also known as Lilial or lilialdehyde) is a widely used fragrance compound found naturally in the essential oil of chamomile. Allergic contact dermatitis caused by Lilial was first reported and well studied in 1983 (Larsen 1983). Currently, this lovely floral synthetic fragrance is used in both elite fragrances and drugstore shampoos, deodorants, tanning lotions, and hairstyling products (Buckley 2007).

Almond-smelling benzaldehyde can be easily derived from apricot, cherry, laurel leaves, and peach seeds, but now is most often made from toluene. In 1977, it was proven that benzaldehyde is a strong contact irritant, but it remains one of the most frequently used fragrance components. Its highest reported concentration of use was 0.5 percent in perfumes. Benzaldehyde is generally regarded as a safe food additive in the United States and is accepted as a flavoring substance in the European Union. Benzaldehyde rapidly metabolizes to benzoic acid in the skin, is absorbed through the skin and by the lungs, and is distributed to all the organs. In 2006, fragrance manufacturers, via the Cosmetic Ingredient Review, assured that benzaldehyde is not a carcinogenic, reproductive, or developmental toxicant at concentrations used in cosmetics (Andersen 2006). However, a new 2007 study determined that "exposure to aldehydes represents potential risks to human and animal health," scientists from ChemRisk in Colorado wrote. They found that this chemical induced formation of stable DNA-protein cross-links in cultured human lymphoma cells (Kuykendall et al. 2007). In plain English, benzaldehyde promoted cancerous cell growth. Today, synthetic benzaldehyde is contained in many popular shaving foams, deodorants, moisturizers, and some "soothing" baby products. As for me, I don't find this information soothing, do you?

Synthetic fragrances may smell like the real deal, but they cannot fool our bodies. The synthetic fragrance molecules aren't recognized by our immune system as safe. Because our DNA has evolved over millions of years, and synthetic fragrances have been in use only since the 1920s, every cell in our body is programmed to accept only truly natural, volatile compounds found in herbs and fruits.

What does our body do when hostile substances attack it? It kicks back, and the outcome of this fight is not beautiful. Asthma, migraines, hyperactivity disorder in children and adults, rashes, depression, and seizures have been linked to synthetic chemical fragrances. New studies linking synthetic fragrances to cancer and diabetes come up daily.

In people whose immune system is constantly alert "thanks" to large amounts of synthetic additives they consume with food, drinks, and cosmetics, every additional chemical triggers a much more acute reaction than in people whose bodies aren't overly sensitized. But it's really hard to get rid of fragrances today. A pretty scent helps sell otherwise no-nonsense laundry detergents, dishwashing liquids, and baby wet wipes. Celebrity fragrances are churned out overnight. For many fashion designers, couture collections serve only to help sell fragrances, shower gels, and body lotions. Our fascination with fragrances grows exponentially: celebrity-fragrance sales have increased by 2,000 percent since 2004.

> Asthma, migraines, hyperactivity disorder in children and adults, rashes, depression, and seizures have been linked to synthetic chemical fragrances.

Here's a bit of harsh reality: British researchers spent quite a bit of money on a massive shopping spree, buying 300 perfumed cosmetic and household products available on the shelves of UK stores in January 2006 (Buckley 2007). They only bought products that listed "parfum," "fragrance," or "aroma" among the ingredients. The results weren't all roses: the top six most frequently labeled fragrances were linalool (found mostly in expensive perfumes, soaps, shampoos, and shower gels), limonene (most frequently found in toothpastes, aftershaves, dishwashing liquids, and detergents), citronellol (found in deodorants), geraniol, butylphenyl methylpropional, and hexyl cinnamal. Other top scents detected in 300 popular cosmetic products were eugenol, hydroxycitronellal, isoeugenol, cinnamal, and oak moss (*Evernia prunastri*) absolute. Hydroxyisohexyl-3-cyclohexene carboxaldehyde (Lyral) was present in large concentrations in almost one-third of the products. Scientists concluded that linalool and limonene, both strong allergens, are the most frequent fragrances inhaled and rubbed into skin by millions of people.

And the list, sadly, can go on and on. A potent carcinogen, methylene chloride, banned for use in 1988, can still be found in shampoos and shoe polish spray; methyl eugenol, also a potential carcinogen in animals, is present in shampoos and men's grooming products; ethyl acrylate, another chemical that killed rats with cancer in 2002, is listed among ingredients in antiaging creams, designer fragrances, and sunscreen towelettes.

When I made a big leap and switched to purely organic scents, the whole picture got clearer and scarier—or maybe my head was working better without all those synthetic vapors? On one side, there is a noticeable interest in truly natural scents. On the other, famous "noses" come up with yet another alluring twist and weave together scents that Mother Nature still has to invent. I can't help but suspect that the fragrance industry may now be acting similar to the tobacco industry in the early 1990s, hiding the truth of the very serious health effects of secondhand smoke and chemicals from cigarettes.

Even perfectly natural and gentle skin products, such as a "98.36 percent natural" carrot moisturizer that I have tested and reviewed recently, contain fragrances. They are used to mask otherwise blunt or even repulsive odors of natural ingredients or to add depth and staying power to scents of essential oils already present in the composition. After years of testing various beauty products, my skin became as tolerant as a celebrity UN ambassador, and I suspect nothing can throw it off balance. But since the phrase "made with pure essential oils" translates to an ingredient list with a small percentage of essential oils, with the remainder being synthetic fragrances, chemical enhancers, and boosters added in an attempt to cut costs, I cannot help but think that a natural herbal scent is in fact a chemical cocktail that is anything but healthy.

Can you really be too careful? Well, you are informed now—maybe scared—and the choice is yours. With a little girl growing up and a family history of allergies and cancer, I prefer to err on the side of caution. If something was proven unsafe once, even in animal studies, I would avoid this ingredient so when new research emerges, I won't be biting my nails (buffed, not polished) over some benzaldehyde-loaded "holy grail" lotion I used diligently over the years. Have you ever heard of a chemical that was considered unsafe for many years being recently declared safe? I haven't. More often, things happen the other way around.

## The Golden Rule of Beauty

When people encounter new scientific information that casts doubt on the status quo, they often can't believe their eyes (or ears). If all this is true, you may ask, why haven't I heard it before? Why do so many dermatologists with perfect credentials endorse beauty products that are making me sick? Could they be doing it to keep themselves busy?

These are all perfectly good questions, and getting the right answers is an important part of your green coming-of-age. To follow all the leads and examine all the underlying reasons may be beyond the scope of this book, but some issues have to be explained. The beauty industry is one of the most profitable of all industries, and as in every business, you may be surprised to find out that the information is governed by the same old Golden Rule: those who have the gold make the rule.

So who has the gold? One of the world's largest and most profitable industries, which will start losing millions of dollars if people start asking uncomfortable questions about what goes into their favorite moisturizers and perfumes. The formulations smell awesome and perform well; they are proven to sell, and the whole process runs smoothly. The financial health of this industry depends on what the public knows about risks associated with many of their products. Like any reasonable business (the cosmetic manufacturers didn't generate this much money by being unreasonable), the beauty industry is doing everything in its power to protect its profits and please its shareholders.

Science and business have long been aware of the links between cosmetics and the meteoric rise of cancer, asthma, diabetes, and a host of other systemic diseases. However, the industries responsible for producing synthetic chemicals have long been seeking, with much success, to downplay or dismiss them.

Things aren't as dramatic as you may think. No one is paying the scientists to shelve the research results. No one is bribing the media. Things are much more subtle. If a cosmetic company buys a certain number of magazine ads, it's very unlikely that the editor-in-chief would be happy to read a story about peanut oil that wasn't mentioned on the label of a sunscreen triggering potentially deadly allergies in hundreds of people, including children—especially since this cosmetic company regularly delivers a boatful of full-size freebies for review and personal use.

Media, government, science, industry, medicine—keeping the status quo is vital for all of them. Too many people would choose profits over health and technology over nature. Using airless packaging that prevents contamination requires fewer investments than spending years in researching and developing another preservative. Thousands of people

## NOT-SO-GREEN FACTS

- Results of the Female Beauty Survey of Great Britain, commissioned by *New Woman* magazine, revealed that only 18 percent of women said they were "happy with their skin," with 44 percent admitting that it was oily, 32 percent saying it was dry, and others complaining of freckles and wrinkles.

- Cosmetic companies spend more on TV advertising than any other group, says the *Townsend Letter for Doctors and Patients*.

- According to Euromonitor International's data, fragrance is the third most dynamic cosmetics and toiletries sector, behind sun and baby care, and posted an increase of 7 percent to reach $30.5 billion.

- In the United Kingdom, the total cost of an adult lifetime of beauty products and treatments was calculated to be £182,528 (US $365,000), or £3,000 a year, of which £600 is spent on facials, massages, and antiaging treatments. About 43 percent of women do not inform their partner of how much they spend, notes *New Woman*'s survey, conducted in 2006.

- The global market for cosmetics and toiletries ingredients will enjoy growth of the ingredients around 5 percent per year through 2010, with color cosmetics to have the highest average annual growth rate, says a 2006 report by the leading information analyst, BCC Research.

- Online sales of cosmetics and fragrances grew by 30 percent, noted Jorn Madslien at BBC News.

would lose their jobs, tons of moisturizers would be left unsold, whole manufacturing processes would have to be revised, a few class-action lawsuits would be filed—and this means millions if not billions of dollars lost. Once a product is on the market, the burden of legal proof required for its removal is extremely high.

The beauty industry is busy beefing up its ego. We believe our life is void if we have cellulite. Our personal life may become null if we have dull hair and lips lacking a lick of shimmery pink gloss. We fear enlarged pores more than job loss. (Otherwise, why would we spend hours in the bathroom applying makeup, even when we're hopelessly late for an important meeting?) As a result, we shop tirelessly, rubbing and sniffing magazine pages and listening to sales blabber, mesmerized and hypnotized by the promise of instant youth in a bottle. After all, if a salesperson is wearing a white lab coat, she knows better, right?

Even if you try to do research on your own, the chances of finding unbiased information are scarce. In the beauty industry, it is almost impossible to examine the long-term health effects of any chemical substance without relying on research conducted by the beauty industry itself. Finding an expert without corporate ties is difficult.

"Show us the dead bodies," cosmetic regulators say when asked about harmful effects of toxic ingredients. "A pinch of glitter cannot kill. Show us the evidence against parabens or aluminum involving humans, not rodents or cells in a test tube." The recent lawsuit filed in California against manufacturers of 1,4-Dioxane-contaminated personal-care products shows that we are slowly waking up to the dangers of toxic beauty. But to win a lawsuit against a cosmetic company for causing your cancer, there must be scientific proof that your disease was caused by your exposure to this exact chemical. To obtain such proof, series of "double-blind" studies on humans must be conducted. But who would participate in them?

All of us are eating, drinking, and breathing a chemical cocktail of pesticides, heavy metals, and plastic compounds. Hundreds of synthetic substances have accumulated in our bodies over decades while we strived to keep our faces youthful and hair shiny. It's impossible to find a perfectly healthy, uncontaminated group of women who would participate in a study proving the harm of 1,4-Dioxane, aluminum, or paraben preservatives. And even if such women exist, I doubt they will agree to rub aluminum and nitrosamines into their skin just to prove how deadly these substances are.

Any solutions? I cannot possibly recommend that you stop washing your hair, brushing your teeth, or wearing makeup. You can still do all those pleasant and rewarding steps of your beauty regimen without inhaling, swallowing, and absorbing toxins. There are many wonderfully effective gentle and safe cosmetic products that won't wreak havoc on your hormones, liver, and lungs.

If you cannot bear parting with your chemical-laden but it-feels-so-good-on-your-skin foundation, you may be surprised to learn that its European-sold version contains much less toxic chemicals. As of September 2004, cosmetics sold in the European market had to be reformulated to comply with the new law banning many toxic ingredients. Now cosmetic manufacturers are required by law to make versions of their products without carcinogenic or toxic substances to meet European regulations. Such versions are not always available in the United States. Can you really expect a hair dye box to carry a label saying "May Cause Bladder Cancer"?

Blaming the system for all our woes is very unproductive and oh-so-out-of-fashion. Remember that through the ages, women happily used highly toxic cosmetic agents such as mercury, lead, or belladonna to make themselves pretty.

So instead of nursing your paranoia and musing over the ugly side of the conventional beauty industry, let's adopt a constructive approach. The first step would be learning how to avoid products that contain toxic, even carcinogenic, ingredients and instead choose products that are made with ingredients less likely to add to your body's toxic burden of harmful chemicals. Such products do exist.

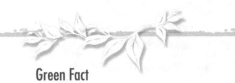

### Green Fact

In January 2003, the European Union passed legislation banning the use in cosmetics of chemicals known to cause, or strongly suspected of causing, cancer, mutations, or birth defects.

## THE TEN COMMANDMENTS OF GREEN BEAUTY

Let's start our journey with some basic guidelines that can help you get through most of the information packed in the chapters ahead. Here are Ten Commandments of Green Beauty. Memorize them and repeat them every time you crave that new shimmery pink blush, dreamily squeeze and sniff a flower-scented lotion at the beauty counter, or read about a celebrity must-have hair mousse in a glossy magazine. Once you learn these commandments, you will gain a better perspective on what you are really paying for at cosmetic counters, and whether any of this can hurt your skin and put you at risk for a serious medical condition in the future.

1. *Thou Shalt Not* buy beauty products that contain phthalates, formaldehyde, phenols, sodium laureth sulfate, coal tar, toxic dyes, and synthetic fragrances.

2. *Thou Shalt Not* buy cosmetics based solely on advertising claims or celebrity endorsements. Very few celebrities actually use the products they advertise. Neither do models whose faces are used in the ads, no matter what models say in interviews. Read the label, scan the ingredients list online using the Skin Deep (www.ewg.com) tool for chemical hazards, read online reviews, and then decide whether this product is worth your money or not.

3. *Thou Shalt Not* believe that just because a cosmetic product is called "natural" it is generally safer. Cosmetics may claim to be "natural" or made with "organic" ingredients, but may still include paraben and formaldehyde preservatives, synthetic fragrances, phthalates, or other toxic ingredients.

4. *Thou Shalt Not* believe that you have to spend a lot of money on organic beauty products. Many inexpensive natural cosmetic lines have

*continued*

wonderful products that perform just as well as expensive ones because most plant extracts, vitamins, and minerals are not exclusive to one company. High-quality ingredients do not necessarily cost a lot more; many cosmetic companies buy ingredients from the same farm or wholesale supplier. There are many organic beauty manufacturers who grow their own ingredients, too. The only difference may be the concentration of these plant juices and extracts, and in the next chapters, you will learn how to choose products that really deliver.

5. *Thou Shalt Not* believe there is such a thing as a magic beauty bullet. There are no secret ingredients that can instantly cure all your skin's woes, but there are many new, effective active ingredients that can do wonders for your skin.

6. *Thou Shalt Not* compare your skin or hair to those of celebrities and spend hours moaning over a pimple, a wrinkle, or a stray lock. All celebrities are humans with their flaws and insecurities, and their picture-perfect skin is not due to the use of some secret potion but rather skillful hairstyling, makeup artistry, and computer retouching.

7. *Thou Shalt Not* share your mascara or lipstick, keep the jar of moisturizer open, lick the tip of your eyeliner, apply face cream with dirty hands, dilute shampoo with water—simply put, contaminate your beauty products and shorten their life span. Never use beauty products when their "best before" date is overdue.

8. *Thou Shalt Not* believe that you need a special moisturizer for hands and another one for the rest of your body; that you need an eye cream and a separate face cream and a really cute neck serum; that you cannot use baby bath gel to cleanse your face; that you should have a different sunscreen lotion for each part of your body. In other words, do

*continued*

not let smart marketers manipulate you. Less is more, especially when it comes to organic formulations. From an oat scrub to a honey mask, the best things in beauty come incredibly cheap, and you don't need to spend tons of money to look great and be healthy.

9. *Thou Shalt Not* believe that if a famous doctor, chemist, dermatologist, yoga guru, hairstylist, or movie star created the formula, it would mean a world of difference. Lots of dermatologists, biologists, herbalists, and even aerospace engineers are involved in whipping up beauty products. It's the juice that counts, not the bottle, as Aubrey Hampton, the pioneer of organic beauty, used to say, and your skin doesn't care whose name is on the packaging. Read the ingredients list, ask smart questions about the concentration of particular ingredients, check reviews, be skeptical, and take everything with a grain of sea salt.

10. *Thou Shalt Not* keep it a secret. Spread the news. Help teenage girls avoid toxic beauty products. If you work in a spa or in a health-care facility, explain the dangers of toxic chemicals to your patients and clients. Phone the companies whose products you use and express your concerns directly. Many product labels carry toll-free phone numbers. Be an informed, vigilant consumer because what you know (and what you don't) can turn really costly in terms of your looks and health.

# READER/CUSTOMER CARE SURVEY

HEFG

We care about your opinions! Please take a moment to fill out our online Reader Survey at **http://survey.hcibooks.com.**
As a **"THANK YOU"** you will receive a **VALUABLE INSTANT COUPON** towards future book purchases
as well as a **SPECIAL GIFT** available only online! Or, you may mail this card back to us.

(PLEASE PRINT IN ALL CAPS)

First Name _____ MI. _____ Last Name _____

Address _____ City _____

State _____ Zip _____ Email _____

**1. Gender**
☐ Female  ☐ Male

**2. Age**
☐ 8 or younger
☐ 9-12     ☐ 13-16
☐ 17-20   ☐ 21-30
☐ 31+

**3. Did you receive this book as a gift?**
☐ Yes  ☐ No

**4. Annual Household Income**
☐ under $25,000
☐ $25,000 - $34,999
☐ $35,000 - $49,999
☐ $50,000 - $74,999
☐ over $75,000

**5. What are the ages of the children living in your house?**
☐ 0 - 14   ☐ 15+

**6. Marital Status**
☐ Single
☐ Married
☐ Divorced
☐ Widowed

**7. How did you find out about the book?**
*(please choose one)*
☐ Recommendation
☐ Store Display
☐ Online
☐ Catalog/Mailing
☐ Interview/Review

**8. Where do you usually buy books?**
*(please choose one)*
☐ Bookstore
☐ Online
☐ Book Club/Mail Order
☐ Price Club (Sam's Club, Costco's, etc.)
☐ Retail Store (Target, Wal-Mart, etc.)

**9. What subject do you enjoy reading about the most?**
*(please choose one)*
☐ Parenting/Family
☐ Relationships
☐ Recovery/Addictions
☐ Health/Nutrition
☐ Christianity
☐ Spirituality/Inspiration
☐ Business Self-help
☐ Women's Issues
☐ Sports

**10. What attracts you most to a book?**
*(please choose one)*
☐ Title
☐ Cover Design
☐ Author
☐ Content

Comments

chapter **3**

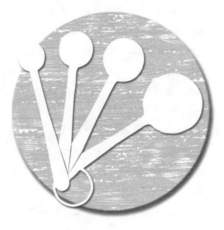

become
an ingredients
list expert

**K**eeping your skin glowing and hair lustrous can cost thousands of dollars, and for many of us, "holy grail" beauty products are the result of a lengthy (and costly) quest filled with hope, patience, and disappointment. Every year, hundreds of products claim to be the newest, cutting-edge, and most effective for everything from acne to wrinkles and everything in between. We constantly look for the magic lotion or potion that will make us look like that porcelain-skinned fifteen-year-old Estonian model.

Since the cosmetic manufacturers are not ready to help us—more likely, they will fill our already confused heads with new fantastic claims—your best bet to protect your skin is to seek out pure and safe skin care products.

When choosing beauty products, the ingredients list should be your number-one reference point. According to new United States and Canadian legislation, product labels must list all the ingredients regardless of their quantity. Often, cosmetic manufacturers will separately list the concentration of the active ingredient, such as "2 percent lactic acid." If you are savvy enough, you will easily spot ingredients you should keep away from. However, sometimes even if you stumble onto a relatively safe and properly formulated product, there's always something that can go wrong, and the search continues. Still, there are certain ways to minimize the money and time wasted.

## Twelve Lessons in Smart Beauty Shopping

Choosing a new beauty product is an exciting, rewarding process. Many of us, including me, buy a new lipstick or moisturizer as a reward. How many times have you bought a lip-gloss to treat yourself for a week-long abstinence from some of life's guilty pleasures (such as ice cream, booze, bickering with in-laws, online gaming, eBay hunting, or too much impulse shopping)? I cannot count how many pretty rose lippies I have collected this way. Each one is like a badge of honor, and I cherish them.

Yet all this excitement and pleasure of finding another age-delaying magic potion can get slashed by the disappointment caused by yet another shattered hope. The shimmery rose lipstick may leave lips dry; the flowery-smelling, green tea–loaded lotion ignites a constellation of pimples right in the middle of a cheek; the sexy, powdery scent of a "most wanted" fragrance will send you (and a few dozen passengers in a subway train) sneezing and wiping away tears. You lost money since you cannot find the receipt to return the irksome stuff. Besides, who has the time and courage to face the sleek cunning of a salesperson who hates to lose her commission?

The truth is, beauty doesn't come in a bottle, and even if it does, choosing what's right for you is not easy. But there are ways to take perfectly good care of your skin. In this chapter, you will find twelve lessons that will help you become a Smart Green Beauty Expert, the good judge of ingredients and aficionado of textures who won't ever get waylaid with false claims or ineffective "snake oil" products; who won't "lemming" the latest celebrity must-have; and who will spend money wisely and remain cool under the heavy artillery of salespeople. More importantly, when you're a Smart Green Beauty Expert, your priorities will be sorted out, which will allow you to treat the avalanche of beauty information with healthy skepticism.

## Lesson 1: Scan Ingredients Lists with Graceful Ease

The best way to shop for skin care products is to become ingredient-wise. You have to stop being afraid of the fine print and learn to read product labels to determine good and bad product ingredients, so you can select skin care products that are most beneficial for you.

Quickly scanning the ingredients list for offending substances is probably the most important skill you have to master. Being able to quickly decipher the ingredients list instead of listening to a salesperson's chatter will save you money, time, and frustration. I have long lost count of how many times a salesperson offered me "completely natural" stretch mark butter or an eye cream, even while the ingredients list was bursting with parabens, PEGs, and formaldehyde preservatives.

Many cosmetic manufacturers don't help us at all. The worse the formulation is, the harder the box is to read. To discourage curious customers from prying into cosmetic secrets, they print ingredients lists in all-capitalized dense letters with very small spaces between lines, so the whole area looks like one grayish square filled with chemical jabber. Often the lavish design masks the most noxious ingredients. Some of them may be hiding under natural-sounding names or abbreviations. Cocamide DEA may sound natural, but in fact it is coconut oil diethanolamine, and we already know that diethanolamine, along with triethanolamine, may be contaminated with carcinogenic chemicals.

Here's a funny thing I stumbled across on the Internet one day. It described two variations of diethanolamine as two completely different substances. "DEA is a clear watery liquid, while lauramide DEA is a rock hard solid. In essence, these ingredients are as different from each other as are apples and automobiles," says Dr. Dennis T. Sepp in the article "DEA, Setting the Record Straight" published on a website that sells "natural" skin care products. Yeah, right—and ice and snow are completely different from water, too. See, one is hard and the other one is fluffy, and they look nothing like water! This is just one example of how cosmetic companies and incompetent experts use to their advantage our lack of desire to question and criticize.

When properly written, the labels can provide you with a lot of useful information. In the United States and Canada, any chemical above 1 percent by weight in the formula is required to be listed in order of concentration. The general rule of thumb is, the higher amount of an ingredient the product contains, the higher position it will occupy in the ingredients list. So pay attention to which ingredient is listed first. Good cleansers and toners start with water, followed by mild detergent or soap at the beginning of the list; toners may begin with water, witch hazel, or alcohol right in the first line. For example, a mediocre toner would list a propylene glycol second in the list of ingredients; a good one will contain floral water, witch hazel, or glycerin. A heavy moisturizer will list mineral oil or petrolatum as its second ingredient, right after water. Such moisturizers will contain many pore-clogging ingredients and therefore will not be suitable for acne sufferers. However, a moisturizer that lists mineral oil somewhere in the middle of the fine print would be less likely to cause breakouts, but nevertheless is less suitable for oily skin than a moisturizer with no mineral oil at all, such as a lotion based on olive oil.

> Good cleansers and toners start with water, followed by mild detergent or soap at the beginning of the list; toners may begin with water, witch hazel, or alcohol right in the first line.

Most often, preservatives, fragrances, and colors are

listed at the end of the list. However, I have seen formulations that listed triethanolamine and paraben preservatives right in the first line, which means that this particular product contained a lot of very questionable substances. But even if there's less than 1 percent of an ingredient contained in the bottle or jar, it doesn't mean that it cannot get any job done. Peptides, enzymes, vitamins, and antioxidants acids are all used in smaller than 1 percent concentrations.

When you think about it, even 1 percent is quite a bit of a chemical. If you imagine 1 percent of a 100 ml bottle, that's 1 ml of a substance, about the size of a tester fragrance vial. Imagine how a guy in a white lab coat takes an ampoule of something that causes cancer in rats and pours it into your body lotion, or worse yet, baby bath. The situation is cartoonish, but you get the idea. Does it look pretty or healthy? It certainly doesn't look good to me.

So resist the urge to scan just the first few lines. Keep reading. Take your time and ignore those spiteful looks from the sales clerk at the counter. It's your money and your health. The girl works on commission, so no wonder she hates you for delaying the decisive moment—you know, the one when she swipes your plastic. And watch her face freezing when you refuse to buy the proffered magic potion.

Sometimes, ingredients lists are not easy to locate—or they are not there at all. In that case, contact the company directly by phone or e-mail. Most companies respond to customer queries about their ingredients, so don't be afraid to contact them if you are unsure about a chemical or it's not listed in any online database.

There are thousands of safe synthetic ingredients that can be used in skin care products. In the next chapters, I will list many natural or synthesized active ingredients that you should look for when buying a new cosmetic product or purchasing online to enrich your existing products. If you want to learn more about each particular ingredient, you can check the safety of a suspicious chemical at the Environmental Working Group website (www.ewg.org) where they have a very comprehensive and searchable database of most existing chemicals used in personal care products.

When you learn the trick of scanning the ingredients list for toxic chemicals and ingredients that can damage your skin, you will never purchase a beauty product just because it looks pretty or elegant, thus falling prey to tricky advertisers and talented product designers. Once you've learned to read the ingredients label and identify marketing scams, you'll be able to avoid wasting money and still take perfectly good care of your skin and hair.

## ANGEL DUSTING: NOT JUST FOR ADDICTS

No worries: I am not telling you how to extract a pinch of illegal substance from ten bottles of herbal shampoo. Angel dusting is the common practice of adding very minute amounts of trendy ingredients just so they can be listed on the product label. These exciting ingredients are being used in very small quantities, so they are physically unable to make any difference in skin's condition. However, the mere presence of "angel dust" on a label generates a lot of interest, making us feel very eager to try the product.

This is how it works: let's take some fantastic ingredient, like "olivoil fifty-peptide," a powerful antiaging molecule similar to palmitoyl pentapeptide but ten times more powerful. A laboratory that developed this magic molecule specified at what percentage "fifty-peptide" must be included in the cosmetics to produce the desired effect. However, this magic ingredient costs $200 per ounce, and it takes a quarter ounce to work its magic.

Therefore, instead of dumping liquid gold into every bottle, smart cosmetic manufacturers would wave a spoonful of "fifty-peptide" over a plopping canister of lotion. Some molecules actually land in the brew. No worries! Now the manufacturer can legitimately list "fifty-peptide" on the label, write a news release about a magic antiaging discovery, and send samples to glossy magazines. Now, because "fifty-peptide" is listed on the label, the antiaging potion sells like hotcakes. Very soon, consumers will be disappointed because fifty molecules are useless and won't repurchase the product. But the "angel duster" would save up to 1,000 percent on the active ingredient without breaking any laws or rules.

While there's nothing harmful in this practice in itself, abuse in angel dusting can be a harmful practice (figuratively and literally) because it deliberately misleads consumers and dissipates the trust in cosmetic innovations. The only way to spot the "angel-dusted" ingredient is to look at the label. Reputable companies always list the concentration of the active ingredient. For example, Prevage by Allergan is made with 1 percent idebenone (a very potent synthetic version of CoQ10), and Strivectin SD by Klein-Becker is made with 5 percent Striadril, a proprietary blend of pentapeptides.

## Lesson 2: Understand What You Are Paying For

Before you ever reach for your hard-earned cash, keep this in mind: of every dollar paid for mass-market skin care, sixty cents goes to the manufacturer and forty cents goes to the retailer. No matter what you buy—a pair of jeans or a lawn mower—the proportion remains pretty much the same.

Manufacturers pay for production, packaging, storage, and transportation. For eighteen cents, they hire smart marketing advisers who tell them how to make women pay $50 for 1 ounce of petrochemicals, preservatives, and synthetic fragrances. These marketing geniuses hire teenage models or starlets to market the product to forty-year-olds. Eleven cents goes toward packaging: a team of artists is picked to design a stylish, expensive-looking bottle. Two cents pays for interest and other boring things, and eighteen cents pays salaries and covers administrative expenses. The retailer pays the rent, designs attractive window displays, and gives gift bags to the media to make them write about the new store event. Forty cents pays salaries to salespeople, bookkeepers, and security guys.

Of every buck you spend on a beauty product, only seven cents will pay the real cost of the ingredients. Another four cents will cover the production—the process of mixing, whipping, and pouring. That's it. The remaining money feeds the army of professionals who do nothing to improve the quality of the beauty product.

I learned this formula from product-development textbooks when I started creating my own skin care line, *Petite Marie Organics*. Since I am a small business, I can avoid many organizational costs and invest the money where it must belong in skin care—in high-quality, organic ingredients.

Let's examine the ingredients list of a popular moisturizer marketed for sensitive skin. The formula is loaded with humectants and film-forming agents that do not penetrate skin. Even though the lotion is called fragrance-free, there are some synthetic fragrances to mask the real (most likely, filthy) scent of the ingredients, and there is a "food-grade" preservative added to extend the shelf life. In my opinion, this is a better formulation, since it contains no synthetic dyes, paraben preservatives, or strong penetration enhancers. It is moderately priced around $9 per generous 16-ounce bottle (almost a half-liter).

So how much would the ingredients cost if you and I tried to recreate the lotion at home? Let's just take a look at the first few ingredients that make up the bulk of the lotion. Water is nearly free, glycerin costs $1.70 per 8 ounces, emulsifier ceteareth-20 costs $2.20 per 4 ounces, another emulsifier and thickener, cetyl alcohol, costs $1.27 per 4 ounces, and macadamia oil—a strong allergen, especially for those with nut allergies—costs $6 per 8 ounces. We will use only a few teaspoons of each ingredient, so the whole formulation ends up costing $1.50, even if you replace some chemicals with more expensive plant oils. Remember, these aren't wholesale prices. We'll be paying this much only if we order 4 or 8 ounces of each component. Cosmetic manufacturers buy ingredients by the tons, and they pay dramatically less.

Any cosmetic product containing beneficial amounts of active ingredients is not going to be cheap. In this lotion, the most expensive ingredient is provitamin B5, or panthenol, and it sells for $2.50 per ounce. Obviously, there isn't a whole ounce of panthenol in 16 ounces of a lotion; this would make the moisturizer extremely potent and most likely very irritating to many people. To keep it safe, cosmetic chemists make a 0.5–3 percent concentration of panthenol. Let's say this particular lotion contains 1 percent, or 0.16 ounce of panthenol. This way, the price of the most expensive ingredient would climb to 40 cents—only if the lotion maker bought panthenol online by ounce, like I do, not by the ton! A little label reading can tell you just how many expensive ingredients are in the skin care product you purchase.

Decent natural cosmetic products may be expensive. You always get what you pay for, and cutting corners isn't the way of ensuring quality. If a product is too cheap, then it very likely contains synthetic, "natural" ingredients such as cocamide DEA or synthetic jojoba oil. You can buy an inexpensive, locally made soap or candle, but when it comes to well-performing facial skin care, ingredients should always come first, and quality ingredients do not come cheap.

When you take a look at the ingredients label of an organic moisturizer for sensitive skin, you'll notice that the natural ingredients, such as *Aloe barbadensis* leaf juice, jojoba esters, calendula extract, or squalene from olive, not shark liver, remain at the beginning of the list. Some ingredients are quite affordable even for an amateur cosmetic chemist: $1.60 for 2 ounces of dried aloe vera extract to $4.50 for 1 ounce of calendula extract, more for certified organic versions and pure juices. Some ingredients, like finely powdered or liquid extracts of Panax ginseng, licorice, white tea, or echinacea, can cost significantly more. But these ingredients contain much higher concentrations because good organic brands aren't mass-produced and do not need to rely heavily on stabilizers, emulsifiers, and preservatives to keep formulations stable, safe, and pleasant to use. Plus, most organic brands do not advertise themselves with massive spreads in glossy magazines. Their fame is due to word of mouth and voluntary celebrity endorsements rather than millions paid to lucky teenagers. That leads us to the next lesson: do not let celebrities judge what's better for your skin.

## Lesson 3: Learn from Celebrities; Don't Copy Them

The celebrity factor is strongest when it comes to beauty. I am no exception. I tried Dr. Hauschka's toner when I first saw it in the movie *Zoolander*; I started buying Jurlique when Madonna said she was using it; I go gaga over Creed perfumes, not just because of their heavenly compositions and staying power, but also because of the royal fleur that oozes from their crystal bottles. And if I, a seasoned beauty reviewer, am not immune to the celebrity factor, let's admit it: people who are not in the business are far more vulnerable. Many women buy lipsticks because they look good on an actress they love, or shampoos because they love her hair. If you are size eight, would you buy a pair of jeans in size two only because your favorite actress wears them? Following celebrities' leads in cosmetics is just as stupid.

Very rarely do celebrities use products they advertise. More often than not, the boatfuls of free products they receive end up in a stylist's bag or are given away as gifts. Not a single celebrity who receives free products—cosmetics, bags, dresses, shoes—will admit that she/he is giving the stuff away. If this information leaks to the company that sends the product, they will stop doing it. The makers of the hottest bag don't want to see their precious creation worn by the actress's nanny or her sister.

> Very rarely do celebrities use products they advertise. More often than not, the boatfuls of free products they receive end up in a stylist's bag or are given away as gifts.

Having a famous face advertise or ultimately design the beauty product is the epitome of marketing efforts for any cosmetic manufacturer. And they spend extravagant amounts of money to achieve this goal.

Hiring stars like Jane Fonda, Eva Longoria, Scarlett Johansson, and Penelope Cruz to face its hair care and makeup campaigns eats a significant share of the $250 million advertising budget of L'Oreal.

If you can't help but snatch a bit of a celebrity style here and there, try using famous women as role models. If you have pale skin, steal some of Nicole Kidman's beauty secrets, such as her complete avoidance of sun and choosing tasteful, pastel hues of makeup. If you have an olive complexion, look at Halle Berry and master the art of wearing foundation that doesn't look ashy or shiny. And even when celebrity endorsement sounds just right, don't forget to scrupulously examine the product, starting at the ingredients list. Only ingredients matter when it comes to taking care of your skin or hair. Remember, bottles and boxes with celebrity pictures on them end up in a trash can. Chemicals and plant extracts end up on your skin and inside your body.

## Lesson 4: Become Immune to Advertising

When a cosmetic company launches a new product, we seem to see it everywhere: on billboards and TV, in every magazine, and on store displays. Very soon, we start to suspect that we are hugely missing out on something if we do not buy this very promising bottle. Even the most critically minded individuals cave under pressure and run to buy a cleanser that will rejuvenate, tone, exfoliate, rebuild, and sing Christmas carols in between.

Open any glossy magazine. What's in the first beauty ad you see? It's the face of a very young girl, often a teenager who stood at the end of the queue when pimples were handed out. She smiles mischievously as if picturing a romantic date she's going to have tonight. We cannot help but think that if we buy the same concealer or lip-gloss she is using, we will also have her skin, hair, and playfulness. Romantic dates will inevitably follow. We see this model every day, on every page, in every commercial break. We suspect that not all of these mediums can be wrong. We are constantly reminded that this product will solve all of our skin dilemmas, and "repetition, repetition, repetition," as every Madison Avenue intern knows, is the most powerful tool at an advertiser's disposal.

Apart from riding high on the image of youth and sexual attractiveness, cosmetic companies are busy maintaining the elitist image of their products. Let's take a look at Estée Lauder ads. All of them feature a model with fine bone structure pictured in the lavish garden of a spacious old mansion. She sends us a subconscious message: Look at me; I swim in old money; I wear only silks and tweeds; I am born for refined living; I have ponies and Labradors; I golf, sail, dine on silver, and sleep on white linen. And we believe and open our wallets.

Just buying a blush in a pretty, blue monogrammed box won't instantly transport you to a summer house in the Hamptons. If you look at the ingredients in Estée Lauder blush, you will soon realize that it is not much different from the Clinique blush that is sold across the department store aisle. The color selection may be slightly different, and Clinique doesn't put its blush in a velvet pouch as if it's some sort of precious piece of jewelry, but the staying power, ease of blending, FD&C colors, and pore-clogging abilities will be pretty much the same.

If you are reading this book, something tells me you are over logo obsession and status purchases. Green beauty has a status of its own. Its value comes not from logos gracing the bottle but from rare herbs, juices, and lack of cancer-causing chemicals inside. Choose effectiveness and safety, not a status statement that will be forgotten in seconds.

Hmmm. Look who's talking now. I spent years raving over holiday collections of makeup, grieving when Chanel discontinued Rouge Noir polish, and declaring those extremely cute Swarovski crystal–adorned lipstick cases as must-haves. Whenever I was feeling down, I headed to the nearest boutique or department store to spend a week's wages on some gorgeous makeup palette. It would come in an awesome box, sometimes with a satin ribbon, in a logo-bearing paper bag and a handful of plastic-packaged samples. Only when I got home would I realize that I had spent fifty dollars on something that I would use twice—and, most likely, would've gotten for free from the manufacturer. The trash bin was full of cardboard and tissue paper, and something deep inside would tell me that fifty dollars could buy me a basketful of organic fruit, wine, and cheese. I would have been much, much happier. And probably healthier.

## Lesson 5: Forget About Brand Loyalty

A very popular and foolproof sales pitch stipulates that to get the very best results, use a cleanser, toner, and moisturizer from the same skin care line. "These products are scientifically formulated in the laboratory to work synergistically," salespeople all over the world chant in unison. "When used together, these products normalize your skin's pH balance, hydrate your skin, erase wrinkles, and fight acne. If you skip just one product, the whole system will be useless." This way, smart salespeople ensure multiple purchases, and nothing is praised more in the sales world than the ability to sell a customer $500 worth of antiwrinkle products when she came for a black eye pencil.

Let me remind you: everyone in the cosmetic business is after your money. This is why it's called business, not charity. The scientist wants to sell his research skills. The advertising agency wants to push its ability to cast bestselling magic on products. The manufacturer and retailer want to sell as much product as possible. The salesgirl lives on commission, so naturally, she wants you to buy a cleanser, toner, moisturizer, and then probably a couple of masks. You want to buy a magic potion that will make you look younger and more attractive. When you are buying a synthetic dream, you end up with the reality of prematurely aging, imbalanced, and fragile skin. When you are buying the reality and judge the product by its formulation, not a bottle, you will end up with healthier, younger skin.

When it comes to natural skin care products, feel free to purchase products from any line. Be creative and don't feel restrained. Many men borrow women's products. Many pregnant moms switch to baby lotions and oils long before the baby is due.

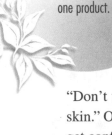

You don't need to be faithful to a skin care line just because you love one product.

You don't need to be faithful to a skin care line just because you love one product. Jurlique makes a gorgeous antiaging product called Herbal Recovery Gel, but it also makes quite average cleansers and very basic toners. If you feel that your skin could use a mild exfoliation every day, why don't you invest in Dr. Hauschka's Cleansing Cream or prepare one yourself?

I understand this shopping style completely contradicts another well-known myth spread by salespeople: "Don't use one brand today and another tomorrow. This confuses your skin." Our skin has no brain of its own. It's unable to convey emotions or get confused. What happens when skin "becomes confused" is a topical allergic reaction or irritation that occurs from using harsh chemicals, such as strong essential oils or highly concentrated preservatives. With well-formulated, mild products, the skin has no chance of "getting confused." The same goes for hair that is reportedly "getting used" to certain shampoos so they stop working. Sometimes I feel that my hair lives its own laid-back life, completely unaware of my humble presence, but shampoos are not addictive substances that hair can get used to and then get cranky as the withdrawal begins.

To keep us interested, most cosmetic manufacturers repackage, revamp, and revise their products approximately every three years. They will reissue it under a different name or maybe add "new and improved" to the old name. As a consumer, I feel intimidated. Why did they make me buy a mediocre product that obviously needed additional research and reformulation? If they thought the old product was safe and effective, why did they have to revise and improve it?

Sometimes cosmetic manufacturers revamp entire product lines as new data regarding safety of ingredients emerges. This way, not just one product is improved, but the whole label adopts a new, greener philosophy. Two years ago, Caudalie, the French beauty brand that uses grape pulp, juices, skins, and even crushed grape seeds in its formulations, reformulated their entire skin care line, which now contains no paraben preservatives. Origins has launched Origins Organics, a line of certified organic cleansers, toners, and body products. That's why it's important to look behind advertising claims. Be informed and remain skeptical. Only a label with an ingredients list will reveal what's really inside the bottle with a familiar name on it.

## Lesson 6: Become a Ruthless Shopper

Salespeople are trained to sell. This is what they do for a living. They master effective sales techniques. Foolproof tactics are used to play on our insecurity. Seasoned salespeople can quickly guess your annual income by your shoes. Too often a salesgirl has critically eyed my bag, which is often stained by leaky baby bottles, smears of carrot puree, and doodles drawn by an eye pencil, and moved to another customer in pretty shoes and well-pressed pants, abandoning me on the grounds that I do not look wealthy enough. Many women put on their best shoes and clutch their priciest bags when they go shopping, hoping to receive a little bit of the personal touch from salespeople.

Luckily, salespeople who work with organic beauty products are less likely to employ brutal sales techniques. They won't tell you that a particular color will solve your makeup dilemmas. But when it comes to buying organic beauty products, they will insist that everything is completely natural and that only the best, purest ingredients are used. Don't take their word for it. Scrutinize, compare, and don't be afraid to reject.

Now it's time to apologize to salespeople out there. Most of them earn minimal wages, and their livelihood depends on how many moisturizers and shampoos they sell. While most of them enjoy what they are doing, they rarely get adequate training to give you honest, trustworthy, unbiased information. When I made my living working in an upscale department store, I knew only two salespeople whose educational backgrounds were related to beauty. One of them, a dermatologist with a PhD from Belarus, was a sales consultant with a seminatural, upscale skin care line, and the other was a talented, professional makeup artist who was selling makeup. The rest received a brief training session by a representative of a brand they worked with, and from time to time they were introduced to new products or makeup collections arriving in the store. To make the sale, they would stretch the truth ("These preservatives are safe—that's why they are called food-grade"), make exaggerated claims ("You can eat this lipstick—it's good for you because it's packed with minerals and vitamins!"), point to your skin problems ("You definitely need an intensive treatment for your acne!"), and reinvent human physiology ("It will make your wrinkles disappear instantly!").

How to withstand the pressure from that side of a store counter? I've found that requesting a box of a product so you can read the ingredient list yourself works best. Strong self-esteem and independent information on what works and what doesn't can save you humiliation and loss of money. Do not let salespeople manipulate you. It's your skin that you need to take care of.

If you hope to find a magic potion that solves all your skin problems, then be ready to face the lies. Salespeople just sense your desperation. But if you ask informed questions, read the ingredients list, and move on to the next product without glancing at a price tag, your chances of buying something really worthy are high.

## Lesson 7: Ask for Samples and Do the Patch Test

Never be shy to request a sample. Of course, most stores don't always carry sample sizes of shampoos, toners, and cleansers. Many will charge you for a mini version of a product. In several countries, I was charged from two to five dollars for little tubes of Dr. Hauschka moisturizers and shampoos, because many stores have to buy samples from the distributor. I would rather spend a small amount of money than bother myself with returning an item (although I am happy to say I have never had to return a single organic skin care product!). Thanks to samples, you are less likely to waste time returning products, airplanes will pollute the air for something more valuable, and the skin care line will save money, too—hopefully for something important, like developing a new, safe preservative.

Many private pharmacies will decant a small amount of a cleanser or a moisturizer in a clear jar. In Sephora, you can also get a product decanted into cute little jars that you can reuse for traveling. Many products reviewed in this book were obtained as samples in stores. Many more were purchased at full price. Not a single product was obtained free of charge for reviewing purposes.

Now that you have your sample, it's time for a little science project. It's called the patch test. Doctors perform patch tests to determine what causes an allergic reaction. They take minute quantities of 25 to 150 mate-

### THE PATCH TEST

Here's how you can perform a simple patch test at home to see if a particular face or hair product is safe for you (assuming that you have already chosen a natural, organic product). Wash a small area on the inside of your arm and wipe it clean. Choose a time when you have just taken a shower so you won't have to wet this area again for some time. Apply a small amount of the cosmetic product you plan to buy, using a spatula or a clean, dry table knife. Cover the area with a waterproof adhesive bandage that has an adhesive area all around the edge, not just at the sides. If the adhesive tapes peel off, the process will have to be repeated. Allow twenty-four hours and then carefully peel off the tape. Any redness, itching, or rash—even a single pimple—indicates that you are allergic to something in this particular product. To be absolutely sure, wipe the area clean and apply the remaining amount of the product from the sample. Cover it with the new tape and wait another twenty-four hours. If the reaction persists, don't buy the product.

rials that commonly cause allergic reactions, make little plastic or aluminum patches, and apply them on your upper back, securing them with special hypoallergenic adhesive tape. Then, after at least forty-eight hours, the patches are removed. Any topical allergic reaction usually indicates that your immune system attacks the substance as hostile. Allergic reactions are so common today that many hair salons in the United States and the United Kingdom now require you to undergo a patch test with their hair dyes two days before your appointment. No patch test, no hair color.

Your olfactory response is another good tool in choosing the most suitable product. If the cosmetic product smells bad to you for no obvious reason, then there's a chance you will develop an irritation to this product.

Some people swear they can train their bodies to accept chemicals they are allergic to. They diligently use the substance for a week or two, no matter how much rash they develop, and slowly the reaction goes away. In the same way, pollen allergy sufferers eat small amounts of local honey in order to prevent spring allergies. I cannot recommend this way of clearing your allergies, because instead of accepting the substance, you may end up with a severe allergic reaction that may require medical assistance.

Don't be afraid or too lazy to return the cosmetic product that gave you an irritation. This way, you will unclutter your beauty routine as well as indicate to the cosmetic company (in a very remote way) that there is something wrong with their product. If a store refuses to refund, ask for the address of the company's headquarters or a local rep and mail them the product with an explanation. Most often, you will receive a check and apologies.

Accept a store exchange if a refund isn't working or you don't want to bother with returns. Take a substitute for a bothersome product if the store has it in stock, or take any sensitive skin product you can use to calm down the irritation.

Many good stores will accept a return and refund your money with no questions asked. Sometimes you will have to demonstrate visible signs of irritation—pimples, redness—to prove your point. Smaller health food stores are less likely to accept returns, so make sure you ask before you buy a new product. Better online stores accept returns and issue prompt refunds. They usually provide you with a voucher for free shipping. If you buy from eBay, you can only return a product if it is faulty (broken, leaked, contaminated, or past expiration date). Not all sellers are happy to issue refunds, so you may need to open a PayPal dispute or file a Visa chargeback in order to get your money back.

## Lesson 8: Choose Sustainable Packaging

Do you really store your cosmetics in the cardboard boxes they came in from the store? Most likely, you don't. So what happens to all that elegant, pretty packaging: sturdy boxes, tissue paper, leaflets, paper bags, satin ribbons, foam inserts? When we get home, we discard the paper bag (hoping each time that we'll find a better use for it than shoving it in a recycled paper bin). We open the box and take out the bottle. We ram that pretty box into the little bathroom waste bin that always looks too small to handle all our boxes and empty bottles. We just wasted about four dollars on making a status statement that didn't impress anyone.

You will probably say, so what can I do? My favorite lotion comes packaged in a neat cardboard box with plastic inserts and tons of leaflets stuffed inside. Maybe they did it for safety, to protect the precious extracts. However, let me ask you this: Do you really think that all these boxes and protective plastic sleeves serve a vital purpose? Do you really believe that without all that protection your newly purchased shampoo/conditioner duo will smash into goo-soaked plastic pieces while you walk or drive home? Or that a cute little glass jar with a half-ounce of cream is so fragile that it has to be wrapped in layers of stiff paper? Many cosmetic brands do not pack their products in boxes, and their products look just fine and work just as well. Did you know, by the way, that full-size samples of Chanel makeup products come packed in plain kraft paper, stuffed in brown cardboard boxes, and these products still look perfect? The same products are sold in department stores bearing eight times their weight in plastic and bleached cardboard.

Overuse of packaging is something that organic and synthetic skin care brands are equally guilty of. Some better brands, like UK-based REN, are ditching cardboard packaging altogether. Their lotions come in airtight pump recyclable plastic bottles shrink-wrapped in recyclable plastic. I also admire Canadian makeup brand Cargo for creating a lipstick range packed in tubes made of corn and sold in boxes that contain real plant seeds. Take out the product, soak the box in water, and plant it to see a new green living creature emerging in a few days. Very smart and very green. Pangea Organics also infuses their

I admire Canadian makeup brand Cargo for creating a lipstick range packed in tubes made of corn and sold in boxes that contain real plant seeds. Take out the product, soak the box in water, and plant it to see a new green living creature emerging in a few days.

cardboard boxes with flower seeds. Joshua Scott Onysko says that the idea came to him during a "psychedelic journey" in Joshua Tree National Park in California.

While wrapping is basically a matter of vanity that adds weight and importance to an otherwise humble jar or tube, packaging is important to keep cosmetics fresh and stable. Sophisticated, technologically advanced airtight pump-style bottles can eliminate the need for preservatives and stabilizers. Granted, excessive packaging and tons of tissue paper may help make a sale, especially during the holidays, but you will always pay dearly for this moment of consumer glory.

When the time comes to buy a new shampoo, conditioner, or cleanser, ask yourself, would you be proud of yourself if this particular bottle was buried with tons of other plastic bottles somewhere between the Bahamas and the Bermudas? Most likely, you won't be. That's why choosing cosmetic packaging made of better plastics, ideally of soya and corn, or at least that's degradable (that decomposes faster than ordinary plastic) or biodegradable (that can be decomposed even sooner), is important.

"Glass packaging ensures not only a sophisticated, sensual experience, but a healthier planet," says Suki Kramer of Suki Naturals. "Our packing uses recycled stock, printed with vegetable ink. For shipping, we buy only organic cornstarch peanuts. We receive hundreds of shipments that contain bubble and Styrofoam. Throwing these materials away or 'recycling' them, which is a very toxic process, would be wasteful, so we reuse them."

An average plastic shampoo bottle needs 450 years to degrade in the landfill. It can swim across oceans to be swallowed by an albatross that would die from hunger since this plastic bottle occupies his stomach and doesn't allow any nutrients to penetrate his body. On the other hand, a bottle made of corn and soya needs thirty to forty days to biodegrade. Even if a beauty-obsessed albatross eats it, all he'd have to digest is some sturdy fiber. After all, fiber is good for digestion.

## Lesson 9: Buy Less, Waste Less

The money you spend on skin care is well worth it when you achieve the results you expect. Many wonderful skin care products cost only pennies to make, while others require hefty investments that may or may not pay off. The truth is, you don't need to spend hundreds of dollars to look good.

"My first advice would be to simplify. There are way too many products available, and the beauty industry encourages you to use way too many products and to spend thousands of dollars on cosmetics," says green lifestyle expert Debra Lynn Dadd, whose beauty routine consists of two products: handmade soap and natural shampoo. "It's not what you put on your skin; it's what you put in your body. People have glowing skin not because they put something on it, but because they glow as human beings."

As you probably figured out by now, I am not going to tell you which natural or organic brand to use. I wish it could be that simple. There are many factors involved in this decision: your budget, your skin type, your need for convenience, your lifestyle, and your personal opinions about your skin—everything matters. Everyone's needs are unique, and it's up to you to prioritize your wishes in order to make smart beauty buys.

So how much do you need to start a reasonable natural skin care regimen? This can range from $20 (a basic system of cleanser/toner/moisturizer) up to $500, if you aim for more expensive organic brands such as Jurlique or CARE by Stella McCartney and include antiaging serums, exfoliating creams, sunscreens, purifying and soothing masks, eye cream, and body and hand cream. Expect your first natural products to last three months. On an ongoing basis, you can expect to pay anywhere from $10 to $100 per product.

Don't let this scare you off using organic products. Do you really need a beauty product for every body part? Many salespeople and cosmetic "experts" insist that you should never use face creams around the eyes because, first of all, they are not formulated for use around the eyes; second, they are "not ophthalmologist-tested"; and third, skin around the eyes is very different from the skin on your face, so you absolutely must use a different cream, even if basic knowledge of human anatomy tells you otherwise.

Let's address the ophthalmologist issue first. When a dermatologist, ophthalmologist, or podiatrist tests a product, this usually means that this particular medical professional reviewed the formulation to see if there's anything in it that can cause problems for the body part he or she is most familiar with. No one will conduct human studies where participants rub the cream into their eyes. Just like face creams, eye creams contain fragrances (even fragrance-free versions contain fragrances that mask or neutralize natural odors of ingredients), preservatives, and potential irritants.

The only reason you may not like using your regular moisturizer under your eyes is because of the texture of your cream. Heavy moisturizers and face oils may creep into the eyes and cause blurred vision and even itchiness, but they won't make you blind. Another myth is that you must use a separate hand cream. Body moisturizer works just as nicely, and it doesn't have to be tested by a "handologist" to be used on hands.

Today's organic skin care products all offer similar ingredients at all price levels. The key is not to buy less but more of a good thing. Invest in a few basic pieces: a moisturizer, a good soap, a sunscreen, a natural deodorant, and a shampoo that doubles as a shower gel. You can blend masks yourself from ingredients in your fridge or kitchen cupboard, and you can treat yourself to a luxurious natural fragrance later, as a reward for being extra good and green.

Unfortunately, not all of the products I will recommend in this book are readily available in your local drugstore or supermarket. While big natural food chain stores, such as Whole Foods Markets, offer a nice selection of organic and natural beauty brands, local health food stores prefer to rely on time-tested Burt's Bees, JASON, and Weleda. In a busy world, convenience can be a significant factor, which is why many of us ditch the idea of green beauty simply because there are not many products available. Luckily, there are many ways to take existing green products and tailor them to our needs. In Chapter 5, you learn new ways of transforming basic cleansers and dull lotions into exciting potions that wipe the floor with their synthetic counterparts.

Since green skin care products contain close to zero preservatives, it's important to use them up quickly. You should expect to purchase at least one cleanser, toner, sunscreen, or moisturizer every month or two. If you don't have time to hit the local Whole Foods Market or there's no good health food store in your neighborhood, buy your basic beauty products online once a month. If you happen to grab a bargain, keep your beauty possessions in a cool, dark place, ideally in the fridge, but not in the freezer.

For convenience and selection, nothing beats the Internet. Many reputable online stores, such as Sephora and Saffron Rouge, post complete lists of ingredients and allow you to choose your free samples. By ordering samples, you don't have to invest in products that may not work.

> You can blend masks yourself from ingredients in your fridge or kitchen cupboard, and you can treat yourself to a luxurious natural fragrance later, as a reward for being extra good and green.

## Lesson 10: Develop a Routine and Stick to It

No matter how you mix and match your cleansers, toners, sunscreens, and antiaging serums, stick to a routine. Cleanse your face every morning and evening, boost the effectiveness of your moisturizers by spraying or padding on some toner, and always put on a moisturizer with sunscreen when you leave home. At night, double-cleanse your skin and dab a little lightweight oil or serum to nourish, not suffocate, your skin when it needs oxygen more than ever.

Be consistent in your quest for green beauty. This means that each product should be natural and contain no synthetic dyes, fragrances, preservatives, or detergents. Not ready for a big green leap? Take one step at a time. One natural product won't mean much of a difference, but it's a nice start. Switch from a foaming cleanser containing several sulfate-based cleanser detergents to a mild olive oil soap. Replace your alcohol-based toner with witch hazel or rose water and dot a few drops of jojoba oil instead of night cream. As you progress with this book, you'll become more knowledgeable and informed in the green beauty trade. You'll be able to compile an easily personalized beauty routine that will perfectly suit your needs. Just keep in mind that several natural products used consistently will produce noticeable results within a few weeks. One product is not a cure-all. Regular use of green beauty products will make a real difference.

## Lesson 11: Clear Up Your Act

Before we discuss green beauty products, let's edit your beauty routine and reevaluate your beauty habits. Take a close look at products you already own. Read the labels. Spot unwanted chemicals. Check expiration dates and get rid of everything that contains one or more toxic ingredients that are listed in the previous chapter.

You don't have to throw out everything right away. Some "holy grail" beauty products are almost impossible to let go of. Can't part with that caviar-based moisturizer that is loaded with paraben preservatives? Don't use it as a hand cream. Your brand-new designer leather bag or butter-soft leather boots can use some fancy massage with posh moisturizer. Just make sure not to treat your suede or soft lambskin bags to oily face creams. You may keep a miracle hair balm if it does wonders for your hair and doesn't cause back or neck irritation. However, I strongly suggest that you double-check all questionable products that sit on your skin for longer periods, such as toners, moisturizers, and serums. Replace them with nontoxic versions as soon as possible. Synthetic cleansers can be the last to get the boot.

I don't expect you to instantly discard all your time-tested beauty treasures. If your heart bleeds, put them in a box and try switching to green, natural skin care for just one month. Give it a try. After one month, if you still feel like it, you can always go back to your chemical skin care. But something tells me you won't want to.

## Lesson 12: Spread the Word

As you gain more knowledge about the principles of green beauty, don't keep it to yourself. Before going to a store for a new lipstick or a shampoo, make it a habit to do a bit of online research. Read unbiased reviews on skin care boards and forums such as MakeupAlley.com. In most cases, the product that caused 75 percent of reviewers to break out will make you break out, too. The same applies to redness, stinging, or flakiness. Post your own reviews and write comments on green blogs. For a deeper insight into cosmetic ingredients, head to the Environmental Working Group's website (www.ewg.org).

If a cosmetic product causes irritation or an allergic reaction, take action. First of all, return the product immediately. Depending on the severity of the symptoms, apply over-the-counter medication or contact your healthcare provider. Call the manufacturer of the offending product and let them know what you have experienced. Most likely, you'll spend twenty minutes on hold before you talk to a call center person, but don't give up—and follow up with an e-mail. If you have suggestions or criticisms, be proactive and speak out: it's the only way to trigger changes.

**the green beauty guide**

*understanding*
green
beauty

If you are reading this book, you are most likely open to exploring alternative ways of treating your skin and hair. Good for you! In fact, it's good for all of us. The world of natural beauty is full of amazing discoveries that will keep you wondering how you could have used synthetic chemical skin care for so long. And as you learn the price you've been paying for conventional skin care, you will no doubt be longing to know if there are any alternatives.

People worldwide are striving to make their lifestyles cleaner and safer. As governments begin to take action against climate change, growing landfill (and sea-fill) sites, and the threatening energy crisis, we can't help but consider lifestyle changes and rethink our purchasing habits. Organic has gone mainstream, and it's no longer just about eating organic food or driving a hydrogen-powered car. Hollywood celebrities are installing solar panels, sharing tips on composting, and driving cars that smell like French fries. They are shopping for organic lettuce and oil made from olives grown at an ancient farm in Tuscany, harvested according to moon cycles and hand-pressed to ensure pure virginity. And the rest of us follow the lead. In the United States alone, sales of organic food have steadily grown by approximately 20 percent every year. In 2006, retail sales of organic foods exceeded $15 billion, compared to only $6.6 billion in 2000. That's double the growth in just six years! Four in ten consumers today buy some type of organic food every time they shop for groceries. Personal care items are among the most popular organically produced goods, along with fruits, milk, and meats.

**Four in ten consumers today buy some type of organic food every time they shop for groceries.**

There are 40 million "green boomers" in the United States today, according to a survey released by AARP, formerly the American Association of Retired Persons. These environmentally conscious consumers make up more than half of the country's 79 million baby boomers, and combined with the younger generation of green-minded consumers out there, this is a very influential consumer group. This is why even a small change in your consumer habits makes a big difference. If you refuse to buy one bottle of toxic shampoo, this means that 40 million bottles remain unsold! This way, corporations have no other choice but to take note.

This book is designed to become your simple yet comprehensive guide to natural, organic, and ecoconscious skin care, hair care, fragrances, and makeup. It will help you make smart choices and mold the principles of organic beauty around your personal style.

Contrary to what some people say, green beauty isn't expensive. My recent check revealed that many organically grown vegetables cost only 10 percent more than their pesticide-laden neighbors. The same with beauty: it's becoming more practical and affordable because many plant ingredients are cheaper to grow than synthesize. Many natural shampoos double as shower gels, so you can get away with using one product instead of two, and they are more concentrated, so you don't have to buy the product as often.

With green beauty, you will be saving some money and becoming healthier. That brings us to the next big topic: what is green when it comes to beauty?

## Green Beauty Decoded

Today, many people associate "green" with eco-consciousness, sustainability, organic farming, chemical-free foods, and low-emission vehicles running on biofuels or electricity. In beauty, green means understanding nature and the human body as a whole, improving your looks naturally and holistically, and abstaining from synthetic, hazardous chemicals.

When I started writing this book, I planned to name it *The Organic Beauty Bible*. In this title, I was thinking about "organic" in its general meaning, as it was used in the beginning of the 1990s before governments started to regulate organic foods and certify producers that meet standards for organic production. Today, organic is better defined and less inclusive. When someone claims their fruits or juices are organic, they must produce proof that it's really so. Back in the 1990s, though,

> Today, organic is better defined and less inclusive. When someone claims their fruits or juices are organic, they must produce proof that it's really so.

organic was still associated with all things holistic and esoteric. So instead of focusing on a few cosmetic brands that use only certified organic ingredients, I decided to come up with "green beauty."

In this book, "green" means that a cosmetic product has been formulated without harmful toxic chemicals—including paraben and formaldehyde-based preservatives, sulfate-based detergents, synthetic penetration enhancers, and artificial dyes and fragrances. Such a product should ideally contain certified organic ingredients whenever possible. It may be packaged in recyclable or recycled boxes and bottles, and it shouldn't contain chemicals that poison the environment, such as phosphate and sulfate detergents, petrochemicals, and phthalates.

Green beauty does not need to be completely plant-derived. Minerals, such as zinc oxide, titanium oxide, mica, and others, as well as vitamins, glycerin, and certain clays make wonderful and very beneficial additions to cosmetic formulations. Other newly developed active ingredients, such as coenzyme Q10 (ubiquinone), kinetin, human growth factor, and various peptides cannot be obtained by simply distilling them from fruits and herbs. These ingredients are derived from natural sources, but undergo complex chemical treatment before they become suitable for use in cosmetics.

Green beauty isn't necessarily certified organic. Many plants cannot be grown in certified organic farms. Many excellent green beauty products use plants that are wild-harvested or grown locally on clean soil without any chemical additives. When you mix and blend homemade masks and hair treatments, you are not exactly doing that according to certified organic standards.

"We use natural ingredients, but this does not mean we use rosemary stems straight out of the dirt and bottle them," says Suki Kramer, the founder of Suki Naturals, favored by Eva Longoria, Jennifer Garner, and Edie Falco, to name just a few ecoconscious celebrities. "We process and refine ingredients down to their essences. Exceptionally powerful and potent ingredients do exist in nature. Science has created more natural sources to create potent active ingredients, and as consumer knowledge grows, synthetic is becoming obsolete. Part of our goal is to teach people that you do not need synthetics to have great, effective cosmetic treatments and great skin."

## Shades of Green Beauty

It's not uncommon to find labels such as "organic," "hypoallergenic," and "cruelty-free" attached to your favorite skin care products. But when you buy green cosmetic products, it's hard to tell whether the word "organic" on a label is a genuine claim. Green claims sound reassuring, but you should be warned that too often they have little, if any, meaning. More often than not, closer inspection reveals that such products contain minuscule amounts of organic herbs, and the rest of the bottle is filled with preservatives and chemicals. The advice in this chapter will help you understand which natural cosmetics on the market really are what they claim to be and which are hyping their products as something they're not. Here are some tips that may help you buy green products that are truly green, not just colored green with synthetic dyes.

### Organic

*Variations:* 78 percent organic ingredients, made with organic ingredients and contains organic extracts.

Some people see organic as a way to reduce the environmental load on Mother Nature. To poetic natures, organic is a return to cosmic harmony and natural rhythms of the universe. Others would rather support a local farmer and shop for local seasonal produce instead of buying organic kiwis shipped on an airplane from New Zealand. The rest—the majority of shoppers—would buy organic because they look for products that contain no harmful chemicals such as preservatives, colorings, or pesticides. Chemical-free, grown in natural conditions, packaged without preservatives, and bursting with more nutrients and vitamins: this is what organic means to us when it comes to food.

As defined by the U.S. National Organic Standards Board, "Organic agriculture is an ecological production management system that promotes and enhances biodiversity, biological cycles and soil biological activity. It is based on minimal use of off-farm inputs and on management practices that restore, maintain and enhance ecological harmony." This means that plants used in organic beauty products are minimally processed without artificial ingredients, preservatives, or irradiation.

"Certified organic" means that an ingredient or the whole product has been grown or produced according to strict government-enforced organic agricultural standards and verified by an approved third-party organization. There are many independent organic certifying organizations. Their standards include the following: no synthetic chemicals, pesticides, or fertilizers; no sewage sludge; no genetically modified organisms; and no animal testing of ingredients or completed products. Organic ingredients must be grown without fertilizers, herbicides, pesticides, or genetic twisting, and processed using natural methods, without chemical ripening. Animals raised on an organic farm must be fed organic feed and given access to the outdoors. They should never be given antibiotics or growth hormones. It's impossible to organically certify water and salt, although many food manufacturers go to extra lengths and use water from springs that flow on organically certified soil.

## Biodynamic

Biodynamic is a forerunner of an organic movement, and it's more holistic in approach. In addition to organic practices, such as crop rotation and composting, biodynamic farms use special plant, animal, and mineral preparations, and the rhythmic influences of the sun, moon, planets, and stars to create a thriving ecosystem. "Biodynamics is a process of healing the skin or the soil, as opposed to replacing the substance or relieving the symptom," says Susan West Kurz, holistic skin care expert and president of Dr. Hauschka Skin Care. "Organic tends to replace synthetic substances with botanicals, but biodynamic asks, Why is there a pest or a weed in the first place. Where is the imbalance? If there are larvae on your broccoli, it tells you that there is something wrong with the health of the soil. So we would apply our biodynamic spray on the plant or on the soil to help it regain balance."

Biodynamic farming is an approach based on the work of Austrian philosopher Rudolf Steiner. In 1924, he believed that the quality of food was downgrading "thanks" to artificial fertilizers, pesticides, and the whole chemical approach to farming. A central aspect of biodynamics is that the farm is seen as an organism and therefore should be a closed, self-nourishing system. "Biodynamic agriculture includes the forces that make food nutritious and that are of benefit to health," says Michael Bate, the head gardener of Weleda. "It is the art of the biodynamic farmer to create a harmonious balance between the various realms of nature. Biodynamic gardening enhances the working of the forces coming via the earth, also through light, air and warmth, and from the influences of planetary rhythms, to create vitalized soil and plants."

The biodynamic method has been controlled and certified by the Demeter International Association since 1928. The U.S. Demeter Association was formed in the 1980s and certified its first farm in 1982. There are several skin care lines that use biodynamically grown plants in their products, such as Weleda, Primavera, and Dr. Hauschka. Biodynamic skin care, according to Susan West Kurz, is based on a process of healing the skin as opposed to removing the symptoms. "We don't say, let's cope with your dryness by putting on a moisturizer," says Susan. "We are stimulating skin's vital functions so it isn't dry all the time. I often ask women why they use night creams, and they say because their skin is dry. Maybe, I tell them, these creams do not work! Why would you need a moisturizer twenty-four hours a day if they were effective? Biodynamics requires a shift in consciousness. We look at the whole process rather than symptoms."

## Hypoallergenic

*Variations:* dermatologist-tested, allergy-tested, nonirritating

These claims are not making a cosmetic product more natural. Company claims that certain beauty products produce fewer allergic reactions often have little ground. According to the U.S. Food and Drug Administration (FDA), there are currently no federal standards or definitions that govern the use of the term "hypoallergenic."

In fact, beauty product manufacturers are not required to provide evidence that their products produce fewer allergic reactions, and products prescribed for sensitive skin often contain chemical and plant-based ingredients that cause skin irritation. It's been proven that all cosmetic products, mild and regular, may cause an allergic reaction in people with sensitive skin. That's why if you are "blessed" with supersensitive skin, you should use beauty products with as few ingredients as possible and consider making your own basic skin and hair care products from organic fruits, vegetables, milk, and cereals, so you are completely sure of what you are using on your skin.

## Cruelty-Free

*Variations:* no animal testing, we are against animal testing

Although the "cruelty-free" and "no animal testing" labels suggest that no animal testing was done on the product or its ingredients, you may be surprised to learn that no legal definitions of these claims exist and no independent organization verifies them. In fact, it is common for manufacturers whose products bear these labels to commission outside laboratories to conduct tests on animals to prove that they themselves do not conduct animal tests. Cruelty-free has nothing to do with green beauty and should not be mistaken for it, even though organic manufacturers steer clear of animal testing in any form.

Animal testing is a big business that kills up to 100 million animals every year, according to the British newspaper the *Guardian* in 2005. And the worst part is that most of them die for nothing. It's true that many groundbreaking scientific and medical discoveries were made thanks to animals, including the development of penicillin, organ transplants, the poliomyelitis vaccine, not to mention the famous Pavlov's dogs, the first cloned animal, Dolly the sheep, and dog Laika, the first animal to travel in space. Finding a new pain-reducing treatment for burn victims or a new flu vaccine is one thing; involving animals in testing a new shimmery base for lip-glosses is another. Besides, more and more scientists today insist that animal testing of cosmetics is indisputably cruel and inhumane and does not always prove the safety of cosmetic ingredients.

During a series of experiments on animals, scientists establish in which concentrations particular chemicals are safe for use. Scientists try to measure the levels of skin irritancy, eye tissue damage, and toxicity caused by various cosmetic ingredients. To test for irritancy, they perform the Draize test, during which caustic substances are placed in the eyes of rabbits to see how much damage can be done to their sensitive eye tissues. This test is extremely painful for the rabbits, which often scream and sometimes break their necks trying to wiggle out of restraints.

Another test performed to evaluate the safety of cosmetics is the lethal dosage (LD) test. During this test, researchers try to figure out the amount of a substance that will kill a predetermined ratio of animals. For example, in the LD50 test, animals are forced to ingest poisonous substances, most often through stomach tubes, until half of them die. Common reactions to lethal dosage tests include convulsions, vomiting, paralysis, and bleeding from the eyes, nose, mouth, or rectum.

What amazes me most is the logic of product developers who order such tests: if they already know that the chemical is irritating, toxic, or lethal, why kill animals and waste time and money to find out how much of this deadly stuff they can legally stuff into a new cosmetic product? If animals develop serious diseases and even die from this substance, why does anyone need to determine whether this chemical is safe for humans if we dilute it with water or another chemical? If you already know it is toxic and/or irritating, why use it in cosmetics at all? There are more than eight thousand chemical substances that are recognized as safe—why continue loading beauty products with yet another deadly chemical cocktail?

Animal tests don't always predict human risks. Each living species reacts differently to various substances. Pet lovers know that certain human foods are poisonous to animals due to their body chemistry. For example, you should not feed pork, onions, grapes, or macadamia nuts to dogs, while aspirin is poisonous to cats. Some substances that are toxic to humans didn't have any adverse effects on animals during tests. One of them, thalidomide (kevadon), a sedative used to treat insomnia, was developed in the 1960s. The drug was put on the market after extensive animal tests didn't show any toxicity. After thalidomide was approved for treatment of depression, it caused severe birth abnormalities. Starting in 1962, there were reports of thousands of children born deformed, and many of them died shortly after birth. The *British Medical Journal* even called it "thalidomide disaster" (Woolham 1962). Today, thalidomide is used in treatment of multiple myeloma and inflammatory diseases, but with extreme caution because we now know it is a strong teratogen.

During tests, researchers use industrial-strength solutions that rapidly cause harmful effects in animals. Basically, any substance used in large quantities can hurt or even kill. Water can be toxic if drunk in gallons at once! Humans are unlikely to encounter high concentrations of toxic substances in real life as they shave, shower, and style their hair. Instead, we use potentially harmful substances consistently in low doses over years and even decades. As a result, systemic effects would be different. It's the same with the sun: when we overdose from exposure to the sun, we get an instant reaction (sunburns) and delayed reaction (premature skin aging, higher risk of skin cancer). Many chemicals we use daily will act slowly, triggering disease after decades of use.

Animals, especially lab animals, live much shorter lives than humans. Many species have been genetically modified so they become more susceptible to cancer or other diseases. Not a single animal test can prove that the chemical in question is safe for use by humans. Such tests can only show that the chemical doesn't cause visible damage over a short period of time. Then the animals are killed, and the cosmetic industry gets a green light to formulate and sell new products using the chemical. Animal tests cannot predict the effect such chemicals have on humans who will encounter these chemicals over prolonged periods of time and in combination with various other chemicals of synthetic or natural origin.

To add injury to insult, animal testing results can be affected by many factors: how well the animals eat and sleep, how stressed they are, and what their living conditions are. Results of the same test can vary from one research facility to another. The LD50 results can be 8–14 times higher in one laboratory than in another, observed the activist group Animal Liberation on their website (http://www.animalliberation.org.au/toxtest.php).

Today, many cosmetic companies develop and refine alternative testing procedures that do not involve animals. Among reliable alternatives to animal testing are tests in vitro, literally "in a tube," when chemical substances are applied to individual cells rather than dropped into a rabbit's eyes or poured into a dog's throat. For example, to study if a certain ingredient irritates the eye, Eytex, a vegetable protein whose molecules have a similar organization as those in the cornea, can be used to study facial skin care, makeup, and hair care. Irritating products make the protein gel appear cloudy, similar to the cloudiness and tears you may experience after applying an eye cream.  Human cornea cells from eye banks can be grown and reproduced in test tubes. After the test chemical has been applied to the human cell culture, scientists examine the number of dead or damaged cells by adding a red dye. Healthy cells take up this dye, but dead or damaged cells do not. The less red dye is absorbed, the more toxic the product is. Finally, to test products that are made of ingredients that are already found to be safe, human volunteers can be used. The greater number of people involved, the more reliable the results. Many well-known cosmetic companies, such as The Body Shop, regularly use human volunteers.

In nonanimal testing, adverse reactions and mutations of individual cells can be accurately measured, recorded, and scrutinized. The results can be measured accurately by a computer, and there's no need to break a rabbit's neck.

The future of animal testing is starting to look dim. The testing of cosmetics on animals is currently banned in the Netherlands, Belgium, and the United Kingdom. In 2009, all animal-tested cosmetics will be banned from sale throughout the European Union, and all cosmetics-related animal testing will be halted. The European Federation for Cosmetic Ingredients, which represents seventy cosmetic companies from all over Europe, opposes the ban.  In the United States, animal testing is still in use.

As consumers, we are partly responsible, too. Each of us can choose not to buy cosmetic products from companies that either practice animal testing or pay other companies to conduct such tests. By voting with your dollar, you can send a strong message to cosmetic manufacturers that testing on animals is cruel, useless, and unacceptable.

The fact that a product is called "herbal" or "natural" doesn't mean it is cruelty-free. Many cosmetic companies claim they do not test their products on animals but buy ingredients from suppliers that either own research labs that perform tests on animals or order such

The fact that a product is called "herbal" or "natural" doesn't mean it is cruelty-free.

tests from independent labs. Still, a logo of a leaping bunny on a box or a tube of a cosmetic product is a good sign that this particular company does not carry out cruel animal testing or at least does not directly support it. In future chapters, I will never recommend using a beauty product made by a company that encourages animal testing in any form.

## Non-GMO

*Variation:* no genetically modified organisms used

A genetically modified organism (GMO) is a natural substance whose DNA has been altered using genetic engineering techniques. A plant's DNA can be twisted up a notch to make it more resistant to pests or a harsh climate, improve its shelf life, or increase nutritional value. Genetically modified plants most commonly used in cosmetics include soya and corn. Soybean oil, corn flour, and potato starch are common ingredients in moisturizers, masks, and makeup. According to Greenpeace, more than 50 percent of the world's soy contains genetically modified organisms. However, no GM labels are required on cosmetics.

The risks of genetic engineering are still unknown. Opponents of GMOs, or genetically modified organisms, warn that any product used on the skin enters the bloodstream more quickly, which increases any potential risk that GMOs may have. "I believe that people should always have the ability to know what they are supporting with their dollars as well as what they are putting on and in their bodies," says Joshua Scott Onysko, the creator of Pangea Organics. "GMOs are man playing god. Companies like Monsanto claim that extensive testing has been done on these new GMO crops, but what does 'testing' mean? How do you 'test' the effects of [genetically modified] organisms on a planet with millions of different species? I believe their stewardship of this planet and its people is as myopic as their business plans."

The practice of genetic modification is not restricted in the United States, although some states and counties, such as Mendocino County, California, banned the production of GMOs in 2004. In general, United States law does not impose mandatory identification of the presence of GMOs in consumer products, whether food or cosmetics, because the FDA does not consider genetically modified food to present any greater safety concerns than other foods do.

Most countries in Europe, Japan, and Mexico declared that genetic modification has not been proven safe. Austria, France, Germany, Luxembourg, and Greece banned the use of engineered corn and rapeseed, but many European countries lifted the GMO ban in 2004. The controversy over genetically modified food in Europe is still going on, even though surveys consistently find that 97 percent of European consumers want clear labeling of all genetically engineered foods and 80 percent do not want genetically engineered foods at all. Currently, the United States is fighting to obtain European Union clearance for the sale of genetically modified seeds, challenging European bans of GMOs in the U.S.-based World Trade Organization.

GM opponents want all food and cosmetic products containing as little as 1 percent of genetically modified organisms to be labeled accordingly, so consumers can decide whether to buy genetically modified products or not. Greenpeace argues that instead of investing in GM plants, governments must support organic farming methods that help repair the damage done by industrial farming and reduce the excessive use of fertilizers, pesticides, and herbicides.

At the very least, produce with GMO ingredients must be properly labeled as such. "The last thing I want to eat is a tomato with fish genes," says Myra Eby, founder of natural skin care line MyChelle. "It is only fair for the end consumer to knowingly purchase products containing GMO ingredients. I feel all manufacturers choosing to use GMO ingredients owe it to us, the consumers, and they should label the products properly so an informed decision can be made. It is shocking to me that the grocery store shelves are lined with produce that contains GMO ingredients without any warnings on them."

So do we have to shun any cosmetics made with soy and corn completely, for the fear of turning into the Bride of Frankenstein? Make sure the product you fancy is made with oils obtained from a certified GM-free source. Today, the identification of GMOs in food products and cosmetics remains voluntary, but it's good to know that all certified organic cosmetics are produced without GMO ingredients. Many ecofriendly, "greener" brands usually indicate that their products are "GMO-free" or "non-GMO" on a visible spot on the product label or box. Many other politically correct brands, such as The Body Shop and Urban Decay, are planning on phasing out the use of genetically modified corn and soya in their products. If in doubt, don't hesitate to contact the manufacturer and ask whether their soy-based products are made of genetically modified plants.

## Fair Trade

*Variations:* ethically produced, fair trade

Fair trade means that a certain product or its ingredients were produced in Third World countries by farmers and manufacturers who obtained reasonable, fair pay for their services and crops. When you see a teal-green round stamp that was issued by the international fair trade certification body FLO-CERT, this means the product was made by a community of workers who received decent pay, with no forced or child labor, and that health and safety requirements were met. Does it make you feel better about using such a product? Absolutely. Does it improve the quality of ingredients? Possibly, since people who work in good conditions and enjoy adequate compensation for their efforts are less likely to make mistakes or intentionally compromise quality, whether fruits, vegetables, cocoa, rice, or coffee.

## Natural

*Variations:* plant-based, botanical, natural botanical ingredients, made with plant extracts, contains natural ingredients, contains essential oils

These claims are most frequently mistaken for organic. Natural and botanically based beauty products are not necessarily formulated with naturally grown plants or their juices, essential oils, or concentrated extracts. Only a few days ago, I was aggressively sold a stretch mark balm that a salesperson touted as "completely natural," even though the label clearly listed triethanolamine, paraben preservatives, and mineral oil among the ingredients. Yesterday, I was drawn to a shelf with Olay products that had green leaves on the packaging and the word "natural" on the label. Since all big cosmetic players are doing mineral makeup now, I was hoping to see an organic line. Not this time. Although the ingredient list contained more natural plant extracts than common drugstore products would, the list was still scattered with PEGs, parabens, and disodium EDTA.

This means that the word "natural" on the product box really means nothing, even when it adorns a pretty label with a bunch of flowers on it. This allows keen marketers to slap the hot word "natural" on the label.

According to government labeling requirements, "natural" means that an ingredient "has not been significantly altered from its original state, nor has anything been removed from it (with the exception of water), nor have other substances been added to it." Nothing in this definition prohibits a company from combining the natural ingredient with the most toxic of chemicals. "Natural" products may contain genetically modified organisms that were grown with synthetic pesticides, herbicides, and fertilizers, small amounts

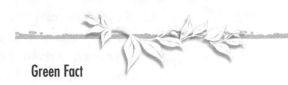

of which seep into our skin. Unlike organic, natural products are not certified by third parties, and their ingredients can still be grown in sewage sludge.

Synthetic beauty manufacturers and affiliated media insist there is no such thing as a 100 percent natural or organic ingredient. To distill an essential oil or collect beeswax, they say, we have to use chemically enhanced machinery and unnatural tools made of plastic and metal. For instance, cocamide DEA is derived from coconut oil. Coconut oil is a perfectly natural source, so what's not natural about it?

Usage of metal machinery and plastic tools should be the least of your concerns when it comes to the difference between synthetic and organic. The truth is, the manufacturing process of cocamide DEA, just like many ingredients with DEA, TEA, and MEA in their names, requires the use of carcinogenic synthetic chemicals triethanolamine (TEA), monoethanolamine (MEA), or diethanolamine (DEA). So even if something comes from a natural source, it doesn't mean it's organic and generally good for you.

This means that skin care products with at least one organic ingredient used in large quantities can be labeled "organic," regardless of the origin of the other ingredients used in them. This is why you should become ingredient-savvy and learn to spot potentially toxic ingredients even if they are tossed between certified organic aloe vera juice and grape seed extract. One organic ingredient doesn't make the beauty product safe and pure, and you are no better off using it than any other conventional product from a drugstore shelf.

"There are many 'hybrid natural' ingredients used in 'green' cosmetics," reminds Debra Lynn Dadd, the proclaimed Queen of Green by the *New York Times*. "For example, sodium laureth sulfate is called a natural ingredient because it's made of coconut oil. But since there are so many chemicals added to it, it's not the same as putting coconut oil on your skin. I could never understand why you have to put artificial colors in a product that is made from oils and juices from a rain forest. I think if a brand is natural, it should be only using natural ingredients. After talking to so many companies, I understood they are not trying to be natural. They take their old formulas and add one or two natural ingredients. While there's nothing wrong with that, people get the idea that these brands are completely natural. As long as the brands are accurate about what they are, I can choose whether to use them or not. The problem comes when a company presents itself as natural while they aren't."

The bottom line is this: a truly natural beauty product should be safe enough to eat. It may not be delicious, but it should be safe and wholesome. Vodka, as harsh as it is, can make a wonderful warming compress that may soothe your cystic acne overnight. At the same time, all you'd expose yourself to is alcohol derived from wheat. It can get you drunk, it can make you perform the chicken dance at a corporate party, but it won't make you ill unless you grossly overdo it or drive under the influence.

If you choose to pick just one piece of advice from this book, make it this: anything you apply to your skin ends up inside your body just as if you had ingested it. So whenever you put something on your skin, think: would I really want to eat this?

> Anything you apply to your skin ends up inside your body just as if you had ingested it. So whenever you put something on your skin, think: would I really want to eat this?

## Are You Confused by Organic Labels?

How many times have you purchased an "organic" shampoo only to discover the same old sodium laureth sulfate, triethanolamine, and parabens among its ingredients? This happens because organic labeling in the United States is pretty much in disarray. Current labeling techniques used by most popular organic personal care products allow placing virtually any claim on the label.

To help define what's truly green when it comes to cosmetic products, the U.S. Organic Consumers Association (OCA) conducted an expansive consumer survey in 2007. The survey was taken by more than 5,500 consumers who regularly purchase organic products. In fact, they said that most or "a good portion" of their personal care products contained organic ingredients.

You may think that such green connoisseurs would know their stuff. Not true! Nearly half of the survey respondents incorrectly believed that a product labeled as "made with organic ingredients" meant that "all" or "nearly all" of the ingredients were organic. In reality, there are no federal regulations requiring personal care products labeled as "made with organic ingredients" to contain any particular level of organic ingredients, and most personal care products using this label are made up of 70 percent or less organic ingredients.

In any store, in any period of time, 95 percent of shampoos, creams, and body washes are not organic enough to meet the criteria required to use the USDA organic seal. These products, which often contain multiple conventional synthetic ingredients, simply list a certifying agency for the organic ingredients contained in the product. Even if a product contains certified organic aloe vera, this doesn't mean that the rest of the ingredients are organic as well! The OCA survey revealed that consumers are confused by the listing of the certifying agency or wording such as "contains certified organic ingredients" and falsely assume that it means the whole product is organic.

One thing seems certain: the overwhelming majority of organic beauty shoppers believe that a product with a derivation of the word "organic" in its brand name should either be 100 percent organic, or, at the very least, should not contain harmful synthetic detergents and preservatives. Many believe that products with only a few organic ingredients in the formulation should also bear a warning: "This product also contains synthetic ingredients."

Many organizations certify organic products and ingredients. They set a number of strict standards for how the plants are grown, harvested, stored, processed, packaged, and shipped. Such standards vary slightly from country to country but are generally the same: the farmer or producer must avoid synthetic chemical additives, including fertilizers, pesticides, and antibiotics, as well as genetically modified organisms and sewage sludge. The farmland must be free from chemicals for more than three years, depending on the country, and all the production stages must be transparent, open for audit and frequent inspections.

Today, only the United States, the European Union, and Japan have clear and well-defined organic standards that are formulated and overseen by governments, so the term "organic" may be used only by certi-fied producers. In the United States, you can confidently buy organic pro-duce when you see the round, green-and-white "USDA Organic" label issued by the U.S. Department of Agriculture. In France, organic certifi-cates are issued by ECOCERT, and in the United Kingdom organic stan-dards are maintained by the Soil Association and Organic Farmers and Growers. In countries that have no established organic laws, certification is handled by nonprofit organizations and private companies.

No wonder we are confused by all these shades of organic and green. Both manufacturers and consumers have been confused. The chemical industry defines "organic" as any compound containing carbon. Apolo-gists of synthetic skin care say that this makes methylparaben perfectly organic, since it is derived from crude oil, which is formed by dead foliage and animal carcasses rotting underground over millions of years. By saying this, they try to nullify the meaning of organic and turn the organic movement into another fad.

Current U.S. legislation allows products that contain at least 70 percent organic ingredients to use the phrase "made with organic ingredients" and to list up to three of the organic ingredients on the label. Processed products that contain less than 70 percent organic ingredients cannot use the term "organic" other than to identify specific ingredients that are organically produced in the ingredients statement. For example, a mois-turizer made with at least 70 percent organic ingredients and only organic vegetables may be labeled as either "made with organic aloe vera juice," or "made with organic plant extracts."

Since February 2008, strict natural and organic certification standards are available for cosmetics, too. The USDA's National Organic Program has been certifying personal care products for more than four years, but the new IOS Cosmetics Standard was created specifically for North America according to existing European, United States, and Canadian regulations and legislations. "With this standard we aim to bring clarity to natural and organic cosmetics producers and create trust among consumers," says Brian Lane, president of Certech, the first North American organization to verify that the claims made by certified cosmetics are proven and supported by facts through a rigorous, unbiased process.

In order to be certified as natural under the IOS Cosmetics Standard, a minimum of 95 percent of the product must be of natural origin. In addition, certified organic beauty products must also use certified organic ingredients that have been grown, cultivated, and stored without the use of chemical fertilizers, herbicides, pesticides, fumigants, or other toxins. The standard also addresses the manufacturing process, which must not use or produce toxins and other harmful substances, and the packaging of the product must be recyclable. The products themselves, as well as their individual ingredients, must not be tested on animals, must be virtually free of synthetic ingredients, and may not contain pesticides, harmful preservatives, artificial colors, or fragrances.

Recently, another organic standard emerged. The OASIS Standard, created by cosmetic industry giants such as Estée Lauder and Hain, is less rigorous than USDA's National Organic Program certification. According to organic produce manufacturers and legislators, OASIS (Organic and Sustainable Industry Standards), which claims to be the first United States "organic" beauty care standard, "deliberately misleads" organic consumers who are looking for a reliable indicator of true, organic product integrity in personal care.

"The OASIS standard allows a product to be labeled outright as 'Organic' (rather than 'Made with Organic Specified Ingredients') even if it contains hydrogenated and sulfated cleansing ingredients like sodium lauryl sulfate made from conventional agricultural material grown with synthetic fertilizers, herbicides and pesticides, and preserved with synthetic petrochemical preservatives like Ethylhexylglycerin and Phenoxyethanol. [Reference: OASIS Standard section 6.2 and Anti-Microbial List]," noted Organic Consumers Association in its April 2008 statement.

Doesn't this seem like a clear case of legitimate organic angel dusting? Today, many products with the word "organic" on the label have as little as 5 percent organic ingredients, and some contain a lot less. Even if a manufacturer uses a 1 percent concentration of organic grape seed extract, it can proudly put "organic" on the product, and now it has an "organic" standard on which to base its claims. Allowing synthetic cleansing ingredients and preservatives to be spiced up by a few "organic" water extracts literally dilutes the whole meaning of organic, since body washes and shampoos are 85 percent water anyway.

Granted, it's impossible to follow the strict guidelines developed for the food industry when you make a shampoo or lipstick. The current list of allowed synthetic ingredients under the U.S. national organic standards was developed specifically for food products. Some beauty products, such as body oils and balms, can meet those food-grade standards, but certain types of skin care and hair care products cannot physically be made without additional synthetic ingredients. Nearly all sunscreens rely on titanium dioxide or zinc oxide to block the sun, and most peptides and vitamins are synthetic. But any organic consumer worth her olive oil body scrub has the right to expect that ingredients in products labeled "organic" are made from organic, not conventional, agriculture, are not hydrogenated or sulfated, and are free from synthetic petrochemical preservatives.

## Green or Greenwashed?

Organic is a hot word in the cosmetic business. Manufacturers constantly look for possibilities of legally placing the word "organic" on the label in any way they can. How about "Totally Organic Experience," a famous slogan of Herbal Essences body and hair products, which contain nonorganic fruit juices and herbal extracts heavily diluted with sodium lauryl and laureth sulfates, cocamide MEA, synthetic fragrances, and coal tar–derived dyes?

Using a drop of organic essential oil to justify the word "organic" on the label is the most common greenwashing technique in the cosmetic industry. Beauty greenwashers usually spend money on promoting themselves as environmentally friendly or green rather than spending resources on formulating toxin-free, environmentally sound products. To jump on the green bandwagon, beauty greenwashers usually change the name or label of a product to give the feeling of nature, for example, by putting an image of a green meadow on a bottle of harmful chemicals or babies playing on a green lawn on a packet of PEG-loaded baby wipes.

Here are the most popular claims that appear on greenwashed beauty products. Let's take a look to see how these claims damage the reputation of all things organic, natural, and ecofriendly.

- Made with organic essential oils
- Contains organic ingredients
- Made with nontoxic ingredients
- 100 percent natural
- Essentially nontoxic

- Earth-friendly
- Environmentally safer

None of these claims ensures that the product is safe and pure. The greenwashed product is just as "organic" as "hypoallergenic" eye cream loaded with preservatives and petrochemical emollients.

Greenwashing ruins the whole green living idea. Environmentally concerned consumers are tricked into buying products they think are good for them and safe for the planet. Green newbies instantly lose trust in organic beauty since it seems to offer no differences. By spending money on greenwashed shampoos or baby products, consumers unwittingly support clever marketers who are hiding behind smart packaging design. When greenwashing is exposed, the whole organic beauty industry suffers a blow. Why should we believe all those important-looking logos and seals if they mean so little? I can't help but question whether my favorite organic products are that pure and natural, considering the newest reports about carcinogens found in "green" bestsellers.

No matter how pure and natural the packaging looks or how promising and ecoconscious the promise sounds, always spot the beauty greenwasher by looking at the ingredients list. It only takes a minute! Many good cosmetic companies are helpful enough to state the percentage of organic ingredients on a label. If they don't, study the ingredients list, where some manufacturers make an extra effort to list which ingredients were derived from organic sources and which were synthesized. Ideally, you want to see organically derived ingredients listed closer to the beginning of the ingredients list rather than at the end of the list. Remember, some ingredients, such as water, cannot be organic, and this is usually reflected on a product label. If you are in doubt, write to the company and ask about the certification of ingredients claiming to be organic. Companies with nothing to hide should be easy to reach and ready to help.

Don't get me wrong: as a consumer, I would rather cheer any effort to take green to the mainstream than support those who churn out yet another brew of petrochemicals and carcinogenic fragrances to "naturally" care for our skin and hair. And while I can sometimes give up and buy a "natural" mascara formulated with parabens, I do not tolerate any harmful synthetics in baby products. Neither should you. Babies cannot vote for green with their dollar, but you can.

## DON'T BE A VICTIM OF
## GREEN BEAUTY MISINFORMATION

Here are some simple steps to help avoid green scams:

**Check the ingredients list.** If the "organic" shampoo is made of sodium laureth sulfate, PEGs, and contains parabens and artificial fragrances, then it's definitely not good for you, no matter how many organic essential oils were used to justify the "organic" claim. There are very few companies that make 100 percent organic beauty products, and even if they use only certified organic plant extracts and herbs, it's impossible to organically certify water, vitamins, and minerals. Still, whenever you buy an organic beauty product, double-check the ingredients list for synthetic chemicals. You will be surprised to find them in many forms, often hiding behind perfectly natural names and neutral-sounding abbreviations. Nobody should get away with false claims.

**Are the green claims relevant?** Sometimes a beauty product may display an environmental certification mark to show that this manufacturer powers its facilities with renewable energy, which is clearly a beneficial environmental feature. However, it doesn't make the ingredients any cleaner or healthier. You could easily be misled by the certification mark to believe that the product is safer or uses safer ingredients than its competitors, when that may not be true.

**Does the packaging back up its claims or green theme?** Try to see more than the natural-looking design of the bottle. "See if the packaging is made of recycled plastic or glass, and if the instructions are printed on recycled paper," recommends Morris Shriftman, one of the founders of Avalon Organics, now a consultant with the brand. "Many companies replant trees that were used in packaging, or otherwise restore the forests." So when you see a new "green" product hitting store shelves, wait a second and ask: does it ring true and sound authentic, or is it obviously hype? Be a vigilant shopper—your own scrutiny of green marketing claims must be one more item to add to your shopping list.

*continued*

  **the green beauty guide**

*Do the benefits outweigh the negatives?* The company may use organic aloe vera or donate a percentage of their profits to eco-friendly charities, but this doesn't make paraben preservatives, silicones, mineral oil, and other synthetic ingredients in a greenwashed product any less toxic. A little selfishness won't hurt: always consider if the product makes you or your children healthier, and only then start worrying about global warming. Make the planet healthier by caring about your own health first.

## Going Green Without Going Broke

The idea of organic beauty products as dusty bottles sitting on the lower shelves of health food stores is very outdated. Just because the treatment is labeled as natural or organic doesn't mean that it has been cooked in a country kitchen. Organic creams today can create an adrenaline rush similar to a pair of designer jeans—and sometimes cost just as much.

Some organic lines were created with pure luxury in mind. Jo Wood, the wife of Ron Wood, the guitarist for the Rolling Stones, developed her line of organic fragrances after years of blending her own oils. In 2005, she came up with an African-inspired line of fragrant oils and mists, Amka and Usiku, whose musky and woody scents captured the hearts (and noses) of celebrities worldwide. Jo Wood's sumptuous creations are a far cry from humble vials of essential oils stocked by health food stores!

Not happy with the selection of organic beauty products in your local health store? Many department stores are becoming greener, stocking Origins, which launched an organic line of products, as well as semigreen Caudalie and Aveda. Some of them have phased out parabens or phenoxyethanol preservatives but still have a few safe chemicals on their labels. Sephora carries Boscia, Korres, and REN seminatural brands.

Another excellent source of new organic skin care lines is eBay, where many spa and organic beauty manufacturers have online stores. If you are open for things new and exotic, you can find amazing natural and mineral-based skin care from Iceland, Hungary, and Israel, as well as herbs and clays for your homemade cosmetic creations. Always check the ingredients list or request one from the seller before buying anything. If you don't have a budget to splash on Jurlique, which has magic potions as pricey as La Mer or La Prairie, I recommend trying simple, affordable, or homemade organic recipes that are tailored to suit every skin's needs.

Already thinking about giving your beauty stash a green makeover? If there's one organic beauty product that you can afford to buy right now, buy a moisturizer. They sit on skin longest, and that's why they should not contain anything toxic. Try a couple of samples and buy a bigger size of the one you especially like. Just make sure to use it diligently since it has to be used up according to its "best before" date. Next, buy a body moisturizer and/or sunscreen. In general, a moisturizer and a sunscreen should be the most expensive things in your beauty arsenal. For a toner, you can get away with rose water or witch hazel, or quickly whip up a simple concoction at home. The last thing to replace should be your facial cleanser. Cleansers should not be expensive to perform well. Ideally, you should adopt a double-cleansing technique using two cleansers (which we are going to discuss in the next chapter), but neither product needs to cost a fortune. For hair care, invest in a good conditioner and stick to an organic baby shampoo. Remember: you don't need to buy more; you need to buy more of a good thing.

Keep in mind that when you switch to all-natural skin care, your skin may start misbehaving. This is because many natural beauty products contain multitasking essential oils that work as spot treatments, antiaging agents, and natural preservatives. Unless you become extremely allergic to one particular ingredient (such as coughing, sneezing, or eye watering), don't quit unless it is absolutely critical. In a couple of days, your skin will adjust.

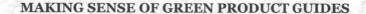

## MAKING SENSE OF GREEN PRODUCT GUIDES

To help you decide which cosmetic product to choose, you will find a Green Product Guide in several chapters. These guides are split into three sections.

**One leaf** is awarded to products that are generally clean and pure, but do contain a few questionable yet generally safe plant ingredients. The concerns are minimal: it could be an overwhelming smell of essential oils or plant extracts that aren't suitable for everyone. Yet none of these products contain harmful chemicals.

**Two leaves** indicate that a product is sensibly formulated, contains nothing toxic, and delivers its promises, yet there's a little "but." Maybe a strong fragrance, less-than-convenient packaging, or maybe the price was hard to justify. In any case, this is an excellent product to try and maybe fall in love with.

**Three leaves** are given to the greenest beauty products. If you already recycle, reuse, drive a hydrogen car, and heat your home with solar energy, then you will go an extra mile or two for that biodynamic body oil. Solutions in this section are likely to be more time- and money-consuming than the rest. You will notice, however, that price point is rarely taken into consideration. All that matters is the efficiency of the product, the purity of the ingredients, and, as a result, the authenticity of the green claims.

How do I award the leaves to the products? To start with, I check the formulation and see how it relates to the latest scientific research about synthetic and natural cosmetic ingredients and their effects on skin. If a product contains an active ingredient, I usually check how much is actually in the product, and if it contains potent plant extracts and essential oils, I will mention the possible risks of allergic reactions or increased sun sensitivity.

*continued*

To see whether a product lives up to its green claims, I take a look at other products in the line. Do they contain questionable ingredients? Does the company make a genuine effort to educate its consumers? If it does, then the green claim is authentic, not hype.

I never base my recommendations simply on my own personal experience. I will not recommend something just because I like the way a cosmetic product feels on my skin. I understand that thousands of other women may feel differently about it. During my years of cosmetic reviewing and reporting, I have tried hundreds of products, but there's nothing like the opinion of a highly independent and discerning panel of dedicated cosmetic junkies, also known as relatives, friends, colleagues, and readers of my websites who offered their help to evaluate and review cosmetic products for this book.

When you see a product guide, simply choose the product that suits your needs most or mix and match as you feel. Whether it's a cure for limp locks or split nails, you will find green and safe solutions for all of your beauty needs.

Only products that fit these criteria are recommended for use in this book. Sadly, many brands that support the green movement and send a strong green message did not make it to the Green Product Guides. Such brands include The Body Shop, most products by Tom's of Maine, Kiss My Face, Derma-E, Jason Naturals, Alba Botanica, and others. As much as I respect the fact that they support fair trade, don't test on animals, or don't use colorants, their "organic" or "natural" products are still loaded with synthetic ingredients with questionable safety records. Some of these ingredients are further discussed in Chapter 5.

Fortunately, many brands reformulate their products to remove synthetic, potentially harmful ingredients, and I look forward to including more green creations in Green Product Guides in the future.

## GREEN BEAUTY CRITERIA

The green beauty product should not contain any ingredient, of natural or synthetic origin, that can poison the environment and cause harm to human health. This includes ingredients that have been proven toxic and mutagenic in animal studies. These include:

- Petrochemicals, including mineral oil and various silicones

- Sodium laureth/lauryl sulfates and other sulfate-based detergents

- Propylene glycol, polyethylene glycol, and various ingredients formulated with PEGs and PGs

- Formaldehyde and paraben preservatives

- Synthetic (FD&C and other) dyes and colorants

- Artificial fragrances of any sort

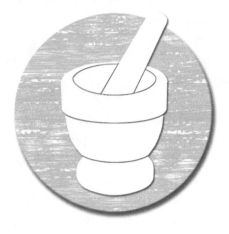

# do-it-
# yourself
## green beauty

**t**ired of talking about natural products? Then why don't you make one yourself? This way, you will know exactly what goes into the jar. You will know why it works; and if it doesn't, you can learn from this experience and improve your formulation. Hundreds of brands, big and small, were conceived in a kitchen, and the best thing is you don't need a gift for cosmetic chemistry or a professional degree to whip up a simple cucumber and clay mask. Once you come to grips with this simple process, you will realize that your homemade cosmetic products are more effective and pleasant to use than commercially available masks sold in pretty tubes and jars. Here are some other benefits of making your own skin care:

1. *Big savings*. You will be able to save up to 80 percent on an advanced antiaging cream if you boost your existing moisturizer with active ingredients that are sold separately. Most scrubs and masks cost pennies when made at home.
2. *Better value*. To put it simply, you are getting the biggest bang for your buck. You are not spending 95 percent of your money on the packaging, labeling, and advertising—so you can get a much better product for a lower cost.
3. *Unique combinations*. You can try combinations that are impossible to find on the shelves. Brands are tied to specific active ingredients (Crème de la Mer uses fermented sea kelp, while RéVive is famous for the use of epidermal growth factor), so it is impossible to find products that have active ingredients marketed by two competing brands, but you can mix them at home very easily.
4. *Custom-tailored strength*. You can adjust the concentration of an active ingredient based on the condition of your skin. By making your own cosmetics, you can be sure that the blend works for you and was not designed to suit a large number of people. If you need a little less of an ingredient, you can more easily adjust the formulation. There is no need to compromise.
5. *Freshness*. You can eschew paraben and formaldehyde preservatives by making a fresh batch of a skin cream or a cleanser at home every month.

6. *Simplicity*. You can save yourself some time and hassle by buying organic base creams and lotions that already contain all the inactive ingredients mixed up in perfect proportions. Some cosmetic products can be whipped up from scratch, but good lotions and shampoos are more complicated to make at home.

7. *Advanced formulas*. By trying new active ingredients, you can enjoy the scientific findings sooner than people who use ready-made products. Conventional beauty lines need two years to introduce new ingredients to the market due to the expense and time to develop new packaging and labels.

## EQUIPMENT AND TOOLS

So how do you get started? First, you need to stock up on the essential tools. To prepare a simple mask, all you need is a stick blender and a glass beaker. To prepare facial oil, you will need more tools, including droppers, beakers, and spatulas. Here's what I use:

- Marble pestle and mortar (I've found that those made of china aren't sturdy enough if I need to smash granules of brown sugar or sea salt for face and body scrubs)

- Enameled simmering pan (for melting waxes and butters)

- Electronic weighing scales (mine are vintage and manual yet precise—for the fun of it)

- Glass measuring glass

- Gas or electric oven (not microwave) for heating, melting, and boiling

- Small stainless-steel cocktail shaker (for no-mess blending)

- Double boiler or a small saucepan with a heat-proof glass cereal bowl that fits inside to create a double boiler (for, well, boiling). Alternatively, you can use a small enamel pan with a wooden handle that would fit into another, larger pan.

*continued*

- Glass cereal bowl (for mixing and whipping)

- Eggbeater or small whisk (for blending)

- Small coffee press (for steeping herbs and teas)

- Wooden spatulas (similar to those used during sugar waxing)

- Antique silver baby spoon (a brilliant local charity shop find, excellent for transferring creams and scrubs into glass jars—silver is a natural anti-bacterial agent)

- Plain medicine glass dropper (for dropping tiny amounts of vitamins and herbal extracts)

- Baby medicine feeder (syringe-style, for very precise measurements)

- Plenty of cobalt blue glass jars, as well as pump and spray bottles (to store, sell, and/or give away)

All this equipment fits nicely into a sturdy medium-sized storage box (mine is from IKEA, complete with a nice lid and a metal window). I frequently sterilize my equipment in a baby bottle sterilizer and store droppers and spatulas in air-tight, biodegradable plastic bags. Whenever I have the urge to try a new recipe, I have everything at hand.

## Choose Sustainable Packaging

I maintain my supply of reasonably priced cobalt blue jars and bottles by purchasing them by the dozen on eBay. I also reuse glass jars from old creams and masks. Mason jars make excellent containers for bath blends and salts. As the jury is out on phthalates leaching into food and water from plastic containers, and aluminum making its way into products from aluminum tubes, I made it a rule to decant all my ready-made and homemade beauty creations into glass containers. Using a pretty container for your homemade goodies is very important, because you are more likely to enjoy using herb-smelling goo from a vintage lead-free crystal jar rather than from a disposable plastic container. Glass containers can be washed, sterilized, and reused, which reduces the amount of plastic that goes to landfills.

Vintage perfume and cosmetic bottles make gorgeous frames for your cosmetic creations. Jo Wood said that luxurious containers were an important part of her organic fragrance collection. "For years I'd been searching for organic beauty products that were beautiful and smelt fabulous; it was important to me that what I put on my skin was just as natural and chemical-free as what I was putting in my body," says Jo Wood. "When it came to packaging, I was hugely influenced by Biba and the Art Nouveau movement, which can been seen in the luxurious black packaging and gold etchings."

## Preserving Your DIY Skin Care

A rule of thumb is to prepare small batches of skin care weekly and store them in the fridge. Refreshing facial toners can be kept in a freezer to give you a quick minilift in the morning. If you use a mild natural preservative, such as my own Silver Vitamin Blend (recipe in Chapter 7) or plain grapefruit seed oil or extract, you may store your products on a bathroom shelf for up to a month. Keep a watchful eye out and discard any product that shows signs of contamination (smells spoiled, develops discolorations, or changes its texture).

While most soaps and shampoos with added parabens, phthalates, or formaldehyde preservatives usually remain fresh for up to two years from the manufacture date (who uses a soap that long, mind me asking?), the shelf life of paraben-free beauty products is much shorter. Mascara, lip balms in pots, and eye creams will remain uncontaminated for three to four months; facial and body moisturizers can last up to six months, depending on the ingredients; shampoos and mineral sunscreens have a shelf life of two years if kept in a cool, dark place; and natural alcohol-based deodorants will stay fresh for up to one year. Anything that has no water in it will remain fresh for longer, but many body oils may go rancid nine to twelve months after being opened or blended. Some essential oils act as natural preservatives, so your citrus-smelling organic products have more chances of staying fresh.

No matter whether you prepare your beauty products from scratch or buy them in a store, make sure you keep them away from direct sunlight. The ideal place to store your organic skin care is a cool, dry cabinet. A refrigerator isn't always the best option, since cold temperatures may reduce the efficacy of certain ingredients.

## Where to Buy Ingredients

Clays, witch hazel, vitamins in pill and liquid forms, herbal teas and extracts, as well as organic sugar and sea salt are available from most good health food stores. Rose and orange waters are available in better supermarkets and groceries. Many online stores sell natural ingredients such as aloe vera juice, borax, citric acid, essential oils, and almond meal for scrubs. You will find some useful resources in Appendix A.

When choosing plant ingredients, ask the seller about the origins of their extracts and juices. "When plants are grown in their ideal region, they contain the optimum amount of nutrients," says Kristen Binder, the founder of Saffron Rouge (www.saffronrouge.com). "Take a cactus and try to grow it in northern Canada. The plant will struggle to survive and therefore be in life and death mode, instead of being focused on flourishing. This plant will be depleted of many vital nutrients because the soil and sunlight are not what it needs. In the same way, if you tried to grow a rose bush in the middle of the desert, the soil wouldn't provide the rose with what it needed in order to make rich oil. I find it so hard to compare lemongrass oil from plants grown in a greenhouse to oil from lemongrass grown on the mountains of Bhutan, where this plant naturally flourishes."

Many organic skin care brands grow their own plants for use in their products. Weleda, WALA (the maker of Dr. Hauschka), and Primavera are famous for their lavish gardens. If they need to use a plant that grows in exotic destinations, these companies support fair-trade communities that grow the plants without the use of chemical additives.

# Active Ingredients: No Rocket Science

Until recently, I had to put up with quite a limited selection of antiaging organic beauty offerings. Most of them were gentle and soothing, but they didn't contain any of the cutting-edge ingredients that were used in synthetic age-delaying creams and serums. Today, thanks to readily available "skin actives," concentrated active ingredients that you can add to your favorite beauty products, I spend hours blending, revamping, and enriching my organic lotions and potions.

If you take a look at the ingredients list of any cleanser or moisturizing lotions, you will notice a long list of tongue-twisting chemical ingredients. Most of them do nothing for the health of the skin. They only serve as a base for the active ingredients, helping them dissolve properly and maintaining the stability of the formulation so that it doesn't become too watery, too thick, or split into layers.

The process of creating high-end, high-performance skin care products is now demystified. Dr. Hannah Sivak, PhD, the scientific mind behind secretive Skin Actives labs, is as blunt as only a scientist can be: you don't need to coat your products with a mysterious air to make them effective. "For example, sea kelp bioferment is a great active, and you do not need to play music or do a light show during fermentation," she says, referring to the famous Crème de la Mer, which contains fermented sea kelp. "The key molecules in this active are the polysaccharides unique to sea kelp, and the music is not going to affect their structure."

The newest active ingredients are naturally found in human bodies and plants. Some of them can be extracted from plants, but others are so rare that it is much more affordable to make them in a lab. To start with, Dr. Sivak recommends two actives, such as epidermal growth factor (EGF), as the signal that tells the skin to go ahead and renew itself, and fermented sea kelp, as a provider of building blocks for the skin to be able to follow the EGF orders. As you become more skillful in mixing, you can add more antioxidants.

Adding active ingredients is no rocket science. All it requires is a tender touch: add one active at a time and mix thoroughly, either with a spatula or a small mixer that fits inside the cream jar. With practice, you will achieve a nice texture that will be pleasant to use. Now, as your skin gets drier, you can adjust the formulation by adding a few drops of rosehip or pomegranate oil to the mix.

While it's possible to replicate any cream or lotion at home using basic ingredients available from most health food stores, the right consistency and even texture can be hard to achieve at home, especially if you are just flexing your cosmetic chemist's muscle. It's more practical to buy simple, "generic" natural lotions and cleansers in stores and use them as a canvas for your own blends.

At your local health food store or online, you can find a multitude of inexpensive, very basic lotions that contain few plant ingredients that are unlikely to interact with the active ingredients you are going to use. You can buy a large bottle of good organic body cream and turn it into several jars of antiaging, antioxidant-rich facial moisturizers. You should look for formulations that contain no irritating ingredients, such as peppermint and eucalyptus oils. Other things to avoid are citrus oils and juices, including those of lemon, orange, grapefruit, lime, and bergamot. Their acidity is not compatible with many active ingredients. Of course, there should be no propylene glycols, parabens of any kind, and artificial fragrances. Ideally, the carrier lotion should contain as few ingredients as possible.

When you come across a good carrier lotion, buy a larger size. It's much easier to make a large batch of an upgraded product and distribute it among friends and relatives than count drops in order to safely blend one ounce of a potent cream. If you have a "holy grail" product you've been using for ages, you can add active ingredients to it too, provided that they mix well.

I like to play with active ingredients, using large bottles of organic body moisturizers or organic unscented face lotions for sensitive skin. By trial and error, I figured out that the strongest players (idebenone, hyaluronic acid, various peptides, and EGF) behave best in Burt's Bees Carrot Skin Lotion and Jurlique Soothing Day Care Lotion. A tiny tube of palmitoyl pentapeptide makes a whopping 8 ounces of Strivectin-strength antiaging lotion—without the steep price.

By all means, do not try to mix too many active ingredients in one product. You may think there isn't such a thing as too much of a good thing, but by trying to beef up your

**Green Tip**

If you try to combine more than three or four active ingredients, you may end up with a product that doesn't blend well, separates after just three days, or is plain irritating. All your efforts go directly down the drain!

cream with every possible antioxidant, you are in fact nullifying their effectiveness. Moreover, too many active ingredients have more chances to interact and synergize in unwanted directions, leading to side effects and irritation. Keep your formulas simple with two or a maximum of three ingredients instead of turning your cream into a fruit salad with high irritation potential.

According to Dr. Sivak, a cream with added actives will last as long as the shelf life of the starting cream. If you add more than three active ingredients, limit the shelf life to six months. Make sure you use good-quality actives. If a botanical extract was not prepared properly, it can add a large load of bacteria and mold to the cream, and no amount of preservatives will be enough to cope with that.

Because a home-mixed product is less expensive, you should not feel guilty when using it often and on areas in need, like hands, neck, and décolleté, which age even faster than the face.

## A Few Words of Caution

Just as you can suffer adverse reactions to conventional cosmetics, natural, homemade lotions and potions can also trigger sensitivity. Avocado oil, essential oils, glycerin, lanolin, a simple tincture of benzoin, sweet almond oil, and wheat germ oil have all been known to cause irritation in some people. Be aware that when you are under stress, your skin may be more sensitive than usual.

With many active ingredients, it's important to use the exact amounts as specified by the manufacturer.

Make sure you use ingredients that are fresh, and, of course, organic whenever possible. As a rule of thumb, discard any ingredient or carrier that has developed an odd smell, discoloration, or has become foggy and uneven in texture.

**Green Tip**

Resist the urge to make the potion more effective by doubling the amount of the active ingredient. You may end up with irritated, inflamed skin.

No matter how you take your green beauty—buying it ready-made, working as a couturier creating your own products from scratch, or being a bit of a tailor, making sure that this particular product perfectly suits your needs—I hope you are keeping it as natural as possible. Exclude all synthetic chemicals, if possible; if not, keep the safe and beneficial ones and ditch parabens and formaldehyde-containing preservatives, as well as mineral oil and other petrochemicals.

## Green Beauty Ingredients

Most green beauty products rely on the same naturally derived ingredients. The only difference might be the amount of hard-to-find exotic plant extracts, triple-distilled extracts, and rare essential oils in a finished product. Once you know what works for your skin, you can make a new beauty product in seconds.

This section describes plant-derived and natural ingredients that are used in popular green cosmetic products and in recipes in this book. I also share with you some of the newest achievements in cosmetic chemistry that shed light on traditional familiar ingredients.

Don't be surprised when you find a synthetic enzyme idebenone next to lemon oil and milk in the next few pages. Many newly synthesized proteins, enzymes, and acids made this list because they meet the green beauty criteria discussed in Chapter 3, "Become an Ingredients List Expert." Some organic ingredients, such as minerals and clays (technically organic, since you cannot organically certify sea salt), are also included. Aromatic chemicals are discussed in Chapter 15, "Green Fragrances." At the same time, many natural plant extracts didn't make this list because they are found to be detrimental for your health.

Now, let's take a look at the building blocks of green beauty products.

### Almond (Sweet) (*Prunus amygdalus dulcis*)

Sweet almond oil is used in moisturizers, hair conditioners, and body oils for its great emollient properties. A green beauty mainstay, sweet almond oil is prized for its high content of fatty acids that appear to be close to skin's own sebum. Almond meal makes a very gentle skin exfoliant rich in minerals and vitamins. Sweet almond oil is commonly available in health stores and online. Beware of bitter almond oil, which has a disputable safety record.

## Aloe Vera (*Aloe barbadensis*)

Aloe has been used as a first aid remedy for wounds, irritations, skin infections, and burns since the era of ancient Egypt. Cleopatra used aloe as a skin rejuvenator. Aloe is rich in polysaccharides, galactose, plant steroids, enzymes, amino acids, minerals, and even natural antibiotics. You can buy aloe juice or extract in health food stores, or you can grow aloe plants at home and squeeze the juice to use in your beauty preparations.

## Alpha-Lipoic Acid (ALA)

Alpha-lipoic acid is also known as lipoic acid. This naturally occurring substance works as a potent antioxidant that stimulates cellular metabolism and protects cells against the destructive effects of free radicals. When taken internally, lipoic acid is effective against liver disorders and diabetic neuropathy. Recently, Thai biomedics found that alpha-lipoic acid could stave off skin cancer by decreasing skin inflammation. Earlier studies showed that alpha-lipoic acid could increase cellular energy, decrease UV-induced damage to skin, and even neutralize heavy metals (Ho et al. 2007).

As a cosmetic ingredient, alpha-lipoic acid is both versatile and economical. It can be added to toners, moisturizers, and sunscreens. It is available in health food stores in capsules and online as a fine yellowish powder. It can be dissolved in most base products in the following proportion: 300 mg of alpha-lipoic acid to 1 ounce of base product, keeping the concentration of alpha-lipoic acid in your preparation under 3 percent. Please note that it may not dissolve easily, so start slowly and blend thoroughly. As with any acid, ALA can sting when applied topically, so if your skin is on the sensitive side, always perform a patch test. Start with a lower concentration of ALA and build it up as you become handy in mixing your DIY products.

## Apple *(Pyrus malus)*

This popular fruit is used in cosmetics in the form of juice or concentrated extract that is a source of alpha hydroxy acid. Apple juice is used in exfoliating peels and masks. Apple juice contains the phenolic compounds quercetin, epicatechin, and procyanidin B-2, which may be cancer-protective, as it has demonstrated powerful antioxidant activity.

## Apricot (*Prunus armeniaca*)

Apricot kernel is rich in oil that is believed to have anticarcinogenic properties. In the seventeenth century, apricot oil was used in England against tumors and ulcers, and Laetrile, an alleged alternative treatment for cancer, is extracted from apricot seeds. Crushed apricot kernel is commonly used in face and body scrubs.

## Arbutin

This glycoside, which is similar to hydroquinone, prevents the formation of melanin and is used as a skin-lightening agent. Arbutin is extracted from bearberry plants, and it is also found in wheat and pear skins. In November 2007, Korean scientists found that a new arbutin compound, arbutin-beta-glycosides, synthesized from bacterium *Thermotoga neapolitana,* inhibits melanin production in melanoma skin cancer cells by up to 70 percent (Jun et al. 2007). However, since arbutin is very similar to hydroquinone, it may pose the same carcinogenic risks. German microbiologists found that intestinal bacteria can transform arbutin into hydroquinone, which may promote the formation of intestinal cancer (Blaut et al. 2006). Until science knows more, it may be advisable to use arbutin-containing compounds with caution.

## Arnica (*Arnica montana*)

I personally have very mixed feelings about arnica. I was introduced to arnica extract when I was looking for a chemical-free topical pain-relieving balm to use postpartum. Arnica extract has been traditionally used to alleviate muscle pain and help heal bruises. Arnica, rich in sequiterpenes, flavonoids, and phenolic acids, is well known for its potent anti-inflammatory and antitumor effects. However, some studies note that the terpenoid helenalin found in arnica is a highly toxic compound. Arnica can be very irritating, and medical science knows quite a few cases of severe allergic dermatitis to this plant. Most often, people who are allergic to chamomile are allergic to arnica as well. Because of its high irritancy potential, arnica is not recommended for use in baby products. My skin tolerates arnica very well, and I find it an effective pain-relieving addition to massage creams.

## Avocado (*Persea americana*)

This tropical fruit contains more fatty alcohols than any other fruit known to man. Avocados are rich in potassium and vitamins B, E, and K. Avocado oil is a highly effective emollient and can be used in many cosmetic products and home recipes.

## Azelaic Acid

This acid is found naturally in wheat, rye, barley, and *Malassezia furfur* (also known as *Pityrosporum ovale*), yeast that lives on normal skin. Azelaic acid is effective against acne when applied topically in a cream formulation of up to 20 percent. "Azelaic acid 15 percent gel represents a new therapeutic option for the treatment of acne vulgaris," wrote acne expert Dr. Diane Thiboudot, professor of dermatology at Pennsylvania State University College of Medicine, in her 2008 study on this exciting new green beauty ingredient, adding that "most physicians (81.9 percent) described an improvement in patients' symptoms after an average of 34.6 days" (Thiboudot 2008). Another important benefit of this plant-derived acid is its activity against excessive pigmentation, including melasma and post-acne brown marks. As if it weren't enough, azelaic acid wards off free radicals, reduces inflammation, appears to be virtually nontoxic, and is well tolerated by most complexions.

## Baking Soda (*Sodium bicarbonate*)

This fine white powder is in natural deodorants for its ability to absorb odors. Baking soda is traditionally used as a tooth whitener because of its abrasive properties. Last but not least, baking soda makes a gentle antibacterial facial scrub, which is especially good for acne-prone skin.

### Beeswax (*Apis mellifera*)

This natural wax is produced in the beehive of honeybees. Beeswax is rich in fatty acid esters and is used in cosmetic products like emollients, thickeners, and emulsifiers. A controlled German study found that a barrier cream with beeswax was more effective in baby care than a commercial product with petroleum jelly (Frosch et al. 2003).

### Beet (*Beta vulgaris*)

Beetroots are rich in the nutrient betaine and red pigments betalains and indicaxanthin. This pigment has been shown to be a powerful protective antioxidant that also prevents the breakdown of alpha-tocopherol, or vitamin E. Beet juice can be used to prepare liquid blushes and lip colors.

### Bentonite

This natural clay has the chemical name aluminum phyllosilicate. Clays are used cosmetically in facial masks for their ability to absorb oil and protein molecules. As aluminum salt, bentonite and kaolin are less toxic than aluminum hydroxychloride, which is used in antiperspirants. However, bentonite clay may be toxic to the central nervous system and detrimental to bones because aluminum competes with calcium for absorption. Currently, cosmetic manufacturers consider bentonite clays safe for use in cosmetics based on a study in which aluminum silicate was applied to human skin daily for one week (Elmore 2003). Long-term effects of exposure to aluminum salt in facial masks and creams are as yet unknown. Keep this in mind when buying clay masks based on salts of aluminum. There are many wonderful aluminum-free clays that have healing potential. Natural muds, such as volcanic fango mud and marine muds from the Dead Sea, are naturally rich in thermal water and minerals. They are used in spa procedures at balneological resorts.

### Birch (*Betula pendula*)

Birch extract has traditionally been used to promote hair growth. Birch bark is rich in anti-inflammatory tannins and saponins, while the leaves contain betulorentic acid, which has anti-inflammatory and anti-HIV activity. Birch extract is used in shampoos, conditioners, and body

  **the green beauty guide**

treatments for cellulite. You can prepare a birch leaf infusion at home to rinse your hair after shampooing.

## Caffeine

This plant alkaloid is found in coffee, tea, maté, and guarana. Known for its ability to dilate blood vessels and purge water from the body, caffeine is widely used in cellulite treatments and eye creams that may reduce puffiness. Recent studies found that caffeine can help protect you from skin cancer. In 2008, scientists of the State University of New Jersey found that topical application of caffeine inhibited the development of sunlight-induced skin cancer in animals, especially when combined with the consumption of green tea or caffeine. Even after intensive UV irradiation for several months, caffeine significantly reduced the formation of skin cancer and slowed cell mutations (Conney et al. 2008). Now, that's a good reason to keep the java flowing!

## Calendula (*Calendula officinalis*)

This plant, also known as marigold, is a traditional herbal remedy praised for its antibacterial and anti-inflammatory properties. Calendula extract is rich in beta-carotene, stearin, triterpinoids, flavonoids, and coumarin, as well as microelements. For this reason, calendula is frequently used in soothing and calming preparations, such as baby baths and creams, and after-sun products.

## Camphor

This alkaloid, derived from the leaves of the camphor plant (*Cinnamomum camphora*), is believed to have an antimicrobial action, which justifies its cosmetic use in topical acne treatments. In large quantities, camphor is poisonous when ingested and can cause seizures, confusion, and mood disorders (Agarwal, Malhotra 2008). According to current regulations, camphor can be used in concentrations of up to 11 percent in cosmetic products.

## Carrot (*Daucus carota*)

Carrot seed oil contains plant antioxidant carotenoids, particularly carotene and luteolin, as well as vitamin E. When applied topically in cosmetic products, carrot seed essential oil has shown to improve sebum production in dry skin, while the antioxidant properties of carotene help it protect skin from UV-induced damage.

## Castor Oil

This plant seed oil is derived from castor beans (*Ricinus communis*). It is rich in ricinoleic, oleic, and linoleic acids. According to Cosmetic Ingredient Review, castor oil can absorb UV light and enhance penetration of other ingredients (CIR Expert Panel 2007). In cosmetics, castor oil is used as an emollient and surfactant in lipsticks, moisturizers, and soaps. Castor oil is also used to make antifungal and antibacterial ointments. Russian scientists reported that castor oil ointment "accelerates the healing and cleaning of infected skin wounds, and produces bacteriostatic action" (Spasov et al. 2007).

## Chamomile (*Matricaria recutita*)

This plant, also spelled as camomile, has been used for hundreds of years in cosmetics for its skin-healing properties. Essential oil from German chamomile is rich in terpene alcohol, also known as bisabolol, which is well-studied for its anti-inflammatory, antimicrobial, and antioxidant effects. During an experimental study in 2008, scientists found that "chamomile extract in the form of rubbing oil had a good potential for acceleration of burn wound healing" (Jarrahi 2008). Please note, however, that chamomile in the form of tinctures, distillates, or essential oils is known to cause contact dermatitis, so if you have a family history of allergies, perform a patch test before adding chamomile to your do-it-yourself beauty products.

## Chrysin

This natural flavonoid is derived from passionflower (*Passiflora incarnate*). In addition to its proven antioxidant abilities, chrysin demonstrated potential as a cancer preventive. In recent studies, chrysin even minimized metastatic spread of cancer after surgery (Beaumont et al. 2008). In green beauty preparations, chrysin appears to protect skin against UV-induced photodamage (Steerenberg et al. 1998). As an active ingredient in Hylexin and many other eye creams that claim to diminish under-eye circles, chrysin seems to activate the enzyme that dissolves the buildup of debris in the delicate eye area (Walle, Walle 2002).

## Coconut (*Cocos nucifera*)

Coconut oil is extracted as a fully organic product from fresh coconut flesh, and it is used as a highly effective emollient in face and body moisturizers, shampoos, and massage oils. Coconut butter, derived from copra, is one of the most stable butters used in cosmetics. Extra virgin coconut oil has been found to be as effective and safe as mineral oil when used as a barrier cream (Frosch et al. 2003).

## Coenzyme Q10

This enzyme is a crucial molecule in the respiration of all living cells. Naturally present in human skin, this enzyme helps maintain healthy energy levels in skin cells, which may help improve the skin's texture and elasticity, improve collagen production, and ward off free radicals. When taken internally, coenzyme Q10 can help prevent diabetes, cardiovascular disease, hypertension, congestive heart failure, age-related deterioration of brain function and vision, immune problems, as well as other age-related health problems (Janson 2006). It is known that levels of coenzyme Q10 diminish with age.

Coenzyme Q10 is a popular cosmetic ingredient, but many antiaging products contain too little of this chemical to make any difference on a cellular level. You may purchase pure synthetic coenzyme Q10, ubiquinone, as capsules or loose powder and use it to create potent yet gentle moisturizers and serums in the following proportion: 300 mg ubiquinone to 1 ounce of a base product. You can add ubiquinone to your sunscreens and moisturizers because it mixes better with oil-based cosmetic products. Coenzyme Q10 appears to synergize well with vitamin E. You may add up to 300 mg vitamin E to each ounce of your DIY preparation to boost effectiveness of coenzyme Q10.

## Collagen

Moisturizers containing collagen and other proteins, such as keratin and elastin, claim to rejuvenate the skin by replenishing its essential proteins that diminish with age. However, the protein molecules are too large to penetrate the skin cells. Collagen may provide temporary relief from dry skin by working as an emollient. When proteins dry, they shrink slightly, stretching out some of the fine wrinkles and providing a temporary lift effect.

## Corn (*Zea mays*)

Cornstarch is used as a thickener in cosmetic products, and more recently as a replacement for talc in natural baby powders. Corn meal, or corn flour, is a cheap facial exfoliator that can be safely used in homemade cosmetic preparations.

## Cucumber (*Cucumis sativus*)

Cultivated for at least three thousand years in western Asia, cucumber is widely used in cosmetics thanks to the high presence of vitamin A, vitamin B6, thiamin, folate, pantothenic acid, magnesium, phosphorus, copper, and manganese, and may have soothing and mild bleaching agents. A small study found that cucumber is rich in phytonutrients and naturally occurring vitamin C (ascorbic acid) that may protect the skin from chemically induced skin cancers (Villaseñor et al. 2002).

## DMAE

Also known by its chemical name, dimethylaminoethanol, this substance is naturally present in human bodies in small amounts, particularly in nerve tissues. It stimulates production of the neurotransmitter choline, which is involved in cell membrane biosynthesis. Synthetic dimethylaminoethanol, an industrial compound commonly used as a paint remover and an epoxy resin curing agent, gained popularity in the cosmetic industry after the discovery that it produces an instant face-lift effect. Topical application of DMAE causes quick and visible swelling of fibroblasts, integral parts of skin cells. Swollen skin cells make the skin look smoother, and for this reason DMAE appears in many antiwrinkle treatments.

But such remarkable results come at a price. A recent study indicates that synthetic DMAE applied topically may pathologically alter the functioning of skin cells. Canadian researchers found that skin cells treated with DMAE died up to 25 percent slower (Morrisette et al. 2006). Skin cells "stop dividing, they stop secreting, and after 24 hours a certain proportion of them die," according to Dr. Francois Marceau of the Centre Hospitalier Universitaire de Quebec in Canada. "I don't want to scare people. The risk is probably not very big, but in my opinion it hasn't been measured accurately."

If, despite the risks, you choose to use DMAE in your DIY skin preparations, you should add it in strictly recommended amounts to any anhydrous fluid, such as glycerin. DMAE can turn any cream containing water into liquid. Conventional DMAE preparations usually contain 1–2 percent of dimethylaminoethanol bitartrate.

## Echinacea (*Echinacea angustifolia, Echinacea purpurea*)

This plant is believed to stimulate the body's immune system and protect against various infections. Echinacea extract is rich in caffeic acid derivative eicosanoids, or prostaglandins, anthocyanins, and phenols that have a strong antioxidant effect. What makes echinacea even more beneficial in green beauty applications is its ability to protect skin from UV damage. Italian scientists found that echinacea effectively wards off free radicals and recommended "topical use of extracts from Echinacea species for the prevention/treatment of photodamage of the skin by UVA/UVB radiation, in which oxidative stress plays a crucial role" (Facino et al. 1995). Echinacea is used in moisturizers and toners for easily irritated, acne-prone skin.

## Eucalyptus (*Eucalyptus sideroxylon, Eucalyptus torquata*)

An essential oil extracted from eucalyptus leaves contains powerful natural disinfectants effective against gram-positive bacteria and *Candida albicans*. Eucalyptus essential oil also has insect repellent properties. For the first time in history, a December 2007 Egyptian study revealed that eucalyptus extracts and oils were toxic to cells of human breast adenocarcinoma (Ashour 2007), but more studies are needed to determine if eucalyptus has anicancer potential.

### Evening Primrose (*Oenothera biennis*)

Essential oil from the seeds of evening primrose contains a very rare omega-6 essential fatty acid, namely, gamma-linolenic acid. This is one of the body's three sources of eicosanoids, which makes evening primrose oil potentially effective for autoimmune disorders, arthritis, and eczema. Gamma-linolenic acid also shows promise against breast cancer. When mixed with antioxidants and applied topically, evening primrose helped decrease UV-induced skin damage.

### Ginger (*Zingiber officinale*)

Aside from being the flavorful heavyweight of Chinese cuisine, ginger plays an important role in green beauty. An extract from ginger root, rich in gingerol, protein, minerals, vitamin A, and niacin, has mild analgesic and antibacterial properties. Ginger is commonly used in creams and hair conditioners for its ability to promote circulation in skin. Ginger also smells fantastic!

### Goldenseal (*Hydrastis canadensis*)

This herb is rich in the natural antiseptic compound isoquinoline. When applied topically, an extract from the whole herb has anti-inflammatory and antimicrobial properties, which make this herb useful in astringents and topical antiseptics for acne-prone skin.

### Gotu Kola (*Centella asiatica*)

An extract of this plant has been traditionally used to stimulate the healing of ulcers and skin injuries, and to strengthen skin capillaries. Calcium, iron, selenium, magnesium, betulic acid, beta-carotene, terpenes, saponins, and the antioxidant quercetin in gotu kola help maintain healthy connective tissue development, speed up the healing process, and improve the barrier functions of the top skin layer. Gotu kola is also a mild antiseptic and anti-inflammatory agent. All of the above more than justifies the use of *Centella asiatica* extract in natural skin care preparations.

  **the green beauty guide**

## Grape (*Vitis vinifera*)

This is one of the strongest players in green beauty formulations. The skin of muscadine and red grapes is exceptionally rich in the antioxidant resveratrol, which has anticancer, antiviral, neuroprotective, antiaging, anti-inflammatory, and life-prolonging effects. Fresh grape skin contains about 50 to 100 micrograms of resveratrol per gram! It has been found that resveratrol may kill cancer cells and acts as a cancer preventive agent (Marel et al. 2008). Other antioxidants contained in grape skin include ellagic acid, myricetin, quercetin, and kaempferol, all with excellent, health-benefiting track records. Proanthocyanidins found in grape skin help preserve collagen and elastin in skin, reduce facial swelling after cosmetic surgery, and can protect from many types of cancer, including skin cancer, according to recent research (Nandakumar 2008; Katiyar 2008). Resveratrol and proanthocyanidins are available in pure form and can be added to homemade cosmetic preparations. I always add grape proanthocyanidins to my sunscreens. They may give the lotion a purple tint, so use it sparingly. Grape seed oil and crushed grape seed are used in cosmetics, too, as an emollient and an exfoliant, respectively.

## Grapefruit

This juicy fruit is rich in sulfur-containing terpene, the antioxidant flavonoid naringin, and a coumarin called begamottin, which is also found in bergamot. This substance is blamed for the negative interaction of grapefruit juice with some drugs. The pink fruit contains lycopene, a potent antioxidant. Grapefruit seed extract is commonly used as a natural preservative. But here's a word of caution: a cohort study conducted by scientists at the University of Southern California in Los Angeles shows that eating grapefruit every day may increase the risk of developing breast cancer by almost a third. Scientists suggest that the fruit boosts the levels of estrogen, which in turn increases the risk of breast cancer among postmenopausal women (Monroe et al. 2007). Until science knows more, it may be wise to refrain from frequent consumption of grapefruit in any form.

## Green Tea (*Camellia sinensis*)

Infusions or extracts of green tea leaves have a plethora of health benefits. Green tea is rich in antioxidants, particularly polyphenols and catechins, which have a wide array of anti-inflammatory, adaptogenic, anticarcinogenic, and antiseptic properties. L-Theanine, a chemical found in green tea, is known to soothe and calm the skin, while caffeine and epigallocatechin gallate, the most abundant catechin in green tea, helps protect the skin from UV radiation-induced damage and skin cancer formation by stimulating the production of interleukins that repair the skin's DNA. In studies, when green tea was ingested and applied topically, scientists noticed that it also helped diminish damage to the immune system by UV radiation (Katiyar et al. 2007; Yusuf et al. 2007; Schwarz et al. 2008).

Pure green tea extract is available in many health food stores, and green tea is a key component in such upscale skin care brands as Teamine and RéVive, but you can prepare your own potent antioxidant green tea blends by adding pure green tea extract to your sunscreens and moisturizers. It blends well with most toners, moisturizers, and sunscreens, and has reportedly been effective for acne and rosacea. This is my skin active of choice that I usually add to my body sunscreens during the summer.

## Honey

Whenever I have a sudden onset of skin rash or a dry patch on my lips, I reach for my tube of pure manuka honey from New Zealand. It makes a wonderful healing facial mask that you can apply as is or mix with your favorite cream to reduce the gluey factor. If you have any sores or chapped patches on your lips, leave on a layer of honey overnight and wake up to the softest, smoothest lips. Since ancient times, honey has been used successfully for treatment of infected wounds because of its antibacterial activity, but modern science has found numerous exciting uses for this golden gift of nature. Honey has proven effective against antibiotic-resistant strains of bacteria and fungi. "Antibiotic-susceptible and -resistant isolates of *Staphylococcus aureus, Staphylococcus epidermidis, Enterococcus faecium, Escherichia coli, Pseudomonas aeruginosa, Enterobacter cloacae,* and *Klebsiella oxytoca* were killed within 24 hours by honey," say scientists from the University of Amsterdam, who used honey to treat skin infections (Kwakman et al. 2008). Honey is successfully used as a wound dressing in many hospitals, including neonatal units (Bell 2007), and even in patients with diabetes (Lotfy et al. 2006).

Honey heals thanks to its ability to stimulate cytokine production when inflammation is present, and kills bacteria due to the low presence of naturally occurring hydrogen peroxide. However, to work its magic (and to minimize the risk of bee pollen allergy), honey has to be medical grade, or produced under controlled conditions, without any added flavorings that local honeys are often praised for. Keep in mind that honey is a strong allergen, and before you use it in pure form or in your DIY preparations, perform a patch test first.

## Idebenone

This synthetic analogue of coenzyme Q10 is currently the most potent antioxidant known to science. It has powerful antiaging effects, as well as anti-inflammatory and photoprotective properties. Idebenone can prevent damage to the skin's immune system by ultraviolet radiation and assist in reversing many other effects of lifelong oxidation. It also boosts cellular activity by improving the functioning of mitochondria, which are like cellular electric batteries. Yet, both coenzyme Q10 analogues, ubiquinone and idebenone, are less effective in preventing UV-related skin damage than vitamins C and E (McDaniel et al. 2005; Tournas et al. 2006).

Idebenone can make a highly effective addition to your DIY mixes. It will push your skin into high gear even at the lowest of concentrations, although keep in mind this is not a natural substance, but is an analogue, and it has more irritation potential. So start with less concentrated solutions. Add 1.5 grams to 5 ounces of base product for 1 percent concentration or to 10 ounces for 0.5 percent concentration and mix thoroughly. Make sure your base product is not acidic in any way. Pure idebenone is bright orange in color, so keep the concentration low to avoid staining your clothes and your bed linens.

## Jojoba (*Simmondsia chinensis*)

Jojoba seeds contain liquid wax, commonly called jojoba oil, which is chemically closest to the skin's sebum. Besides its emollient action, jojoba liquid wax has mild anti-inflammatory action, which can be very beneficial in treatment of acne and sunburns (Habashy et al. 2005). This odorless, colorless, and very stable substance is a great moisturizer and carrier oil for natural fragrances and massage oils. In beauty preparations, jojoba liquid wax also acts as a penetration enhancer. In natural hair care, jojoba wax makes a wonderful conditioner for straightened, dyed, or otherwise chemically damaged hair.

## Kinetin

This plant hormone promotes cell division. Kinetin, whose chemical name is N(6)-furfuryladenine, exists naturally in the DNA of almost all organisms, including human cells. Vigorously tested since the 1990s, kinetin is a popular cosmetic ingredient that has powerful antiaging effects in human skin cells and other body systems. Recent studies indicate that kinetin may have antitumor activity in animals, and kinetin as 0.1 percent lotion helps restore skin barrier function, which is important in the treatment of rosacea.

## Kojic Acid

This natural whitening substance is produced by the fermentation of malted rice with the Japanese fungus *Aspergillus oryzae*. Kojic acid is used in cosmetics to lighten skin since it inhibits melanin production. Kojic acid also has antibacterial and antifungal properties. Studies conducted in 2007 in Japan confirmed that kojic acid does not have tumor-promoting or genotoxic properties, as suspected earlier (Higa et al. 2007). However, please note that kojic acid is still not recommended for long-term use. There are many other natural and botanical extracts, such as licorice, niacinamide, yeast derivatives, and polyphenols, that can effectively lighten skin tone without potential toxic effects.

## Lavender (*Lavandula angustifolia*)

This ubiquitous plant is used in green cosmetics as an essential oil and flower infusion. Essential oil of lavender has antiseptic and anti-inflammatory properties. Lavender oil is traditionally used as an acne remedy, especially when diluted with rose water or witch hazel. An infusion of lavender is claimed to repel insects, as well as soothe and heal insect bites. In aromatherapy, lavender is used to calm and promote natural sleep. However, these wonderful qualities come with a price: studies in vitro have shown that lavender oil mimics estrogens in the body and has antiandrogenic activities. There has been a report that three teenage boys developed gynecomastia (breast tissue growth), which coincided with the topical application of products that contained lavender and tea tree oils (Henley et al. 2007). In another disturbing report from Japan, medical researchers from the School of Dentistry at Meikai University, Saitama, found that essential oils of lavender and rosemary enhanced free radical damage and decreased the stress hormone, cortisol, which protects the body from oxidative stress (Atsumi, Tonosaki et al. 2007). Until science knows more, it may be advisable to avoid using sunscreen products heavily scented with lavender and avoid aromatherapy with lavender oil during pregnancy and breast-feeding.

## L-Carnitine

This amino acid, commonly contained in energy drinks and weight-loss supplements, was recently found to promote hair growth. Scientists of the University of Hamburg have discovered that L-carnitine stimulates hair growth by increasing the energy supply to the hair matrix and can be used to treat alopecia and other forms of hair loss (Foitzik et al. 2007).

## Lemon (*Citrus limon*)

Lemon juice and lemon essential oils have many uses in natural beauty. Lemon juice is a natural astringent and may lighten skin when applied top-ically. Lemon oil, rich in terpenes, is a well-known antibacterial and insect-repelling agent. It is frequently used in aluminum-free deodorants for its ability to inhibit the growth of odor-causing bacteria. Lemon juice can work as a mild hair bleach that yields very natural results: to lighten your hair with sun-bleached highlights, simply spread some lemon juice over your dry hair in streaks before you step outside during summertime. Lemon juice has a certain stickiness in it, so you can easily use it as a natural, nutri-tious hair gel. Don't use the hair bleaching with lemon as an excuse for baking under the midday sun: a mineral sunscreen is still a must!

## Licorice (*Glycyrrhiza glabra*)

No, I am not advising you to rub your face with those yummy gummy sweets. Licorice has much more to offer than pleasing our taste buds. Licorice root has been used in Europe since the ancient Greek era, and modern science offers new uses for this delicious plant extract. A new flavonoid isolated from licorice root, licochalcone A, is known to have anti-inflammatory and potentially anticarcinogenic effects on animals, while glycyrrhizin, the main chemical found in licorice, may offer protection from the damage induced by UVB radiation. Licorice gel has been traditionally used in herbal medicine for dermatitis, eczema, pruritus, and cysts. In green beauty, licorice is used as a skin-whitening agent and shows promise in the treatment of hyperpigmentation.

## Linoleic Acid

This omega-6 essential fatty acid influences skin physiology on a molecular level, improving eicosanoid production, membrane fluidity, and cell signaling. This polyunsaturated fatty acid is an excellent emollient and emulsifier that helps in the treatment of acne, psoriasis, and sun-damaged skin. Linoleic acid also speeds up wound healing. Recent studies demonstrated that this nonirritating acid is also a natural penetration enhancer and can be used in cosmetics instead of propylene glycol. Last, and certainly not least, linoleic acid can help you stay younger for longer. "Higher intakes of vitamin C and linoleic acid and lower intakes of fats and carbohydrates are associated with better skin-aging appearance," concluded British scientists as they performed research for Unilever in 2007. According to them, higher intake of linoleic acid, naturally found in flaxseeds, evening primrose, pumpkin and mustard seeds, wheatgerm, spirulina, and green leafy vegetables, may reduce dryness and atrophy of aging skin (Cosgrove et al. 2007).

## Lycopene

One of the most potent carotenoid antioxidants, bright red lycopene is found primarily in tomatoes, watermelon, papaya, and red bell peppers. Lycopene is the most powerful destroyer of singlet oxygen, which is produced during UV exposure and is the primary cause of skin aging. Lycopene offers 100 times better protection from singlet oxygen than vitamin E. Lycopene is sold in health food stores and online. You can add powdered lycopene to your skin care preparations, but beware: it can instantly turn any cream or lotion bright pink!

## Milk

Cow and goat milk are rich in saturated fat, protein, and calcium, as well as a host of vitamins. The green cosmetic industry uses whole milk as an emollient due to its high fat and protein content, and milk acid, also known as lactic acid, for its mild exfoliating properties. Yogurt, kefir, and sour cream make excellent, quick, and nourishing skin exfoliating masks.

## Myrrh *(Commiphora myrrha)*

The sap of myrrh is used frequently as an antiseptic in natural mouth-washes, gargles, and toothpastes for the prevention and treatment of gum disease. Myrrh is currently used in healing balms to treat abrasions and minor skin irritations, and it has proven effective as an ingredient of healing balms for chronic wounds, alongside honey (Lofty et al. 2006).

## N-Acetyl Glucosamine

A major component of hyaluronic acid, glucosamine is making news in natural cosmetics due to several beneficial effects on the skin. Glucosamine works as an anti-inflammatory substance that triggers synthesis of hyaluronic acid in skin, accelerates wound healing, improves skin hydration, and decreases wrinkles. It also safely lightens skin tone by inhibiting melanin production, which makes it a godsend for people with hyperpigmentation, age spots, and uneven melanin distribution.

## Olive (*Olea europaea*)

Olive leaf extract is rich in hydroxytyrosol, one of nature's most powerful antioxidants, which strengthens the skin's immune system and protects it from the oxidation effects of UV radiation and tobacco smoke. Plain olive oil is a traditional skin emollient, while squalene, which is derived from olive oil, is an excellent natural moisturizer that quickly penetrates the skin, does not leave a greasy film, and blends well with active ingredients.

## Orange (Sweet) (*Citrus sinensis*)

Petals of the orange blossom are used to prepare orange water, a natural skin refresher rich in vitamins and volatile oils that has mild antiseptic action. Orange essential oil is rich in flavonoids, rutin, beta-carotene, and aromatic terpene d-limonene, which is classified as toxic or very toxic in several countries. It's inadvisable to use pure orange oil in cosmetic products.

## Peppermint (*Mentha piperita*)

This aromatic herb is rich in manganese, vitamin C, and vitamin A, and contains trace amounts of iron, calcium, folate, potassium, tryptophan, magnesium, omega-3 fatty acids, riboflavin, and copper. Recent studies discovered antioxidants and free radical scavenging activities in peppermint leaf extract, while peppermint essential oil has been proven effective against the herpes simplex virus, even against acyclovir-resistant strains. Peppermint oil can be irritating, but toxicity reports found peppermint oil and extracts safe for use in cosmetics.

## Pomegranate (*Punica granatum*)

Antioxidant-rich pomegranate fruit is one of the newest kids on the antiaging block. Pomegranate bursts with anthocyanin and hydrolyzable tannin, which explains its cancer-prevention abilities. Studies have shown that pomegranate extract, both taken internally and applied topically, can greatly reduce photoaging and prevent formation of UV-induced skin cancer. Pomegranate seed oil, when used in a 5 percent concentration, also significantly decreased skin tumor incidence in animals, which makes it a very promising, safe, and effective natural agent against skin cancer. Pomegranate seed and fruit extract are used in many green beauty lines, particularly in Juice Beauty organic moisturizers, and you can add this valuable ingredient to your own lotions and potions.

## Propolis

Along with beeswax, bees use propolis to build their hives. In natural skin care, propolis is used to relieve skin inflammations, ulcers, superficial burns, and scalds. It has shown local antibiotic and antifungal properties, and there is some evidence that propolis may actively protect against caries and other forms of oral disease. Propolis is sold in most health food stores and can be applied topically or added to skin care preparations and mouthwashes. Propolis can also be used as a natural preservative in green beauty products.

## Protein Peptides

We know these power players as palmitoyl oligopeptide, palmitoyl pentapeptide, and palmitoyl tetrapeptide. Peptides—amino acids held together by peptide bonds and attached to palmitic or acetic acid—are hot talk in skin care. Two amino acids make a dipeptide, three a tripeptide, five a pentapeptide. Argireline is acetyl hexapeptide, comprising six amino acid molecules linked to acetic acid. They work to release wrinkles by inhibiting the release of neurotransmitters. The skin becomes stiff, as after a Botox injection. However, there are no independent clinical studies proving the safety of this ingredient. Matrixyl is palmitoyl pentapeptide that links five amino acid molecules. This synthetic peptide imitates the action of matrikines, small peptides formed when the dermis proteins are damaged and degraded. These cell messengers prompt the skin to start repairing itself and heal wounds, leading to increased synthesis of collagen and other skin molecules. Matrixyl is better researched for safety and effectiveness than other peptides: one study found that this molecule is effective in repairing skin photoaging, and more recent studies note that it helps thicken the skin, thus relieving wrinkles. No side effects have been reported, thus making Matrixyl a promising addition to your DIY antiaging preparations.

## Rose (*Rosa damascena, Rosa centifolia*)

This gorgeous flower is used in many green beauty preparations. Rose petals are steam-distilled to produce essential rose oil. The hydrosol portion of distillate is used to make exquisite rose water, a highly emollient and soothing fluid. Essential rose oil, also known as attar of rose and rose absolute, contains more than 300 compounds, among them citronellol, geraniol, linalool, farnesol, pinenes, terpinene, limonene, and many others. In recent studies, citronellol has demonstrated antioxidant and antimicrobial activity, probably due to the presence of antioxidant quercetin, discovered in rose petals by German scientists in 2006. This makes rose oil and rose water valuable ingredients in any green beauty preparation.

## Saffron (*Crocus sativus*)

Although traditional herbal medicine used saffron for centuries, modern medical science only recently discovered cancer-suppressing, mutation-preventing, and antioxidant-like properties in this ancient spice. Medical studies have demonstrated that crocin, the main ingredient of saffron extract, may prevent the development of chemically induced skin cancer.

## Sage (*Salvia officinalis*)

Common sage is used in infusions that make great deodorants and mouthwashes with a soothing and mildly antiseptic effect. However, sage is known to inhibit milk production and therefore is not recommended for use during breast-feeding.

## Sea Buckthorn (*Hippophae rhamnoides*)

This bright orange berry is a rich source of unsaturated fatty acids, phytosterols, carotenoids, and flavonoids, and it is filled to the brim with the powerful antioxidant proanthocyanidin, which can protect skin from different types of free radical attacks, including ionizing radiation. Thanks to its antioxidant and antimicrobial effects, sea buckthorn extract can serve as a natural preservative in green cosmetic products.

## Sea Salt

Sea salt usually has a higher mineral content than table salt. It is commonly used in bath preparations, physical exfoliants, and hair-styling products for its ability to temporarily evict water from hair shafts, making hair stiff and curly.

## Shea Butter

This natural butter, extracted from shea nuts (*Butyrospermum parkii*), is an exceptionally good moisturizer and emollient with anti-inflammatory properties. Shea butter is great on its own and truly shines when used in preparations for fading scars, and alleviating eczema, burns, rashes, acne, stretch marks, and even psoriasis. Shea butter provides natural UV protection of approximately SPF6, but you should never rely on shea butter alone for sun protection! You can buy pure shea butter and use it as a face and body cleanser and moisturizer, or you can mix it with active natural ingredients to suit your needs.

## Silver

Colloidal silver is a water suspension of ionic silver. Since medieval times, silver has been used as a bactericidal agent that helps heal skin abrasions and burns. Colloidal silver has been approved by the Environmental Protection Agency for disinfection purposes in hospitals. Colloidal silver sprays are commonly used to treat burns and throat infections. In natural cosmetics, colloidal silver makes a safe and nonirritating preservative with an added anti-inflammatory bonus.

## Soy (*Glycine Soja*)

Soy is one of the mainstays of green beauty, and it's the only basic ingredient that should always be certified organic or GMO-free if you find it in an ingredients list. Soybean oil is made of linolenic, linoleic, oleic, stearic, and palmitic acids, which make it a great emollient, and soybean protein isolate can nourish and moisturize skin and hair. Yet, soy is rich in isoflavones, called genistein and daidzein, which are potent phytoestrogens. Women with current or past breast cancer, as well as those with a family history of breast cancer, should be aware of the risks of potential tumor growth when using soy-rich cosmetic products for a prolonged period. At the same time, women in Japan and China, where soy is a dietary staple, have significantly less severe menopausal symptoms and enter menopause at a later age. Soy may have a protective effect on the brain and cardiovascular systems. However, until science knows more about what effect phytoestrogens have on humans, I recommend refraining from using cosmetic preparations containing high concentrations of soy isoflavones.

## Witch Hazel (*Hamamelis virginiana*)

An extract from the bark and leaves of this plant is highly astringent and antiseptic. Witch hazel is traditionally used for the treatment of sores, bruises, swelling, hemorrhoids, and postpartum tears of the perineum. In cosmetics, witch hazel extract is commonly used in cleansers and toners for acne-prone skin, in aftershaves, and in topical treatments for insect bites. To prepare your own witch hazel toners, look for steam distillates of witch hazel, also called hydrosols or hydrolats, rather than conventional witch hazel, which contains alcohol.

# Take Your Vitamins

We all know that taking vitamins orally provides important nutritional benefits. Hundreds of well-designed studies validate the power of vitamins: they make us healthier by boosting our immune systems, control free radicals, and even protect against cancer and heart disease. There are so many health benefits for taking vitamins, especially if you opt for more expensive natural vitamins that contain more bioavailable substances than conventional synthetic pills.

There's a common notion that rubbing vitamins into the top skin layer of cells will not improve your skin in any way because (1) only low concentrations are used in cosmetic products; (2) the stability of most vitamins decreases as soon as they are exposed to the air and light; and (3) the form of the vitamin molecule (an ester or a mixture of isomers) may not be absorbed or metabolized effectively by the skin. However, recent scientific findings prove that vitamins A, C, D, E, and K are indeed very effectively absorbed by the skin and deliver a host of benefits for healthy skin, hair, and nails.

## Vitamin A *(beta-carotene, retinol)*

Vitamin A exists in many forms: as an alcohol (retinol), an aldehyde (retinal), or an acid (retinoic acid). Provitamins, or natural precursors to vitamin A, include alpha-carotene, beta-carotene, and beta-cryptoxanthin. In cosmetics, vitamin A as a retinol and beta-carotene is used to help repair and reverse sun damage and to inhibit collagen and elastin breakdown. Some other benefits of beta-carotene include its ability to combat and prevent skin disorders, such as acne, psoriasis, and eczema. Beta-carotene is effective as a protective measure against melasma because it changes the chemical mechanism of skin pigment cell production.

Vitamin A is available as retinol, retinyl palmitate, retinyl acetate, or beta-carotene packed in softgels and is sold in health food stores and online. Retinol is most effective but most irritating, while beta-carotene, retinyl acetate, and retinyl palmitate are better tolerated by sensitive skin. Vitamin A mixes well with most creams and lotions in the following proportion: 10,000 IU per ounce of base product. Do not exceed the recommended dosage. Since beta-carotene is fat-soluble, it accumulates in the fat tissues in our body, and excessive vitamin A intake (more than 10,000 IU a day) can lead to dangerous side effects.

## Vitamin B3 (*niacin, or nicotinic acid*)

Deficiency in vitamins of the B group can result in many beauty woes, not to mention other serious consequences. Lack of vitamin B1 may lead to edema (swelling of bodily tissues); vitamin B2 (riboflavin) deficiency causes chapped lips, seborrheic dermatitis, and high sensitivity to sunlight; not getting enough vitamin B3 (niacin) and vitamin B6 (pyridoxine) may cause dermatitis; while deficiency in vitamin B5 (pantothenic acid) can result in acne.

Among vitamins of the B group, only one has been proven effective when applied topically. Vitamin B3, or niacin (nicotinic acid), is a potent skin rejuvenator. A 2007 study in Tucson, Arizona, reported that when applied topically to photodamaged skin, niacin repaired the skin barrier by increasing the stratum corneum thickness by approximately 70 percent and decreased water loss through the skin by approximately 20 percent while increasing the rates of skin cell renewal (Jacobson et al. 2007). Earlier studies have proven that niacin can smooth out wrinkles, reduce inflammation in acne and rosacea, and even hold back the development of UV-induced skin cancers.

Niacin is used in cosmetics for its antiaging and skin-whitening properties. Niacinamide is a key ingredient in such upscale antiaging creams as Hylexin and Shiseido Future Solution. Niacin is often sold in pharmacies and health food stores, but it may contain fillers and anticaking agents. You can prepare your own niacinamide-rich skin cream by adding one teaspoon of pure niacinamide (sold online) to 4 ounces of cream or lotion.

## Vitamin C *(ascorbic acid)*

Of all the topical vitamins, ascorbic acid probably has the best track record. Vitamin C in its various forms protects us from free radicals that form during sun and pollution exposure. Ascorbic acid is also necessary to synthesize collagen, and it is known to inhibit the synthesis of the skin pigment melanin, probably by preventing skin cell damage before melanin synthesis can be triggered by UV exposure. (You will learn more about the sun's effects on skin in Chapter 10, "Green Sun Protection.")

Numerous studies have demonstrated that ascorbic acid, especially in combination with vitamin E, can even repair past damage to your skin by age and sun. Ascorbic acid and its derivatives promote wound healing and reduce inflammation and skin swelling. The latest findings regarding vitamin C suggest that it can be a very effective skin lightener, similar to hydroquinone, but without the side effects. Another important quality of vitamin C is its ability to stabilize sunscreen ingredients, making sun-protective formulations even more effective.

To use vitamin C in your DIY preparations, look for L-ascorbic acid, not calcium ascorbate. You can buy pure ascorbic acid online or use powdered vitamin C, such as Philosophy Hope and a Prayer. The most effective topical form of vitamin C is anhydrous, or waterless. During a study on human skin, scientists found that vitamin C has the greatest healing potential when applied to damaged skin in dry form (Heber et al. 2006). But we all know that vitamin C stings like crazy. Pour a drop of lemon juice on a fresh wound and see what happens! For this reason, you can dissolve vitamin C in pure vegetable glycerin, glycerin-rich organic personal lubricant, a pure dimethicone such as Monistat Chafing Relief Powder Gel, or a very oily cream like Weleda Skin Food in the following proportion: ½ teaspoon of vitamin C to ¼ cup of base product. Use the preparation quickly and watch out for a yellowish tint that signals vitamin C oxidation and loss of efficiency. Vitamin C serums can be irritating, so always perform a patch test before using. Nonirritating forms of vitamin C include tetrahexyldecyl ascorbate and magnesium ascorbyl phosphate, both available online.

A blend of vitamins C and E truly shines as a skin protector: these vitamins support each other and deliver a double whammy against free radicals (Burke 2007). Vitamin C blends really well in vitamin E–rich facial oil.

## Vitamin D

This important vitamin, which is synthesized in our skin during sun exposure, has been proven to reduce the risk of many autoimmune diseases, but topical use of vitamin D is still under investigation. Dermatologists at the University Hospital Leuven in Belgium found that topical vitamin D in the form of calcipotriol is helpful in psoriasis treatment (Segaert, Duvold 2006).

## Vitamin E

This is the most common vitamin used in skin care. Vitamin E in the forms of tocopherol and tocotrienol is a fat-soluble antioxidant found in our bodies. Since it's fat-soluble, it helps protect fatty components of cells from free radical damage that builds up over a lifetime of pollution, sun, and cigarette smoke exposure. This vitamin also offers a protective barrier for the skin when used topically. As a skin care ingredient, it helps heal skin wounds, nourish the skin, and prevent stretch marks. To reap the benefits of vitamin E, use the natural form of this vitamin, which contains both tocopherols and tocotrienols, even though it may cost more than the synthetic version. Vitamin E mixes well with most cleansers, creams, and lotions. One or two standard-size gelatin-packed softgels will make an excellent addition to your lotion or body oil, and you can add vitamin E to lip balms to heal your lips tortured by too much wind, frost, or sun. Just pinch a small hole in a softgel, squeeze out the oily substance, and blend with the base product in the following proportion: two 400 IU vitamin E softgels per ounce of lotion or oil. Do not increase the amount of vitamin E or it will leave a yellowish cast on the skin and stain your clothes and bed linens. Use up the product in one month because vitamin E becomes unstable when exposed to air. You can apply vitamin E oil or squeeze vitamin E from the capsule on your lips whenever you have a bout of dryness, some nasty sores, or plain chapped lips. Works like magic, but I prefer my manuka honey!

*chapter* **6**

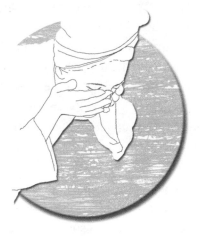

*green*
# cleaners

In previous chapters, you learned about the functioning of your skin, the dangers of synthetic skin care, and the principles of green beauty. Now it's time to address green beauty in detail and develop natural, pure beauty routines for your face, hair, and body.

A green skin care routine includes five steps: cleansing (face, hair, and body), exfoliating (face and body), toning (face and hair), moisturizing (face and body), and protection from the elements (face, body, optionally hair). Each step plays its own important role. Skip one, and the results will be far less impressive. If time is running low, you can use multitasking products that will take you through two steps in one simple move.

So what is green cleansing? As we wash our face, we get rid of daily grime, makeup, dead skin cells, and oxidized sebum using a gentle cleansing agent formulated without sulfate detergents, penetration enhancers, harsh acids, synthetic preservatives, or synthetic fragrances. Such agents can be liquid and foaming or milky and nonfoaming, depending on your skin's needs.

I think that most people, especially women, tend to overdo it when it comes to facial cleansing. For some reason, we believe that if we rub our skin really hard, it will be cleaner and automatically healthier. However, if you revisit Chapter 1, you will recall that human skin, thanks to sebum, is perfectly able to cleanse itself. If it wasn't for makeup, environmental toxins, and city dust and grime, you could keep your skin clean with a cotton ball and some warm water.

Unfortunately, not all of us are blessed with the opportunity to spend lazy days in a seaside cottage on a remote beach. City life is ruthless to our skin, and a good cleanser is essential for a clear, healthy complexion. Do we really need a heavy-duty cleanser to make sure that our skin is truly, deeply clean? Not at all! All we need is to get rid of the dirt that accumulates on our face during the day. Remember, our faces are the most exposed yet fragile part of our bodies. If the weather is harsh, you can wear gloves or mittens to cover your hands, and you can wrap a scarf around your neck, but you cannot hide your face under a knitted mask—unless you plan on robbing a bank.

Every beauty book and skin care–related magazine article declares that neither dirt nor chocolate can contribute to skin problems. Well, it depends on what we call dirt. Dirt does not necessarily mean smudges of mud or streaks of dust on a sweaty face. Most often, dirt on our faces consists of airborne particles of soot, smoke, dust, dried sweat, and residue from makeup, sunscreens, and skin care. These fine particles pile on the surface of your skin, clogging up the pores and forming a sticky nonbreathable film on top of your skin. As a result, congestion forms deep under the skin's surface, resulting in visible blackheads, an uneven, dull complexion, allergies, and acne. The solution: you must eliminate the dirt without overcleansing, which may cause skin irritation. In this chapter, I will describe the correct way to double-cleanse your skin using products and techniques designed specifically for each skin's needs.

There's no such thing as one "perfect" skin type.

## Forget About Skin Typing

Combination oily, dehydrated sensitive with oily T-zone, mature yet acne-prone—the cosmetic industry comes up with endless variations on skin typing. Some cosmetic brands have developed complex facial "mapping" techniques that put a label on each square inch of our face and assign a separate product to tackle every zone, no matter how small it is. Other companies would use computers and complex questionnaires, not to mention well-versed salespeople who seem to decipher your unique skin needs at first glance. The skin care industry tries to convince us of two things: (1) there is one ideal skin type, and that's a "normal" skin: flawless, dewy, wrinkle-free, like the one you had when you were six years old; and (2) none of us have it. Of course, the sales pitch continues, we can correct our imperfect skin if we buy the right products.

Let's take a minute to challenge this concept. There's no such thing as one "perfect" skin type. Our skin undergoes constant changes. It can be drier at the end of the day, yet shine like a disco ball by midday, and all this is the perfectly normal way our skin functions. When we are at peak condition, our endocrine glands command sebum glands to produce more oil, but as we are getting tired and ready to go to sleep, our body systems, including the sebum glands, slow down and take a break. As a result, it's almost impossible to define our skin type once and for all. Here are the main reasons you should stop being guided by a skin type and start choosing cosmetic products based on your skin's unique needs.

**The climate and environment we live in have a great impact on our skin.** If you live in Toronto with its breathtaking winter winds and humid, hot summers, you will have different skin care concerns than a person living in the hot, dry air of Los Angeles, even if you are both labeled as combination-dry skin types.

**Women tend to overachieve when it comes to skin care.** We think that if we use a cupful of cleanser, followed by another cupful of a toner, and then cover our face with a thick layer of cream, we will stay young forever. As a result, we use too many cleansers, toners, scrubs, chemical exfoliants, and acidic "rejuvenation" serums. Our skin is overloaded with various chemicals that are busy interacting with each other rather than keeping our skin youthful and clear. Strong chemicals or concentrated essential oils can trigger allergies, while heavy moisturizers can aggravate breakouts. Your current skin care routine can create more problems than it's trying to solve.

**Gender matters in skin care, too.** Men's skin is thicker, more rigid, and less fragile. Thanks to a different hormonal constitution, men's skin is less prone to premature aging but can develop acne more easily. Also, the oily skin of a woman who uses ten products every morning will be dramatically different from the oily skin of her partner who uses two products: a shaving gel and an aftershave lotion.

**Health problems, such as allergies, digestive problems, thyroid disorders, and polycystic ovary syndrome greatly influence the skin's condition.** Hormonal fluctuations during the monthly cycle can make a woman's skin drip oil one day and feel taut and dry the next.

**Identifying your skin type is a very subjective issue.** Most women think they have oily or combination-oily skin just because their face develops a bit of a shine by the end of the day. We get one blemish and we instantly label our skin as acne-prone. We notice a tiny wrinkle at the corner of the eye, and we rush to buy the newest, most expensive antiaging serum for dry, mature skin types.

**Skin problems take time to reach the surface, so the skin that you see in the mirror today won't be the same tomorrow.** Signs of sun damage may not become visible until you are forty, yet sun protection is vital for everyone. Dry skin doesn't happen overnight: it takes weeks if not months of skipping moisturizers, worrying too much, smoking, tanning, and drinking more bubbly than water. Acne blemishes also need weeks to reach the skin's surface. It takes consistent, diligent efforts to handle skin dryness and acne, and treating only what you can see (dry patches, tightness, flakiness, pimples) worsens your skin's condition. What you see on your skin's surface should not dictate what kind of cosmetic products you need. Always look at the bigger picture.

**Some "experts" will determine your skin type based on your age.** This is according to the theory that most young women have oily or combination oily skin; most women in their thirties are combination or combination-dry; and all women over forty are in the dry skin category. While our skin indeed changes with age, "older" or "younger" skin works the same way. Women over fifty can suffer from acne and oily skin, and twenty-somethings can have dry, dehydrated skin at risk for premature aging. However, all women with mature skin are prescribed creamy cleansers and emollient, heavy moisturizers, while all women under thirty are being aggressively sold harsh liquid cleansers, alcohol-based toners, and lightweight, "shine-controlling" moisturizers. All women, no matter how old they are, need gentle, nonirritating products formulated with as few chemical ingredients as possible.

**Skin typing serves as a powerful marketing tool.** Instead of helping women choose products that help solve their skin problems, cosmetic marketers label products based on traditional skin types. Salespeople can start their endless song about how you're not using the right product for your skin type, which creates problems and can actually destroy your skin. The moment we learn that our skin is anything but normal, we open our wallets and buy whatever is sold to us so our skin will be back to normal again. In fact, using products that are "wrong for your skin type" cannot destroy your skin. Your skin can be damaged by careless tanning, using synthetic chemical skin care, and smoking, but not by using a creamy cleanser if your skin is "combination oily."

In fact, *all of us have combination skin*. The middle section, or T-zone (the T-shaped area around the nose, forehead, and chin) will usually seem shiny by midday. It will feel drier in the evening and oilier in the morning. It will become sensitive in the winter and acne-prone, with a few blackheads, in the summer; but it can become fragile and dehydrated if we spend too much time in the sun without sunscreen.

Most of us have all four skin types at the same time: oily in the T-zone, combination to normal on cheeks, dry at the neck and around the mouth, and sensitive around the eyes.

There's little use in choosing skin products based on your skin type, simply because our skin is much too complicated to be labeled by only one of four types. If you choose a cleanser based on your skin type, you can end up using a product that is too harsh or too mild. For example, if a cosmetic salesperson looks at your midday skin and tells you that you have some blackheads and an oily T-zone, she'll sell you a whole routine for oily skin that will include a drying bar soap, a harsh alcohol-based toner, and a salicylic acid–based moisturizer "to clear blackheads." Instead of normally functioning combination skin, you create an oily, sensitive, and easily irritated skin that develops new pimples daily.

When you choose cosmetic products based on your skin type, you assume that once you've been told you have oily or dry skin, it's going to stay that way forever. That is not going to happen. Your skin is a living organ with a complex life. Climate, hormonal fluctuations, stress, lack of sleep, and certain medications can instantly change your skin type, making it oilier or drier. A perfectly good product can become plain wrong for you the very moment the hormonal roller coaster hits its peak or you have had a tough day in the office.

Instead of picking cosmetic products based on the skin typing theory, I suggest that you tune in to your skin's own voice and focus on your skin's needs. This way, you will be able to choose ingredients and textures that are able to satisfy these needs. An effective skin care routine should be based on the current condition of your skin, not on the assumption that it should "get back to normal" in a few days because you use a heavily advertised beauty product.

It couldn't be simpler: pay attention to what's going on with your skin today and adjust your skin care routine accordingly. Whenever your skin feels different, the cosmetic industry suggests that you need to spend a fortune on an entire new set of cleansers, toners, and moisturizers, but you can get away with much more subtle yet effective changes. If your skin feels dry, wash it as usual, but add a drop or two of facial oil underneath your usual moisturizer. If your skin feels oily, don't try to cleanse it excessively or soak up the oil with a new drying, alcohol-based toner or moisturizer. Just carry around blotting papers and use them frequently. In the evening, apply a clay-based mask to absorb excess oil and debris from pores, drink a cup of soothing tea, and use a lightweight serum instead of your nighttime moisturizer.

If your skin suddenly starts behaving oddly, it may be that it is reacting to a new product or, sadly, developed an allergy to something you've been using for quite a while. Carefully reevaluate your skin care routine, checking for possible irritants; pare down your morning and evening skin care regimen; and use soothing baby care products until the condition improves. This way, you will only need a few additional products: a pack of blotting papers and a clay mask for oilier days, a soothing and hydrating serum for sensitive days, and a lightweight, possibly homemade facial oil blend for days when your skin feels dry and tight. Spend less, waste less—this is one of the main principles of green beauty.

## Green Cleansing Essentials

For some people, the condition of their skin starts improving once they master the art of cleansing. Surprisingly, this is very simple. Here are essential tips for getting a good facial cleansing.

### Pick the Green Product

And we aren't talking color here. There are many great natural and organic cleansers available, from traditional foaming gels suitable for heavy makeup users to soothing cleansing milks and waters that do not lather and are great for those makeup-free days. There are newer types of cleansers such as self-foaming cloths and pillows that are both convenient and very effective. For a double-cleansing technique that leaves skin truly clean, use lightweight cleansing oils. They are becoming a very hot trend.

Your skin condition is the key to choosing the right texture of cleanser. You should avoid abrasive scrubs with scrubbing particles if you have any kind of skin irritation. Pimples, sunburns, and rashes should not be scrubbed because tiny particles break the protective cell layer and increase inflammation.

If your skin is dry, keep away from cleansing creams that do not require rinsing because they will block the pores and leave an impermeable film on the surface of your skin. Your skin will retain more moisture but won't absorb any beneficial ingredients from moisturizers and serums you may use after cleansing.

## Use the Right Tools

Ideally, you should use only the fingertips for facial cleansing. Do not use any kind of sponges, Buf-Pufs, or abrasive pads on irritated skin for the same reason you shouldn't use scrubs. During a double-cleansing, a clean muslin cloth is very handy for rinsing off the oily cleanser after the first step. Cotton balls can leave behind annoying fibers that can get into your eyes and make life miserable. After rinsing your face with tepid water, pat it dry with a clean towel. All this hardly takes a second but makes a lot of difference to your skin.

## Cleanse Twice a Day

No matter if you use layers of makeup or your cosmetic bag contains just an odd jar of lip balm, make a habit of washing your face once in the morning and once in the evening. Wash or at least wipe your face after any vigorous activity that makes you perspire, like exercise.

The morning cleansing should be gentle. Work the cleanser of your choice in circular motions, starting with your forehead and moving down to your cheeks and nose. Work the nose area well. Don't forget to wash your chin, throat, and the jawline area, especially under your ears. If you are using a medicated cleanser, for example, with salicylic or glycolic acid, leave it on for only a few minutes before rinsing.

You should double-cleanse your face in the evening. In general, the evening cleansing is more important than washing your face in the morning (which doesn't mean you can skip the morning wash!). Make it a new habit to double-cleanse in the evening. It takes slightly longer than a basic rub-rub-rub, splash-splash, but the results are nothing short of remarkable.

**Green Tip**

Exfoliating cleansers are useful when you have relatively clear skin, especially if you spend a lot of time in a room with central air-conditioning or during the summer since dry air speeds up the cell-shedding rate.

**the green beauty guide**

# How to Double-Cleanse

Double-cleansing is making news, although this technique is nothing new. Some sources claim that the double-cleansing method originated in European spas, while others argue that facial cleansing oil has been a staple of Asian skin care rituals for a very long time. No matter where it comes from, double-cleansing can make a whole world of difference, if correctly used and adjusted to your skin's needs and its current condition.

During the first step, use an oil-based cleanser to get rid of the surface dirt, which, as we already know, consists of airborne particles, dust, makeup, sebum, dried sweat, dead bacteria, and residue from moisturizers and sunscreens. The higher the content of oil, the better the cleansing power. All you need is to massage the cleansing oil onto your dry face with dry fingertips to dissolve the makeup gently. Some cleansing oils will stick to your face and be hard to wash off. To speed things up, use a soft muslin cloth, available from many health stores. Eve Lom was the first cosmetic manufacturer to sell her cleansing balm complete with muslin cloths.

Contrary to popular belief, oily cleansers will not aggravate acne or cause new outbreaks because they are much gentler to the skin than conventional cleansers with sulfate-based surfactants. When stripped of the skin's own sebum and further irritated by antibacterial agents and penetration enhancers found in synthetic cleansers, some skin may experience dryness, and to compensate for this dryness, your skin will secrete more sebum. Some people may experience whiteheads a few days after they start using the cleansing oil. This happens when you use a second cleanser to complete the double-cleansing ritual or when you do not remove the first cleanser properly.

**Green Tip**

Cleansing creams may feel oilier to the touch, because of the low emulsifier content, but they are much safer on sensitive and acne-prone skin.

As I mastered the art of double-cleansing, I found that many good cleansing oils and creams do not effectively tackle the task of removing mineral makeup, which is not oil-based. They want to get hold of oil, but there isn't any. If you are, like me, a diligent user of mineral makeup, you are far better off with a plain bar soap cleanser.

Bar soap regularly gets a bad rap from cosmetic experts. They claim that solid soaps often contain pore-clogging fats and harsh surfactants that can wreak havoc on human skin. While this is true about conventional animal tallow–based bar soaps, traditional olive and coconut oil soaps are not damaging to skin. They contain natural ingredients, such as saponified olive, coconut, jojoba, or hemp oil, and none of these is pore-clogging or sensitizing. I especially like the naturally scented French-milled olive soaps that I purchase online from a small factory in Provence. Another indulgence is Santa Maria Novella soaps, cooked according to ancient techniques. I also like the feeling when blackheads and tiny bumps of congested pores are melting under my fingertips as I massage the lightweight foam into my skin. Call it conditioning, call it Spartan upbringing, but I have it embedded deep in my mind that only soap can bring true cleanliness.

As for pH, the issue is more complicated. You have probably heard that good cleansers won't alter the skin's natural alkaline balance, or pH. The pH of a substance is a measure of its acid or alkaline content. Science ranks pH on a scale of 0–14, with pH 7, the natural acidity of water, being neutral. The further below 7 a pH value is, the more acidic the substance; the higher above 7, the more alkaline.

Our skin is naturally acidic. The pH of healthy skin is 5.5. This level of acidity helps ward off certain microorganisms from the skin's surface. Opponents of soap used to say that soaps, which are very alkaline (the opposite of acidic), remove too much natural fatty acid from sebum covering the skin's surface, thus leaving it tight, dry, and vulnerable to bacterial attacks. However, research dating back to the 1980s says that our skin has excellent self-protecting capacities that can neutralize even the most alkaline substances in soaps, but not sulfates and other synthetic chemicals that make up the bulk of those fragrant bars that we traditionally associate with bar soaps. At the same time, plant-based soaps formulated without sulfates are proven safe for the most intolerant skins. This is why it's very important to check the quality of the ingredients in the cleanser you plan to buy or prepare yourself: natural ingredients with their naturally balanced pH levels will give your skin all the protection it needs.

When you have melted the dirt and makeup using oil or soap, rinse your face and apply the second cleanser. This time you purify your skin, not remove makeup. If you were using oil, you should now use a gentle foaming cleanser to remove the oil residue. If you were using soap, choose a soft, milky, nonfoaming cleanser to remove soap residue and soften your skin. The second cleanser may contain additional benefits, such as oil-absorbing clay, herbal astringents, soothing infusions, or exfoliating particles that will cleanse your pores and deliver a treatment of your choice deep down where it's needed. Work your cleanser in a circular motion for no less than one minute and rinse thoroughly with lukewarm tap water. Finish with a cool rinse with tap, filtered, or better yet, mineral water with essential magnesium, such as Volvic, Vichy, or Evian.

After you're done cleansing, gently pat your face with a facial towel. Don't use your regular bath towel. Don't rub, either—this may cause unnecessary pressure and increase irritation. Be as gentle as possible.

Most people with acne think that frequent and vigorous cleansing with abrasive or antibacterial washes will reduce the oiliness and keep skin clear and healthy. However, no scientific evidence proves that the lack of washing is associated with skin problems or that frequent washing improves the condition of skin. Instead, intense cleansing and scrubbing can worsen the inflammation in acne breakouts, and synthetic antibacterial agents such as Triclosan and chlorhexidine do not affect acne bacteria.

## Green Cleansing in Detail

Single- or double-cleansing, I simply love washing my face! I believe that facial cleansing is the most underestimated step of a skin care routine. In Chapter 2, we talked about various synthetic chemicals used in beauty products. Many of these chemicals may be or are already proven to be toxic to your skin, and by removing these chemicals from their products, cosmetic manufacturers are reluctantly acknowledging the fact that they were doing something wrong. We already know that many conventional skin care products contain such chemicals despite the factual evidence arguing against their use. However, I still believe that cleansers, even when made entirely of synthetic chemicals, can only do relatively minor damage compared to toxic sunscreens or foundations.

How do we use cleansing gels and milks? We apply them, briskly rub our faces, snort and spit the obnoxious foam, and quickly rinse it off in less than a minute. A cleanser's penetration may be improved by added acids (lactic, ascorbic, or salicylic), warming actions ("self-heating" masks and gel cleansers are becoming popular), or exfoliating particles. Some cleansers employ all three big guns in order to achieve prime cleanliness. Unfortunately, not all synthetic cleansers deliver remarkable results, or any results to justify the use of toxic and potentially carcinogenic substances. More often than not, they are made of ingredients that are not physically capable of thoroughly cleansing our skin. Most nonfoaming milky cleansers, labeled as cleansing lotions, milks, and creams, are made of water, mineral oil, beeswax, stearic acid (a highly comedogenic substance made of animal tallow), synthetic wax ozokerite, and glycerin or propylene glycol, plus minuscule amounts of herbal extracts, vitamins, and fragrances. Foaming cleansers usually contain water, sodium laureth/lauryl sulfate, propylene glycol, triethanolamine, or the more "natural-sounding" cocamide DEA, MEA, or other ethylene amines. Most likely, these cleansing gels and lotions contain synthetic colors and dyes, all striving to please us. Would you use a cleanser that has a "clean water smell" and color that is "pure as ocean water" or an organic substance that smells like whipped tomato oatmeal and looks even worse?

All cleansers, whether biodynamic gels for your face or basic liquid soap for your floor, function in the same way. Nonfoaming cleansers (oils, milks, and lotions) contain a lot of fatty acids that lift oils in makeup, cosmetic products, and daily grime. Foaming cleansers contain surfactants, or substances that persuade oil and water to mix so they can be washed away together, grabbing all dirt and other solids along the way. The stronger the surfactant ingredient in a soap, the more residue it can remove.

Ideally, an effective facial cleanser washes the daily amount of dirt, oxidized sebum, and dead skin cells off your face while leaving behind enough of the skin's own oil (sebum) to naturally moisturize your skin. If a cleanser, used alone or in a double-cleansing ritual, leaves your skin feeling dry, it is removing too much of this natural moisturizer. If it leaves your skin feeling greasy and sticky, either it isn't removing enough oil or it contains heavy emollient and film-forming ingredients that clog pores.

What's different about green cleansers? With plant oils, it's simple: the most natural facial cleansing oils contain pure or organic cold-pressed oils and herbal extracts grown without toxic chemicals. Olive and sunflower oils are suitable for almost every skin, while avocado and wheat germ oil offer additional nutrition and protection. Sage, geranium, rosemary, and gentle citrus oils, such as mandarin or bergamot, can be added. Read the labels carefully and ask for a complete list of ingredients if you are unsure.

Organic plant soaps are based on saponified organic olive, jojoba, or hemp seed oils, and sometimes contain crushed fruit kernels, seaweed, and oatmeal for exfoliation. Foaming gels or milky cleansers are usually formulated with foaming agents derived from coconut oil, lauric acid, and plant sugars. Such ingredients include cocamidopropyl betaine, cocoglucoside, lauryl lysine or sarcosine, decyl glucoside, and glycolipids. Cleansers may also contain emulsifiers derived from coconut (cocoglycerides), vegetable glycerin (glyceryl linoleate), and a few plant-based antimicrobial agents to preserve the product, such as amino acids, sodium hydroxymethylglycinate, plant-derived potassium sorbate, citric acid, and grapefruit seed oil.

"Soap is my number-one beauty secret," says Debra Lynn Dadd. "I use lots of different handmade soaps to cleanse my face and my body. I can spend five or six dollars on a bar of soap. Some people would think this is outrageous! These are not perfumed soaps. They don't have anything toxic in them, just wholesome, pure ingredients like chocolate and fragrances like lavender—it's really good!" When traveling, Debra buys unusual, exotic soaps in bulk and savors them as some may savor wine or perfume.

We already know that choosing skin care products based on your skin type is very outdated. Instead, look for ingredients that are helpful for your current skin condition. If your skin feels congested and you have noticed tiny little bumps on the cheeks and blackheads around the T-zone area, you can benefit from soaps containing green and white clays. As a double-cleansing technique, use a soap or lightweight oil first, and follow it with a clay-based cleanser, which will absorb the remaining oil as well as dark matter clogging your pores.

If you have noticed a few breakouts, use olive oil or glycerin soap followed by liquid cleanser formulated with lavender, tea tree, geranium, or chamomile oil. In the morning, use a foaming cleanser with essential oils or baby soap formulated with calendula, chamomile, lavender, or geranium plant extracts.

If your skin feels dry, use oil-based balms and milks for double-cleansing or pure plant oils (avocado, grape seed, virgin olive oils)

### Green Tip

Avoid using peppermint, balm mint, wintergreen, or any other "minty" ingredients that smell and feel refreshing but can burn and sting. These extracts are better for deodorizing your feet than combatting pimples!

for a thorough massage before a second cleanse. For an additional skin cell removal use mild abrasives such as jojoba granules, finely grated seaweed, or oatmeal.

Sensitive skin needs an extremely gentle approach: you don't want to go to bed in your makeup, but you still hate all that itchiness and rashes. This is when baby body washes and baths come in handy. Use organic baby oil as a first step of your double-cleansing ritual and follow it with an organic baby body wash. In the morning, freshen up with a drop of foaming organic baby wash. There is no need to excruciate your skin in the morning.

Virtually all naturally based skin cleansers on the market work quite well, depending on your skin's condition, but don't expect expensive products to be more effective than those bought at the local health food store. What's most important is to find green products that you enjoy using and that suit your skin's current needs.

## The Green Product Guide: Cleansers

No matter how exciting the product looks and how green the label reads, choose products that are packed in pump bottles or at least in bottles with a narrow spout. Even the best formulation will quickly go rancid if packed in a jar that leaves the product exposed to less-than-clean fingers, humidity, and the warmth of your bathroom. The following are my recommended cleansing products, rated from one to three leaves, with three being my favorite.

### Cleansing Oils

**L'Occitane Apple Almond Cleansing Oil:** This lightweight blend of sweet almond and sunflower oils, as well as vitamin E, rosemary, and apple fruit extracts, comes in a convenient pump bottle. It washes off easily thanks to a few safe synthetic emollients.

**Trevarno Lavender & Geranium Cleansing Oil:** This rich, emollient, organic cleansing oil leaves just enough oily trace to double as a moisturizer for late nights when all you can do is take off makeup. The wide-necked bottle makes it hard to pour an exact amount of cleanser, so expect some oily mess.

**Laventine Olive Forte Water-Soluble Facial Cleansing Oil:** Rich and satiny, this organic olive oil blend in a handy pump bottle washes clean without leaving greasy residue.

## Bar Soaps

**DHC Mild Soap:** This transparent glycerin soap is enriched with olive oil extract and honey, so it's nondrying yet not pore-clogging. It's fragrance-free and preservative-free.

**Weleda Calendula Baby Soap:** This is a classic baby product formulated with saponified coconut and olive oils, as well as chamomile, rice, and calendula extracts. Fragranced with essential oils, but the scent is very natural and not strong at all.

**Dr. Bronner's Organic Bar Soap:** The range boasts dozens of fragrances, including classics such as lavender, rose, and tea tree oil, but the unscented Baby Mild version has just enough plant scent to entertain the senses. This olive and coconut-based moisturizing cult soap is enriched with vitamin E, plant glycerin, and jojoba oil.

## Foaming Cleansers

**Desert Essence Thoroughly Clean Face Wash with Organic Tea Tree Oil and Awapuhi** is a liquid castile (olive oil) soap enriched with ginger, tea tree oil, bladder wrack, and chamomile extracts. This gel cleanser contains a tiny amount of peppermint oil, which doesn't seem to increase its overall irritation potential.

**REN Mayblossom and Blue Cypress Facial Wash:** This gentle foaming cleanser is recommended for oily and sensitive skins, but I found it gentle enough for daily use on my normal skin thanks to sugar-based foaming agents, soothing extracts of lavender, mild exfoliating salicylic acid from willow bark, and amino acids from oat. However, the fragrance may be too strong for sensitive noses.

**Juice Beauty Cleansing Gel:** This is a soothing, therapeutic blend of plant extracts and certified organic juices, including sweet cherry, grape, and aloe, among others. It is very gentle and not too foaming, leaving behind a subtle herbal scent. It may not be suitable for irritated or damaged skin because of the high content of lemon juice and citrus oils.

**Suki Lemongrass Cleanser** is a gently foaming, creamy cleanser that uses fruit acids and sugar to exfoliate the skin with zero irritation. Formulated with organic sugar and rice flour in a handmade olive soap base, this cream cleanses thoroughly and is suitable for all skin conditions and all seasons. The fresh scent of lemongrass adds a finishing touch to this truly divine experience!

### Nonfoaming Cleansers

**Burt's Bees Lemon Poppy Seed Facial Cleanser** makes a wonderful second cleanser for colder months when skin can use some extra moisture. Thick and rich, this stearic acid–based cream cleanser contains citrus oils, as well as sugar enzymes and exfoliating crushed poppy seeds. It is made of natural but not certified organic ingredients. The cleanser is packed in a wide-neck jar that can turn the product rancid fairly quickly.

**Aubrey Organics Sea Buckthorn & Cucumber with Ester-C Facial Cleansing Cream** doubles the richness of the coconut creamy base with the cleansing abilities of castile soap, a combination that performs a really thorough cleansing. It contains a plethora of vitamins, beneficial herbs, and reasonably measured amounts of essential oils, but unlike vitamins in gel cleansers, the wholesome ingredients of cream cleansers are likely to remain on your skin longer. Also, this cleanser smells wonderful, which is not typical for this otherwise brilliant organic beauty brand.

**CARE Stella McCartney Gentle Cleansing Milk** is the only cleanser that can convert a foam junkie like me into a milk cleanser aficionado. Its satiny, lightweight texture dissolves impurities while doubling as a gentle moisturizer rich in organic lemon balm, apricot extract, carbohydrates, and vitamins E and A, packed in a sensible pump bottle that looks great in the bathroom.

## Making Your Own Cleansers

When you buy cosmetics, you rely on the expertise of many experienced chemists. When you create your own cosmetics from scratch, you may not achieve truly elegant results, but you will know exactly what goes into the product, and you can twist and tailor the formulation to suit your needs. Few of us have time to rely exclusively on home-made creations, but making your own products saves money and is definitely fun.

"A good cleanser will remove grime deposited on the skin, and that can be very important in the city, without removing the lipids that are vital to the role of the skin as a barrier from the environment," says Dr. Sivak of Skin Actives, who recommends blending a no-nonsense cleanser by combining sea kelp bioferment, some nice plant oils, and a small proportion of a mild surfactant, such as castile soap.

## GREEN BEAUTY SHOPPING LIST

When I do my weekly grocery shopping, I make sure to pick up some staples that can be used in homemade cosmetics:

- Avocado (for instant facial packs and masks)

- Baking soda (quick face and body scrub)

- Eggs (for masks)

- Epsom salts (for soothing baths)

- Chamomile tea (for baby diaper wash, toners, masks, and hair rinses)

- Lemons (for facial exfoliants, hair rinses)

- Cornmeal (great filling agent for masks and scrubs)

- Milk of magnesia (indispensable for acne, canker sores and irritated skin)

- Organic mayonnaise (a great moisturizer and foot mask)

- Milk (used in masks, baths, hair packs)

*continued*

- Oranges (to be used in a flavorful bath; peel can be used, too)

- Green tea (makes great toner, goes into masks, eye compresses, baby diaper wash)

- Honey (a luxurious mask on its own, can also be added to hair treatments). "I always tell people to spread honey all over their faces," says Suki Kramer of Suki Pure Skin Care. "Works for so many things!"

- Sour cream (a wonderfully nutritious exfoliant)

- Sea salt (makes a great body scrub)

- Extra virgin olive oil for hair masks and body scrubs, extra light olive oil for facial cleansers and moisturizers, both preferably organic

- Strawberries (useful for bleaching teeth and making a nourishing whitening mask)

- Oat bran and oatmeal (scrub, cleanser, bath bomb—you choose)

- Tomatoes (great for invigorating hair packs)

- Greek-style plain yogurt (makes a great mask; can be added to cleansing creams)

- Powdered milk (can go in many lotions, potions, and bath preparations)

- Sugar (choose organic brown sugar that can be used in facial scrubs, hair treatments, and hand exfoliants)

Try the following original recipes to discover how easy it is to create organic cosmetics in your own kitchen.

## Just Olive Cleansing Oil

2 ounces organic extra-virgin olive oil

1 ampoule of vitamin E (a blend of tocopherols and tocotrienols)

1 drop of essential oil of chamomile

*This is a green replica of conventional cleansing oil formulations, but when you make your own, you can skip all those mineral oils and paraben preservatives. This gentle cleanser will stay fresh for up to three months when stored in a pump bottle on a bathroom counter.*

1. Pour the oil into a stainless steel shaker; add the vitamin E and essential oil. (If you have acne outbreaks, replace the chamomile oil with one drop of tea tree or geranium oil.)
2. Shake vigorously for 30 seconds.
3. Pour the contents into a pump bottle. Thanks to the antioxidant action of vitamin E and chamomile, this blend has a long shelf life in dry, cool conditions.

**Yield: 4 ounces**

## Eye Bright Layered Makeup Remover

1 ounce pure organic green tea (without any added flavors)

1 ounce sweet almond oil

½ ounce vegetable glycerin

*Do not add any essential oils to the mix. This cleanser is deliberately left unscented so it can be used on the sensitive eye area. Apply with cotton ball, gently wiping in a circular motion around the eye, from the inner corner outward and back into the eye toward the nose. Keep this lotion in the fridge and use as a soak and a compress to soothe tired eyes and reduce puffiness. To extend the shelf life of the lotion, replace the sweet almond oil with wheat germ oil, which acts as a natural preservative.*

1. Prepare green tea by steeping it in a teapot or in a cup from a teabag.
2. Combine all ingredients in a wide-neck bottle, shake-shake-shake thoroughly, and watch lavalike shapes form. Eventually the mix will settle into two layers. This cleanser can be stored in a refrigerator for up to ten days, so prepare smaller batches and use them up quickly.

**Yield: 5 ounces**

## Carrot Cake Cleansing Cream

½ ounce organic semolina

⅓ ounce muscovado (fine brown) sugar

1 ounce organic orange water

½ ounce coconut oil

⅓ ounce vegetable glycerin

⅓ ounce unrefined beeswax

10 drops rosemary leaf extract

5 drops carrot seed extract

3 drops vitamin E

**Yield: 4 ounces**

*Originally, I wanted to create a duplicate of Burt's Bees Poppy Seed Cleansing Cream, but the recipe got tastier and tastier, so I ended up with something delicious enough to put on top of a muffin.*

1. Lightly grind the semolina and muscovado sugar in a mortar.

2. Carefully heat the orange water in a stainless steel saucepan and set aside.

3. Using a double-boiler method, melt coconut oil, glycerin, and beeswax until liquid.

To melt ingredients using double-boiler method, place them in a clean stainless-steel saucepan with a wooden handle (for easier handling) and set it over a bigger saucepan filled with very hot but not boiling water. Make sure the water is not boiling, as droplets of water may fall into your melting ingredients and make clumps. For the same reason do not cover the top saucepan with the lid because droplets of water may condense under the lid and drip into the melting mass. Place the large pan on very low heat. As the ingredients begin to melt, stir them carefully with a wooden spatula. When the ingredients are liquid and mixed well, remove the bowl from the heat.

4. Pour the hot orange water into the melted oils, beating in the ingredients with a fork until fluffy and uniform. Blend in the sugar and semolina mix, carefully adding the rosemary leaf and carrot seed extracts and vitamin E.

5. Mix thoroughly, transfer into a jar, and resist the urge to eat. Instead, apply daily as your morning cleanser, especially in winter. This blend can be stored up to two weeks in a cool, dry place or refrigerator.

## Day in Provence Cleansing Powder

1 teaspoon loose organic green tea

1 teaspoon dried rose petals

1 teaspoon dried calendula (marigold) petals

1 teaspoon dried lavender florets

1 uncoated aspirin tablet

1 ounce white clay (bentonite)

1 ounce rice bran

3 capsules of vitamin C

**Yield: 5 ounces**

*This second-step exfoliating cleanser works particularly well if you have congested or acne-prone skin. For emergencies (such as pimples, dullness, overall uneven complexion), leave on up to five minutes as a mask. You can store it up to three months in an airtight twist-cap bottle.*

1. Crush the green tea, rose and calendula petals, and lavender florets in a mortar. Add the aspirin tablet, crush it, and blend with plant particles. Add the clay and blend thoroughly. Add rice bran. Twist open capsules of vitamin C and add them to the mix.

2. Transfer to a wide-neck glass bottle and shake vigorously so the ingredients form a homogeneous mix.

3. Use daily by pouring a teaspoonful (size of two quarters) into a dry hand. Add a few drops of water, form a dense paste, and rub into face, avoiding the eye area.

## Sunshine and Lollipops Soap

200 g (1 cup) finely grated pure olive soap

30 mg (1 ounce) dry organic milk or organic baby formula

15 mg (½ ounce) vegetable glycerin

2 teaspoons Manuka honey

5 drops mandarin essential oil

3 drops neroli essential oil

2 drops rose essential oil

1 drop chamomile essential oil

Molds: vintage soap dishes, jelly or cookie molds, milk cartons cut in half. You can always form balls of soap by hand.

Small dried flowers for decoration (marigolds, violets, chamomile)

Yield: 4 ounces

*Milk, especially when used in baby formula, acts as a wonderful source of fatty acids, while olive soap serves as a great neutral base for essential oils. The scent is adorable, and you can use it to cleanse your face, body, and hair.*

1. Put the grated soap and milk in a bowl over a simmering pan of water, stirring occasionally until melted and runny.

2. Add the glycerin and honey and stir until completely dissolved with no cloudy particles left.

3. Add the essential oils when the mixture has cooled.

4. Transfer the soap using a clean spoon into molds or form soap balls. Press some dried flowers on top.

5. Set aside in an airy place until completely dry and hard.

6. To polish the soap, lightly moisten a muslin cloth with water or olive oil, and then buff the soap.

## Yummy Mummy Oatmeal Cleanser

1 cup organic oatmeal (not the instant type)

1 teaspoon sweet almond oil

2 tablespoons full-fat organic milk

1 free range egg

1 tablespoon organic brown sugar

Yield: 5 ounces

*Use this cleanser on your face, neck, and chest before a special occasion to give your skin a festive glow.*

1. Grind up the oatmeal in a food processor or in a mortar.

2. Add the remaining ingredients and blend well until the mixture becomes the consistency of a mayonnaise sauce. Add some water if the mixture is too thick.

3. Step into the shower and massage the scrub all over the face and neck for two to three minutes. Rinse with a washcloth and warm water.

## Skin Rescue Cleansing Cream

½ ounce cocoa butter

½ ounce olive oil

4 teaspoons non-GMO soybean wax

2 teaspoons vegetable glycerin

1 drop chamomile essential oil

1 drop clove essential oil

1 drop eucalyptus essential oil

1 drop tea tree oil

**Yield: 4 ounces**

*This is a green duplicate of the famous and outrageously priced Eve Lom Cleanser, which is a blend of mineral oil, lanolin, cocoa butter, essential oils, and a mighty dose of paraben preservatives. Instead of hops oil, we will use tea tree oil that has additional antibacterial properties.*

1. Melt the cocoa butter, olive oil, and soybean wax using the double-boiler method described previously. Whisk until the mass becomes uniform without lumps.

2. Add the glycerin and whisk the mixture until it thickens.

3. Add essential oils and set aside to cool.

4. Pour into a glass jar. You can store this balm in the fridge for up to one month. If you want to prolong the shelf life, add contents of one capsule of vitamin C to the balm while it's still hot.

## Quick Green Cleansers

Organic full-fat milk is the ultimate quickie cleanser. Just pour some milk on a cotton wool ball and wipe off the eye makeup and refresh the skin. There is no need to wash off the milk. Top it off with your regular moisturizer or leave it as it is and enjoy a mild exfoliation as milk sours and gives your skin a natural glow. Plain Greek-style yogurt also yields excellent results, especially when left on skin for a few minutes and then rinsed off with tepid water. Dried milk powder (or a baby formula) and finely ground almond meal, mixed in equal proportions, make a great natural scrub. The lactic acid in yogurt, especially when joined by the antibacterial properties of honey, makes an excellent antibacterial cleanser. Simply blend two great natural foods with a fork or stick blender.

Oatmeal makes a wonderfully gentle buffing cleanser. You can use it plain with a few tablespoons of hot water, but make sure not to scald your face! Hot water is needed just to soften the oatmeal. You can mix cooked or steeped oatmeal with another great natural exfoliator: organic mayonnaise. If you need an even stronger cleanser, mix one tablespoon of organic oatmeal with two tablespoons of plain low-fat yogurt. Apply to dry skin, wait for five minutes, and rinse off.

When out of your regular eye makeup remover, saturate a cotton ball or a cotton wool disk with virgin olive oil or grape seed oil and gently wipe off mascara and eye shadows.

Many baby cereals work as wonderfully gentle cleansers. Just mash the leftovers from your baby's breakfast with a few drops of olive or sweet almond oil and spread over your face, massage a little, and rinse off.

When my skin feels like staging a riot over all those sleepless nights, I cannot find a better second-step cleanser than milk of magnesia. Use the plain variety, without added sugar or strawberry flavors. Apply milk of magnesia with a cotton ball after you've removed makeup with facial oil or soap. Leave the liquid for a few minutes and rinse off.

When it comes to nonabrasive scrubs, nothing comes close to juicy, ripe papaya. Papaya skin contains an enzyme called papain that helps to remove dead skin cells and impurities. With regular use, papain helps fade postacne marks and blotchiness caused by sun damage. After cleansing your face, peel a ripe papaya and rub the inner side of its skin directly all over your face, avoiding the eye area. Leave on for five to ten minutes and rinse with tepid water.

Got a great all-natural homemade cleanser recipe? Drop me a line and share your bit of green knowledge with the world at www.thegreen beautyguide.com.

### Green Tip

When out of your regular eye makeup remover, saturate a cotton ball or a cotton wool disk with virgin olive oil or grape seed oil and gently wipe off mascara and eye shadows.

# chapter 7

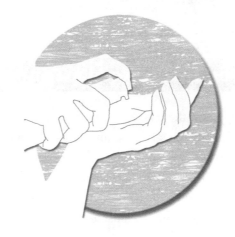

*green*
# toners

**b**eauty experts seem to have mixed feelings about toners. Some say that this beauty category is so yesterday, it should be sold as a collectable antique item at auction. Some say toners are so versatile and beneficial that you should have a separate one for each of your body parts. I believe that, unlike sunscreen and moisturizers, toners are optional, but they can greatly improve the overall condition of your skin.

## Do You Really Need a Toner?

You may know them under a variety of names: astringents, fresheners, clarifying lotions, facial mists, and floral waters. First, let's define what we mean by "toner." No matter what they're called, toners are fluids or lotions designed to remove surface skin cells, soap residue, and oils from the skin. When you wipe a cotton ball soaked in a toner, your skin feels fresh and vibrant. Some men use toners as an aftershave splash.

Most conventional toners are alcohol-based liquids loaded with petrochemicals, artificial dyes, and synthetic fragrances, sometimes with a drop of witch hazel and glycerin, usually sold with a cleanser to "shrink your pores" and "remove cleanser residue." Toners cannot shrink your pores. As you already know, skin is a very complex organ with delicate and intricate workings. The way it functions and the size of its vital parts, such as the pores, cannot be altered by a single lick of a cotton ball. The size of our pores is both hereditary and the result of years of exposure to the sun, makeup usage, and general skin care habits. If you double-cleanse, a toner does not need to become an additional cleansing step.

A good toner conditions, nourishes, soothes, calms blemishes, and delivers active ingredients to freshly cleansed skin. A mild toner also works as a weightless

**Green Tip**

Alcohol-based toners irritate skin, making it swell, so that the pores look slightly smaller. As soon as the alcohol evaporates, the swelling goes away, leaving behind irritated, dry skin.

moisturizer, and sometimes in the evening, you can get away with a rich oil-based cleanser and a moisturizing toner, skipping the moisturizer and letting your skin breathe and heal itself during the night.

Toners also make a great multipurpose beauty product if you are on the run. For example, instead of carrying a whole beauty kit to the gym, pack a mini spray bottle of toner of your choice. Spray your face frequently after strenuous activity that makes you sweat, and finish your shower with a dab of toner to soothe your skin and prep it for a moisturizer. Toners are indispensable during air travel, but make sure to pack them in small containers according to airline specifications for onboard fluids.

Some toners make a very lightweight yet potent mask: saturate a thin gauze mask with exfoliating or hydrating toner and apply it to the skin for a few minutes. This is a great way to apply a treatment toner while in the bath! You can also mix your clay-based dry mask with a little bit of toner so you enjoy double benefits from two products working in harmony.

There are three types of toners available today. Mild, hydrating toners are called face fresheners or facial mists. They contain no alcohol and are water-based, sometimes with added glycerin that hydrates skin by helping it retain moisture. Mists and fresheners usually come in spray bottles. Spraying a toner from a vaporizer bottle is a very hygienic and economical way to use a toner since not a drop is wasted on a cotton ball or your fingertips.

Skin fresheners, or classic toners, usually contain a small percentage of alcohol. They are most suitable for use in warmer months or if you feel that your skin is becoming oilier. Contrary to popular opinion, alcohol-based toners do not dry out pimples and do not decrease oil production. In fact, they can increase the production of sebum because the removal of oil from the skin can lead to excess oil production as the skin tries to compensate for this and prevent moisture loss.

Astringents are the heavy artillery. When used recklessly, they can cause more problems than they solve. Astringents usually contain a high percentage of alcohol (up to 60 percent), antiseptic ingredients, oil-absorbing clays, and essential oils. To prevent dehydration and premature skin aging, astringent toner is best applied only to problem areas of the skin, such as acne. Don't overindulge in astringents in your pursuit of clean skin. Such potent alcohol solutions can lead to severe dehydration and premature aging of the skin.

The most common application of a toner is with a clean, pure-cotton pad, but the most economical way to use a toner is to spray or spritz it on your face. Hold the atomizer or spray bottle about ten to twelve inches from your face, close your eyes, and mist it over your face two or three times. Massage the liquid into your skin. And if some of the toner gets into your hair, don't worry—it's good for your hair and scalp.

Consider making a toner a part of your daily skin care regimen. A well-formulated and correctly chosen toner can hydrate, remove dead skin cells, help prevent acne, fade brown spots and postacne marks, as well as soothe sunburns or skin irritations and even slow down aging.

## A Word About Alcohol

If a toner contains alcohol, it should be grain alcohol (ethanol), not petroleum-derived isopropyl alcohol (propan-2-ol), which is considered poisonous. Isopropyl alcohol, or rubbing alcohol, used in many conventional toners, is made of the known toxic chemical acetone, the alcohol denaturant methyl isobutyl ketone, and around 70 percent ethanol. It is cheaper than grain alcohol, but it's not the safest substance for use in cosmetics.

SD alcohol, often used in natural preparations, stands for "specially denatured" alcohol. It's often combined with a bitter substance, denatonium benzoate, to prevent some hungover individuals from drinking the product. European products often list denatured alcohol as "Alcohol Denat." Most often, denatured alcohols used in beauty products are listed as SD Alcohol 23-A, SD Alcohol 40, and SD Alcohol 40-B. The numbers indicate which substance was used to "denature" the alcohol.

Witch hazel, rose water, and orange water are traditional facial tonics that have been used safely for many centuries. Calendula, licorice, green tea, and lavender suit all skin needs, while lactic, pectic, and tartaric fruit acids perform mild exfoliation. Zinc gluconate, hyaluronic acid, seaweed extracts, and squalene from olive oil add antiaging benefits. If you have acne, your best bet is a toner with salicylic or glycolic acid. Such toners are best applied with a cotton ball, not with a vaporizer. You don't

### Green Tip

For use during colder winter months, you may want to choose a toner with added glycerin, which attracts moisture from the air and draws it to the skin.

need any glycolic acid in your eyes! You may also use a mild acidic toner if you like to double-cleanse with an alkaline-based foaming cleanser that may leave the skin's natural pH off balance. A mild acidic toner will neutralize the alkalinity and return the skin's acidic balance to normal.

The best toners I have tested are formulated with floral water. They are essentially a mix of distilled water with a small percentage of plant extracts. Mineral water by itself can make a wonderful and inexpensive toner. A really good toner I once stumbled upon contained seawater as its main ingredient. Unfortunately, the same toner contained too many synthetic and even toxic chemicals to consider adding it to the Green Product Guide. For your homemade toners, choose mineral water with a high content of magnesium, which is very soothing.

Some companies advertise their toners as "irritant-free." This doesn't mean that you must blindly obey and skip checking the product's ingredients list. If you notice any ingredients that bother your skin, find another toner. Common irritants include menthol (menthol, menthyl acetate, and menthyl PCA), citrus oils and juices (orange, grapefruit, bergamot, lemon, lime), ylang-ylang, jasmine, arnica, camphor, and many fragrance components.

As with all skin care products, don't use any toner, organic or not, that makes your skin burn, sting, redden, swell, flake, or break out. Nor should the toner leave your skin feeling dry, tight, and irritated. Return it to the store where you bought it and try a different product. If any skin reaction lasts longer than three weeks, consult your doctor.

## Green Product Guide: Toners

When you buy a new toner to replace your less-than-green astringent or add a specialized toner to clarify blemishes or soothe a sensitive complexion, it's always better to err on the side of caution. Let your cleanser, exfoliating cream, and moisturizer do the major work. Let your toner complement your skin care efforts and gently soothe your skin after a day at the office or vigorous activity. Do not make toner the heavy-hitter in your beauty regimen. The following are my recommended toning products, rated from one to three leaves, with three being my favorite.

*Santaverde Pure Aloe Vera Spray* is a versatile green creation that can double as a lightweight moisturizer for acne-prone skin. Apart from the juice of aloe vera (grown and harvested by Santaverde) and salicylic acid–rich black willow extract, it contains synthetic, albeit safe, levulinic acid, which is used during photodynamic therapy for acne. This acid is normally produced from refined petroleum, but it can also be made from starch by boiling it with diluted hydrochloric or sulfuric acids. If not for this acid, this toner could well earn two or three stars.

*Burt's Bees Garden Tomato Toner* is a perfectly "green" astringent you may like if you have acne blemishes or use foaming soaps and cleansers. This acidic toner is a potent blend of grain alcohol and extracts of tomato, bilberry, and sugarcane, all natural sources of alpha hydroxy acids. To soothe the skin, this toner employs green tea and cucumber. I found that with daily use this toner helps fade postacne marks, thanks to the parsley and cucumber, both traditional skin lighteners. Last but not least, it smells like freshly tossed green salad.

*Dr. Andrew Weil for Origins Plantidote Mega-Mushroom Treatment Lotion* is a luxurious multitasker. It soothes, moisturizes, fights blemishes, and prevents wrinkles. Formulated for Origins by the guru of integrative medicine, this useful addition to the Mega-Mushroom line contains magnesium-rich mushroom extracts, soothing and antioxidant cordyceps, ginger, basil, and turmeric plus. The water-based, slightly slippery toner does not come cheap, so the savviest way to use it is to splash it on your face with your fingertips—don't waste a single drop with a cotton ball! The only drawback is the scent: the toner contains too many essential oils, such as lavender, orange, patchouli, geranium, and mandarin, which can be a problem for those "blessed" with sensitive, fragile skin.

For dehydrated skin, **Aubrey Organics Rosa Mosqueta & English Lavender Facial Toner 1**, a green cocktail of witch hazel, flowers, and plants, delivers a healthy dose of nourishment. Aubrey Hampton, the creator of the line, uses whole organic chamomile, calendula, lavender, peppermint, and extracts of linden, sage, clematis, Saint John's wort, burdock, bladder wrack, horsetail, cucumber, and elder flower, enhanced by rose hip seed oil (Rosa Mosqueta) and rose oil. However, lemon juice, as well as arnica and peppermint, may be too irritating for sensitive types. I found that this toner does deliver a good deal of moisture, especially if you have overindulged in the sun or spent a winter day outdoors.

🍃🍃🍃 If you can buy just one organic beauty product, it should be **Clarifying Facial Toner by Dr. Hauschka.** A cult celebrity and makeup artist favorite, this alcohol-containing, witch hazel–based toner with kidney vetch, calendula, echinacea, horse chestnut, daisy, and rose is surprisingly gentle even on sensitive, post-beach skin, while another of Dr. H's toners, plain Facial Toner, contains much fewer beneficial herbs and a bit more alcohol. Dr. Hauschka's experts recommend using toners and nothing else when you go to sleep, but I found that if your skin feels tight, this toner is best combined with lightweight oily serum.

## Making Your Own Toners

To prepare a toner, you will need a bottle of mineral or spring water, preferably with a high content of magnesium. You can purify mineral water by passing it through a jug filter, such as Brita. You will also need a glass spray bottle. Plastic bottles with vaporizers are fine, but why spend time creating purely organic products only to pack them into petrochemical plastic? Besides, glass bottles look so much better on your bathroom counter. Buy bottles in bulk on eBay or specialized online stores that cater to small cosmetic businesses. Homemade toners, especially with pretty, handmade labels and perhaps a dried flower or two floating inside, make wonderful holiday gifts.

### Green Garden Moisturizing Toner

4 ounces purified mineral water

2 drops carrot seed oil

1 drop sandalwood oil

1 drop chamomile oil

**Yield: 4 ounces**

*This is a homemade duplicate of the famous Burt's Bees Carrot Seed Complexion Mist, but the potentially irritating balsam peru, ylang-ylang, and vetiver oils have been replaced with gentler alternatives. This toner has a long shelf life. You can also use it to refresh your hair and to seal mineral makeup foundation.*

1. Pour the water in a glass bottle of your choice and add all essential oils.
2. Shake vigorously and use any time your skin needs refreshment.

## Apple Cider and Aspirin Toner

½ ounce organic apple cider vinegar

3 ounces mineral water

5 plain aspirin tablets, uncoated

*Apple vinegar is helpful when it comes to clearing up acne scars, while salicylic acid from aspirin works as a powerful exfoliating and astringent agent. If you like the way it works, you can experiment with the concentration of apple cider vinegar in your toner. Some people swear by applying vinegar directly on skin, but this might be harsh for more delicate skin types.*

1. Dilute vinegar in the following proportion: eight parts water to one part vinegar.

2. Crush aspirin tablets with pestle and mortar and add the mixture to the water and vinegar mix.

3. Apply the toner sparingly only to the areas where you usually have acne or enlarged pores.

Yield:
5 ounces

## The Rose Witch Toner

3 ounces witch hazel

2 ounces rose water

1 teaspoon calendula tincture

1 drop rose oil

1 drop geranium oil

*The smell of witch hazel is not exactly like roses, which is why it's combined with rose water and other pleasant-smelling plant tinctures, making it softer, too.*

1. Blend all the ingredients in a stainless steel shaker and shake vigorously.

2. Pour into a glass bottle and use within one month. You may also soak a few cotton disks and store them in a glass jar in the fridge, making a month's supply of astringent pads without any chemical gunk in them.

Yield:
4 ounces

## Green Chai Toner

3 organic green tea bags

5 drops organic tea tree oil

2 drops geranium oil

1 drop eucalyptus oil

1 mg green tea extract

1 mg Acai extract

*This toner makes a great soothing potion for blemishes that tend to pop up overnight. According to studies, Acai berry extract contains more antioxidants than red grapes, which makes it an excellent inflammation quencher. It's also thought to have cancer preventive properties. Acai berry is harvested in Brazil rain forests, so make sure to buy an extract that was ethically harvested.*

1. Steep the green tea stronger than you'd usually drink (for about ten minutes). Let the tea cool until it's lukewarm. Keep the cup covered to preserve the steam that may carry beneficial volatile compounds of the tea.

2. Blend well. Remove the teabags and add all the oils and extracts.

3. Store this toner in the fridge for up to one month, but do not freeze.

**Yield:**
5 ounces

## Silver Vitamin Blend

10 drops colloidal silver

400 IU vitamin E

2 ml beta-carotene

1 g ascorbic acid

*This blend is a powerful antioxidant with clinically proven anti-inflammatory action. It can be used as an antimicrobial base for your homemade cleansers and masks. This blend prolongs shelf life of oil-based creams for up to six months, and keeps water-based preparations fresh for up to two months.*

1. To make a concentrated solution that you can use in your homemade green beauty preparations, combine all ingredients in ½ ounce of purified water. Add the blend to 4 ounces of the finished product.

2. Alternatively, add the ingredients one by one to the DIY preparation of your choice.

3. To prepare a soothing toner for daily use, combine all ingredients in 3 ounces of purified water.

**Yield:**
5 ounces

## Fresh Summer Cucumber Water

4 ounces (½ cup) cucumber juice

4 ounces (½ cup) purified mineral water

½ ounce orange water

1 drop peppermint oil

1 drop melissa oil

1 drop tea tree oil

1 drop grapefruit oil

**Yield:
5 ounces**

*Cucumber doesn't keep well unless preserved, especially in summertime. Use citrus oil and colloidal silver as mild preservatives. The toner may be frozen to make a refreshing, lifting treatment or poured into small spray bottles and carried wherever you go. Use organic cucumbers for this toner.*

1. Mix all the ingredients together.
2. Strain through a coffee filter to remove cucumber pulp that may clog the spray tube.
3. Pour into a spray bottle and use as often as needed.

## Green Valley Toner

4 ounces purified mineral water

2 teaspoons dried elderflower blossoms

2 teaspoons dried chamomile blossoms

1 teaspoon dried calendula blossoms

½ teaspoon dried lavender florets

1 teaspoon vegetable glycerin

5 drops carrot seed oil

5 drops rose hip seed oil

**Yield:
4 ounces**

*This is a soothing lotion for skin that has been attacked by the wind and sun. The prepared toner may be frozen in ice-cube trays and defrosted as needed.*

1. Bring the water to a boil, then pour over the dried elderflowers; cover and set aside to cool.
2. Add the remaining ingredients, mix well, then cover and leave for six to eight hours.
3. Strain the mixture through a coffee filter. Freeze in metal ice-cube trays or store in a frosted glass bottle.

## Layer Cake Clay Toner

1 ounce white clay

½ ounce witch hazel

1 teaspoon chamomile hydrosol

2 drops cedarwood essential oil

1 drop frankincense (optional)

1 drop oregano essential oil

**Yield:**
**5 ounces**

*This is a double-phase toner that has to be shaken, not stirred, before use. It can soak up excess oil from dilated pores.*

1. Combine all the ingredients in a stainless steel shaker and shake well to blend thoroughly for not less than one minute.

2. Store in a dark-colored glass bottle in the cool, dark bathroom drawer or medicine cabinet for up to two weeks. Alternatively, you can keep this blend in a refrigerator for up to one month. Shake before use.

## Quick Green Toners

Apply plain witch hazel straight from the bottle onto your face with a cotton ball. Let it evaporate. You may pour the witch hazel into a spray bottle so it can be misted directly on the skin after cleansing. Make sure not to aim at the eye area.

Squeeze half a lemon and add it to one cup of water. Strain off the pulp and seeds and pour into a small plastic bottle, shake well; apply to the face with a cotton ball. Use a spray top on your bottle to spray the toner on the skin. Let evaporate. An added benefit to this toner is that the citric acid helps to fade postacne marks and brown spots over time.

Chamomile tea can be applied directly to the skin. You may also rub a tea bag in an upward motion to help clear the pores and soothe any inflammation.

Green tea is a wonderful toner rich in antioxidants that helps soothe any inflammation and shrink puffiness. Steep an organic green tea bag in a cup of hot water, let the tea cool, and then transfer it to a glass bottle with a spray top. To prolong the shelf life of your green tea toner, add a capsule of vitamin C or a few drops of the Silver Vitamin Blend.

chapter 8

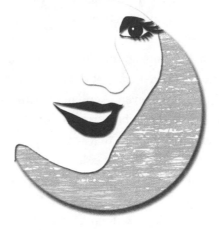

green **home
facials**

s you saw in Chapter 1, your skin is constantly on the move. Skin cells are born deep in the skin's lower layers, migrate to the surface during a period of two to four weeks, and then serve as part of the thick and dense keratinous layer before being sloughed off.

For many reasons, cells in the horny layer don't always shed as regularly and completely as they should. Sometimes sebum becomes stickier, so skin cells clump together after they reach the surface. Sometimes new bacteria and fungi on the skin's surface make skin cells more prone to excessive shedding, so they form a thicker layer on top of the skin. This dry and weathered crust of old cells starts to crack and peel, and the skin looks dull and uneven. Acne may erupt at this point, because dead skin cells, teaming with bacteria and oxidized sebum, clog skin pores, triggering an inflammation that forms zits.

Will getting rid of old skin cells save your skin? Not likely. Cosmetic companies make us believe there's a gorgeous, clean, and clear new skin just a few dead skin layers away  and that exfoliating a few skin cells (they are dead anyway!) will unveil a brand-new face. Keep in mind that shedding your outer layer of dead skin cells a few nanometers thick (that's one billionth of a meter) will not magically clear all your skin problems. Prudent exfoliating won't stimulate your skin to produce new cells, nor will it give you a blemish-free complexion. Clear skin takes a little bit more than that.

So why do we pay so much money for expensive exfoliating lotions, at-home microdermabrasion kits, and spa facials? Because most of them really work and can make our skin look healthier and feel less congested. Exfoliating facials remove the dead layer of skin cells so that new, healthy cells can enjoy all the goodness of the new, perfectly organic moisturizer or mask. This moisturizer, and especially a mask, will absorb a lot better because dead skin cells won't cling like a plastic wrap to our skin's surface (and we know that Mother Nature designed our skin to be waterproof, even when we trick it into absorbing more chemicals than it needs). Microdermabrasion, an intense scrubbing with mineral particles and special rotating tools, sheds dead skin cells at a much greater rate. Spa facials use intensive scrubbing and steaming, complete with extraction procedures, when a skillful aesthetician removes pore blockages manually, which results in smoother, less irritated skin.

Unfortunately, most spas and high-end skin care clinics use chemical skin care products loaded with petrochemicals, synthetic preservatives, penetration enhancers, sodium laureth/lauryl sulfates, artificial fragrances, and dyes. Even when the spa reception area smells heavily of lavender and chamomile, chances are high that you'll be treated with synthetic skin care "inspired" by essential oils. When essential oils are used, they may contain preservatives and artificial fragrance enhancers. This doesn't help in your quest for green beauty, but you can recreate the spa experience at home and enjoy virtually the same procedures—minus the chemical junk.

## Deep-Cleansing Routine: Masks and Scrubs

To schedule a facial, you need to call the spa; you need to wait a few days until they see you, depending on how busy the particular establishment is; and then you waste an hour, possibly two, to get a really good facial rub, a facial steam bath, a massage, and a clay-based mask. They may also pluck your eyebrows and apply a light makeup, possibly at additional cost. And they will always, always try to sell you their products and feel insulted when you pass on their offerings.

It's not that I am against spa facials. I enjoy all those lunchtime peels and minifacials. I love the way my face looks after manual extractions, especially when they are done by a merciless aesthetician. They really know how to get to the root of that annoying blackhead!

Imagine if you could get a facial every week, without waiting, commuting, and the steep price? Sounds good, right? Achieving spa results at home is quite possible, and there are a few benefits, too—no waiting time and almost no money spent. Granted, there is some elbow grease involved, but this is easily offset by the fact that you are using completely natural products with zero preservatives, zero dyes, and only natural fragrances.

Regular exfoliation is your first step toward sparkling skin. Facial scrubs should become an important part of your facial care routine. Many gentle scrubs can be used as a second-step cleanser in a double-cleansing routine. If your skin behaves, you don't need to use the scrub every day, unless you really want to.

There are two types of exfoliating products available today: abrasive and nonabrasive. Alpha and beta hydroxy acids exfoliate by dissolving the very top layer of dead skin cells with glycolic acid from sugarcane, lactic acid from sour milk, tartaric acid from grapes, malic acid from apples, and pyruvic acid from citrus fruits. Malic and tartaric acids are more commonly used in exfoliating body products, as they are more potent.

Abrasive exfoliating products remove dead skin cells by physical friction, using synthetic or natural particles, such as jojoba beads, crushed fruit kernel, seeds, salt, or sugar. Nonabrasive exfoliating products use alpha and beta hydroxy acids to dissolve the top layer of dead skin cells. Many exfoliating products combine both principles, offering a double action against dead skin cells, but such products can be irritating if you have fair, delicate, or easily irritated skin.

**Green Tip**

Scrubs are best to use when you have uneven or flaky skin and no visibly inflamed areas.

A word of caution: if you have inflamed acne lesions, an irritation, or a sunburn on your face or body, you should never use abrasive scrubs, no matter how natural or gentle they feel. Grain and beads in the scrub will further damage the fragile skin in the area of inflammation, so the irritation gets worse and all your efforts to speed up the healing process will go down the drain along with the scrub. You may use a scrub as part of your daily double-cleansing routine as a second step after removing makeup with your first wash. You can also use abrasive scrubs in your weekly home spa regimen before applying a nourishing, whitening, or deep-cleansing mask.

Rule of green thumb: when buying a new scrub, squeeze a little from the tester tube and rub it into your hand, applying as much pressure as you usually do when pressing cell phone buttons (very light but focused). Do you feel the gritty particles? Then the scrub is too harsh for your face. Try finding a nonabrasive alternative. If none is available, make a new shopping list: you are going to cook a new scrub at home.

No need to despair, as there are many wonderful and natural exfoliating creams and lotions available today. Most of them are very gentle, and they can be used daily as cleansers on their own. Mild abrasive particles are usually buffered with rich oil and beeswax blends so the risk of scrubbing too hard is minimal.

The best time to apply the scrub is when you have just stepped out of the shower or are taking a warm bath.

Apply the scrub with small onward and outward movements. Roll and press on your skin, rather than rub the scrub into it. Avoid the delicate eye area. You can leave the scrub to double its efforts and work as a mask before you rinse it off with tepid water.

Make green scrubs and nonabrasive exfoliating lotions a part of your daily skin care routine. After just one use, you will feel that your skin is literally coming back to life. Ideally, an exfoliation with a chemical or physical scrub should be followed by a clay- or charcoal-based mask that will deep-clean pores you have already opened with a scrub. Here are a few sumptuous techniques to enjoy a spa-grade exfoliation and deep cleansing at home.

**Green Tip**

Add a drop of cedarwood or jasmine oil to your bathwater. These oils smell wonderful and help open up the pores.

## Green Product Guide: Exfoliants

How do you know that you have the right exfoliating product that suits your skin's needs? This is not a case of "no pain, no gain." If the scrub feels uncomfortable or hurts when you're using it, stop immediately. Some redness is normal for chemical exfoliating lotions, which may leave your skin feeling hot or inflamed. If your skin's condition looks suspicious, trust your guts and act accordingly: rinse off the product, apply a soothing toner, steep a cup of green tea to spray all over your face, or better yet, soak a clean cotton towel, apply to your face, and relax. Wait several days to give your skin time to recover. If the irritation persists, call your doctor. The following are my recommended exfoliants, rated from one to three leaves, with three being my favorite.

### Scrubs

**Jurlique Daily Exfoliating Cream** is a nongranular, rich, daily scrub that uses almond meal, oats, and honey to gently get rid of dead skin cells. Please read the ingredients list carefully to make sure that the current version of this product contains only natural ingredients.

🍃 🍃 **Green People Organic Body Spa Sensuous Sugar Scrub** is made of organic raw cane sugar and a plethora of antioxidant and healing oils, including calendula, jojoba, rose hip, pomegranate, cranberry, avocado oils, and olive leaf extract. Designed for the body, this incredibly soft scrub is gentle enough for your face and hands. The scrub is packed in a recyclable plastic jar.

🍃 🍃 🍃 **Dr. Hauschka Cleansing Cream** is a product with a cult following, and it has rightfully earned three leaves. This almond meal–based cream is rich in essential oils, organic plant extracts, and juices. It's very nourishing, too, because according to Dr. Hauschka experts, you do not need a moisturizer at night, so the cream doubles as a lightweight hydrating lotion, and its oils are not removed by the toner applied afterward. The only drawback is the small size of the tube.

For proper cleansing you need approximately one inch of the cream, and you have to massage it into your face for up to five minutes if you have acne. (The cream is so soft, you won't damage your healing zits.) I found that one tube usually lasts for about two weeks, significantly increasing the cost of my monthly skin care routine. But I am willing to put up with this extra expense because my skin looks luminous and flake-free, no matter the season.

## Nonabrasive Exfoliants

🍃 **Ecco Bella Leave-On Invisible Exfoliant & Blemish Remedy** is formulated with a potent blend of lemon and lactic and salicylic acids. Its high content of antioxidants (alpha-lipoic acid, vitamin E, carotenoids, lutein, and lycopene), and organic extracts of oat, calendula, and licorice make this fluid lotion a good lightweight moisturizer that can be worn day and night under a moisturizer or a sunscreen.

🍃 🍃 **Juice Organics Apple Exfoliating Peel** has all the fruit acids you could think of: malic acid from organic apples, citric acid from organic lemons, glycolic acid from sugarcane, tartaric acid from . . . no, not from steak tartar, but from organic white grapes, plus aloe, glycerin, organic algae (!), and vitamins E and C. It smells heavenly and leaves skin looking even better. No preservatives, no colorants, only the fruity goodness.

🍃 🍃 🍃 **Dr. Hauschka's Cleansing Clay Mask** is a definite winner. Its formulation is simple: clay, cornstarch, witch hazel, Indian Cress extract—but results of its use are dramatic. To use, you mix a teaspoon of dry powder with any carrier you like: a toner, rose water, purified water, even green tea. The shelf life of the mask is virtually indefinite. The mask is very ecoconsciously packed, too: a solid glass jar for first-time buyers and simple cardboard bags as refills when you repurchase. Buy less, waste less.

## Making Your Own Scrubs

Even the most expensive professional treatments can be duplicated right in your kitchen for a fraction of the price and without any unwanted chemicals. With homemade scrubs, you can alter the intensity of the exfoliation based on your skin's condition. You can add new healing and soothing ingredients, and when you become confident with essential oils, you should be able to whip up a week's supply of antiacne, antiwrinkle scrub in no time.

We will not be using any essential oils in our scrubs or masks. This is done to minimize irritation. When you rub the scrub into your skin, you cannot help but damage it, at least a microscopic bit, and the mask has to be soothing and gentle. So save your aromatherapeutic concoctions for your toners and cleansers.

Scrubs may be made in bulk, stored in glass jars in the bathroom, or, better yet, the fridge, and mixed with water or a toner as needed.

## Almond Milk Scrub

4 tablespoons of very fine almond meal

4 tablespoons white clay

1 tablespoon organic milk powder

**Yield:**
**4 ounces**

*Almonds are very softening to the skin, and fine almond meal makes this scrub gentle enough to use as a regular cleanser.*

Add all the ingredients to a glass jar and shake well to mix the contents. To use, pour 1 tablespoon in the palm of your hand, massage gently into the skin, rinse off with lukewarm water, and pat your skin dry.

## Breakfast Yogurt Scrub

20 g of brewer's yeast in powder or tablets

2 teaspoons plain organic yogurt

2 teaspoons almond meal

1 teaspoon Manuka honey

*Yeast stimulates the circulation and is rich in vitamin B6, while honey disinfects and calms the complexion. Prepare enough scrub for one application, and to make the most of the concentrated nurturing ingredients, leave the scrub on your face for a few minutes before rinsing off.*

1. Grind the tablets of brewer's yeast (if using tablet form) in a mortar.
2. Add remaining ingredients and mix together. Use the scrub immediately, and do not store in the refrigerator.

Yield: 5 ounces

## White for Sake Scrub

1 organic green tea bag

5 grams white willow bark extract

120 mg of gingko biloba extract

1 cup rice bran or baby rice flakes

½ cup oatmeal

Juice of 1 ripe papaya

5 drops of grapefruit oil

Optional: 2 tablespoons sake

*This mild peel, originally a creamy green version of the famous Dermalogica Daily Microfoliant, can also be prepared with sake (Japanese rice wine) for even stronger whitening results. If using sake, you will need to use the prepared mixture immediately because sake will ferment the rest of the ingredients into a smelly mush.*

1. Steep a green tea bag in ½ cup of boiling water for 10 minutes.
2. Meanwhile, crush the aspirin tablets, crack open the gingko biloba extract capsule, and blend with rice bran or baby rice flakes and oatmeal.
3. Squeeze the papaya juice into the mixture and add the green tea to form a soft, but not runny, paste.
4. To preserve the mixture, add 5 drops of grapefruit oil. If using sake, add it just before you are ready to use the scrub.

Yield: 4 ounces

## Sugar Mommy Scrub

1 tablespoon sugar

1 tablespoon olive oil

3 drops rose oil

1 drop vanilla extract

*This scrub will impress you with how well it works. There is a commercial product just out on the market that has sugar and olive oil as the only ingredients. The cosmetics company is charging $32 for a 10-ounce jar. However, this recipe costs pennies to make! The scrub has no shelf life and should be prepared fresh before use. Sugar babes just have to be high maintenance, don't they?*

1. Whisk all the ingredients in a glass bowl.

2. Massage the mixture all over the face and neck for 2 to 3 minutes. Rinse with warm water and a washcloth to eliminate the oil residue. Follow with a toner of your choice and moisturize.

Yield:
5 ounces

## Making Your Own Masks

While it's complicated to replicate a shampoo or a moisturizer at home, masks are simply crying out to be homemade. Make sure you use fresh, organic ingredients and store the mask in the fridge only for a week. If making a mask from fresh fruit, vegetables, and milk or yogurt, prepare them as needed and keep in the fridge for no longer than twenty-four hours. Do not freeze masks.

To preserve the mask for longer storage, you will need to add a least 500 mg of vitamin C and several drops of colloidal silver or grapefruit seed oil, although this last ingredient may irritate your skin.

## Clay Your Eggs Mask

2 tablespoons white clay

1 tablespoon corn flour

1 organic free-range egg white

1 drop chamomile oil

This mask works as a temporary lift while deep-cleansing and drawing out impurities from the skin. It is most suitable when you can use additional nutrition for your skin.

1. Blend the ingredients in a china bowl. Mix well to dissolve the egg white completely.

2. Apply to clean, dry face. If the paste is too thick, dilute the mixture with freshly brewed chamomile tea. Allow to dry and wash off with tepid water.

**Yield:**
**5 ounces**

## Kinky Oatmeal Mask

1 ounce purified mineral water

3 tablespoons plain organic oatmeal

1 medium onion, peeled

Onion acts as an anti-inflammatory agent and inhibits the overproduction of collagen in acne scars, while oatmeal penetrates deeply into pores, cleansing the excessive cell buildup and clogged pores.

1. Boil the water and pour it over the oatmeal, letting it steep for five minutes.

2. Finely grind the onion in a food processor, making a smooth puree. Add it to the oatmeal while it is still warm.

3. If the mask is not thick enough, add some honey or green clay until the mask is thick enough to sit comfortably on your face. Store the mask in the fridge for one week.

**Yield:**
**4 ounces**

## Ozone Aloe Whitening Mask

½ peeled, sliced cucumber

2 tablespoons plain aloe juice

1 tablespoon whole-fat condensed milk

1 tablespoon honey

*Yield: 5 ounces*

*The name of this mask comes from the fresh, sea-breezy scent of a fresh cucumber. I recommend using organic cucumber in this mask. When you start using organic fruits and vegetables in your home cosmetics, you will be amazed how rich and vivid the scents are. Experts say that the concentration of antioxidants, vitamins, and minerals is higher in organic veggies, too.*

1. Blend the cucumber in a blender or food processor. Add the aloe juice, milk, and honey.

2. If the mask is too runny, add some kaolin clay until the mask forms a comfortably thick paste.

3. Apply to clean, dry face and leave on for 15 minutes or until dry. Gently wash off with tepid water.

## Lemon Cheesecake Whitening Mask

2 tablespoons honey

4 teaspoons lemon juice (freshly squeezed or bottled)

3 teaspoons plain or Greek-style yogurt

1 egg white

*Yield: 4 ounces*

*In this mask, the antibacterial properties of honey are boosted with the antifungal and whitening properties of lemon. Both lemon and yogurt work as excellent natural peels, helping fade postacne marks. Egg white adds proteins that help strengthen the skin's own defenses, while lemon and vanilla create a comforting, soothing cocoon while you linger with the mask in your bath. You can store this mask in the fridge and use it up within one week.*

1. Combine all the ingredients in a bowl and whisk until the mask thickens.

2. Apply to clean, dry face and let set for 15 minutes. Gently wash off with warm water.

# Custom-Tailored Facial Routines

Even after you establish a healthy routine of daily double-cleansing and effective toning, your skin needs a regular dose of high-performance special treatment. Just a half-hour a week can mean a huge difference!

Please find below several home facial routines that you can custom-tailor to your current skin condition.

## Rise and Shine Facial

*This is a weekly facial routine that you can enjoy on a Saturday morning, after a long Friday night. You can also submit your skin to this intensive care if a sudden pimple pops up before an important event.*

1. *Cleanse.* Wash your face with your regular cleanser. Rinse thoroughly with lukewarm water and blot dry with a fresh towel.

2. *Exfoliate.* Apply a homemade or organic exfoliating treatment based on your skin condition. Massage the scrub or peel in circular motions for two minutes. Rinse clean and pat your face dry.

3. *Steam.* Prepare an anti-inflammatory facial steam bath: boil some filtered or mineral water, pour it into a ceramic, glass, or metal bowl (careful: the bowl may get hot!), and add one drop of each of the following essential oils: chamomile, eucalyptus, rosemary, and tea tree oil. Skip rosemary and use lemon oil instead if you are pregnant. Cover your head with a clean cotton towel and bend over the bowl. Let the vapors envelope your skin. Close your eyes and breathe slowly. Added bonus: your sinus condition will heal faster, too. Continue steaming for five minutes.

4. *Exfoliate.* When your face is still wet, apply another portion of a scrub and massage gently for two minutes. Rinse and pat the face dry.

5. *Deep-cleanse.* Apply a thin layer of a clay-based homemade or charcoal mask. Leave on until dry. Rinse clean with cool mineral water and pat the face dry. Follow with your regular toner and a moisturizer.

## Acne Freeze Facial

*The following technique has a lot of shock value in it. Treat your freshly erupted pimples to this intensive procedure before an important event.*

1. *Cleanse.* Wash your face with your regular cleanser. Rinse thoroughly with lukewarm water and blot dry with a fresh towel.

2. *Freeze.* Crack or crush several ice cubes and wrap them in clean gauze or a washcloth. Apply ice to the acne zit. Hold it in place for as long as you can stand the cold but no longer than 10 minutes.

3. *Treat.* Remove the ice and dot on your homemade acne medication containing lavender or tea tree oil. Repeat every four hours or so until the blemish has diminished in size and is no longer red.

## Salt Facial Lift

*This temporary face-lifting facial works especially well if you have only five minutes to look five years younger. You will need some sea salt and a freezing cold bottle of mineral water.*

1. *Cleanse.* Wash your face using the gentlest cleanser in your beauty arsenal. Avoid using oily cleansers or exfoliating scrubs.

2. *Salt It.* Boil a cup of mineral or filtered water. Add a teaspoon of sea salt and make sure it dissolves completely. The water must be warm but not so hot that it will burn you. Saturate a cotton ball or gauze square in the mixture, press out excess, and apply to your face, avoiding the eye area. Let the salt remain on your skin for five minutes.

3. *Tone.* Now saturate a cotton ball or gauze in ice-cold mineral water and apply to your face with very gentle pressure for 30 seconds. Blot dry.

4. *Repeat.* Repeat these steps several times, depending on how much time you have or until wrinkles and puffiness have diminished.

# chapter 9

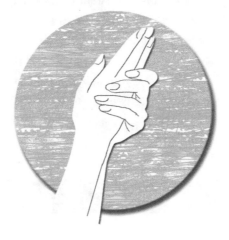

## green moisturizers

now that we have learned about some of the best green cleansers and toners, and how to create natural cosmetic products at home, we are ready to seal the results with the right moisturizer. For many people, moisturizer is the most important—and most expensive—cosmetic product they own. When our skin feels unusual, we would rather replace the moisturizer than a cleanser or a toner. Many of us are on a constant quest for the "holy grail" moisturizer, and when we find one, we tend to stick to it for years, despite the changes occurring in our skin. This simply doesn't make sense. Just as your favorite set of underwear isn't made to last for five years, the same is true of your moisturizer: your skin changes as your body does, and not a single skin care product is made to meet the ever-changing needs of human skin.

## Do We Really Need a Moisturizer?

No matter what your skin's condition is, you need a moisturizer, which today serves more purposes than simply keeping your skin hydrated. For oily, blemish-prone skin, moisturizers deliver antibacterial and soothing agents. For mature, wrinkled skin, they add an extra dose of softening and antioxidant ingredients. All of us benefit from sun-shielding mineral components and antioxidant enzymes, vitamins, and oils that protect our skin from a less-than-pure environment.

How do moisturizers help? They form a film on your skin that reinforces the barrier ability of the epidermis, helping to prevent transepidermal water loss. They contain certain ingredients that attract moisture from the environment, and they contain healing substances that soothe irritations and neutralize free radicals.

Some moisturizers can actually prevent and reverse wrinkles. Just a few years ago, such a notion would cause a few eyebrows to skeptically rise, as many experts argued that moisturizers applied to the top layer of the epidermis do not change the physiology of the skin and do not prevent wrinkles from forming deep inside. While a simple moisturizer can relax fine lines caused by facial tightness, many advanced ingredients such as coenzyme Q10 and its synthetic and more potent colleague, idebenone, as well as certain peptides, plant extracts, and amino acids, can relax wrinkles and even reverse them. This is especially true when these ingredients are used diligently in effective concentrations and in conjunction with the meticulous use of sunscreens, a smart diet, and positive lifestyle changes. Classic components of antiaging moisturizers, such as alpha hydroxy acids and vitamins, can also help to stave off premature aging.

## How Moisturizers Work

Every good moisturizer is made of five ingredient groups: *emollients, humectants, emulsifiers, penetration enhancers,* and *active ingredients.* It's good to know and understand how these ingredients work so your expectations of your moisturizer will be reasonable, and the next time you buy a new hydrating lotion or serum, you'll be armed with the latest knowledge.

Traditionally, moisturizers were believed to work by slowing down water loss from the epidermis by locking it in with film-forming agents. Water originates in the deeper skin layers and moves upward to hydrate cells in the stratum corneum, eventually being lost to evaporation. Every day we lose up to one pint of water through the pores! The higher the water content in the epidermis, the more pliable and wrinkle-free the skin will be. Moisturizer is the most important antiaging step and must be used consistently, no matter how old you are. "Take care of the skin you have; it is meant to last a lifetime," says Anne Dolbeau, the founder of organic spa line Inara.

Moisturizers work together with the skin's own hydrators, such as natural moisturizing factors and sebum, to maintain the skin's protective barrier. They increase water content, reduce water loss, and preserve skin's youthful appearance. Moisturizers also hydrate by providing water directly to the skin.

## Emollients

Emollients, the biggest group of ingredients in moisturizers, soften, heal, and hydrate skin by preserving the water content of the epidermis. They also lubricate by creating a "skin slip," the feeling of smoothness following moisturizer application, and eliminate that dry, tight-feeling skin. Emollients fill the cracks between clusters of dead skin cells with molecules of fatty acids and alcohols. Let's take a look at some of the best natural emollients. You will need to know them to make informed choices when buying a new cream or lotion.

Phospholipids are contained in living human and plant cells. Along with cholesterol, they preserve the integrity of the skin cell membranes. Lecithin, derived from eggs or soybeans, is an excellent emollient phospholipid. Ideally, lecithin should be obtained from non-GMO sources.

Many people think that plant oils moisturize the skin. That's not exactly true. Oils seal the cracks in the skin's upper layer and lock in the moisture, but they do not deliver any moisture directly. Plant oils can also repair a damaged skin barrier. Some oily emollients penetrate skin better than others. Look for olive oil and squalene from olive oil, as well as castor, jojoba, and coconut oil.

Mineral oil and petroleum jelly are often used to mimic the action of natural emollients. Once a cure-all for skin disasters from burns to wrinkles, the glory of Vaseline (the commercial name for petroleum jelly) is fading, even though many celebrities attribute their glowing skin to this medicine chest staple. Instead of penetrating between dead skin cells, petrochemicals form a waterproof plastic film on top of all the debris on the skin's surface, locking in the bacteria, dead skin cells, sweat, and sebum. No wonder acne thrives in such conditions!

## Humectants

Humectants are the next most important ingredients in moisturizers. They attract moisture from the air by bonding with water molecules and then releasing water gradually. Glycerin and sorbitol (sugar alcohol), when derived from natural sources, are the best green humectants. Sugars are able to attract water in two ways: they enhance water absorption from the lower layers of the skin into the epidermis, and in humid conditions, they also help the skin absorb water from the external environment. Unlike petrochemical propylene glycol, which is not recommended for use on damaged skin, all naturally derived emollients and humectants have low potential for irritation (Johnson, Cosmetic Ingredient Review Expert Panel 2001).

## Emulsifiers

Emulsifiers hold together all moisturizer ingredients. Normally, oil will not mix with water, but beeswax, when heated, turns oil and water into a smooth mixture. Green emulsifiers include lecithin; plant-derived waxes cetearyl alcohol, cetearyl glucoside, and cetearyl olivate; coco caprylate/caprate from coconut; cholesterol; and algae extract.

## Penetration Enhancers

Penetration enhancers allow the active ingredients in the moisturizer to be absorbed into the skin. The best natural penetration enhancers are water and essential oils, such as menthol and chamomile, glycerol, cod liver oil, squalene, linoleic, oleic, and arachidonic acids.

## Active Ingredients

Today, moisturizers do much more than preserve the delicate water balance in the epidermis. They protect our skin from photodamage using sunscreen ingredients and antioxidants; they increase cell turnover with mild alpha- and beta-hydroxy acids; they heal blemishes and curb inflammation with antibacterial additives such as tea tree oil, zinc oxide, or various plant extracts that have antibacterial effect; and they can actually reverse damage done to our skin and prevent premature aging using novel ingredients such as peptides, human growth factor, cytokines, and good old vitamins and minerals. Many active ingredients multitask. For example, zinc oxide acts as a physical sunscreen while helping to prevent acne blemishes. Green tea extract prevents skin aging on many levels. Many active ingredients synergize, or act in sync to provide a combined effect. For example, vitamins C and E work better together than separately, and catechins from green tea improve the sun protective qualities of mineral sunscreens.

## FABULOUS GREEN MOISTURIZERS

A good green moisturizer should contain the following:

- **Emollients**: beeswax, squalene from olive oil, jojoba and other plant oils, shea butter, cocoa butter, plant-derived silicones. Beware: thickening agents like triglycerides, palmitates, myristates, and stearates may be pore-clogging.

- **Humectants**: hyaluronic acid, glycerin, or sorbitol.

- **Emulsifiers**: beeswax, non-GMO soybean wax, vegetable waxes identified by "caprilate," "caprate," or "cetearyl" in the name, lecithin, cholesterol, or algae.

- **Penetration enhancers**: vegetable squalene, linoleic acid (rosehip oil), oleic acid, peppermint extract (if your skin tolerates it well), or chamomile extract (if you don't experience a skin reaction to it). Avoid propylene glycol and tetrasodium EDTA in your moisturizers.

- **Active ingredients**: **physical sunscreens** (zinc oxide, titanium dioxide); **soothing extracts** (bisabolol, allantoin, aloe juice/extract, licorice root, green tea, and chamomile extracts); **antibacterial** tea tree oil, and **antiaging** components such as peptides, hyaluronic acid, *Boswellia serrata*, CoQ10 and/or idebenone. Universally appealing **antioxidants** include green tea, Acai and pomegranate extracts, grape polyphenols, beta-carotene, vitamin C esters, and vitamin E. For **nighttime use** you may choose a moisturizer or a serum with alpha- and beta-hydroxy acids, but keep in mind, wearing them during the day is not recommended since even mild acids may increase facial pigmentation and result in uneven skin tone and brown spots.

When buying a new moisturizer, you should always check a product's ingredients; when in doubt, test it on a patch of skin first to make sure it doesn't cause any adverse reactions. Also, be aware that just because a product has a certain ingredient listed on a label, that doesn't necessarily mean it has enough of it to produce visible results.

## What About the Texture?

When we choose a moisturizer, we can't help but think in terms of skin type. Younger skins need gels, while combination skins can use lotions. Dry, mature skin requires a heavy artillery of creams and serums. As before, let your current skin condition be your guide. If you feel that a lightweight cream can do a much better job for your face, then go for it. Some thick creams are less heavy and occlusive than oil-rich lotions.

All creams and lotions are called cosmetic emulsions. Lotions are oil-in-water emulsions, while creams are water-in-oil emulsions. There are more complicated emulsions, such as oil-in-water-in-oil, serums, gels, sprays, and milks.

Moisturizing lotions tend to be thinner and more suitable for daytime use, especially if you wear makeup. Creams are generally made with heavier fats and waxes and are often applied at night.

## How Many Moisturizers Do We Need?

In general, any product that hydrates the skin on your face will do the same for the rest of your body. However, better facial moisturizers usually contain a higher concentration of active ingredients. Even if you choose to improve your existing moisturizer, would you waste $100 worth of colloidal gold to dilute it in ten ounces of body lotion and get a concentration that will nullify all the goodness of this precious extract, or would you rather infuse your facial cream with this potent ingredient and see real results?

Of course, you can use many body products on your face and vice versa. You can take a perfectly green body lotion—the one without preservatives, synthetic fragrance, and mineral oil—and turn it into a powerful facial cream by adding antioxidants and soothing plant extracts. Be creative. Your only limitation may be the price (the ingredients in facial creams are probably too expensive to lavish on your entire epidermis) and texture (many body moisturizers, especially those for hands and feet, are too heavy; extra oils could travel into your eyes or even clog your pores).

It's impossible to stock a moisturizer for every condition of your skin. This way, you will need an artist's brush and loads of time to precisely apply an oil-absorbing, pore-tightening gel on your nose, an antiaging, lightening serum and a coating of SPF on your cheeks and forehead, a rich antiwrinkle cream around your mouth and on your neck, and a light-weight antioxidant serum under your eyes. Who has the time or money to do that daily?

I firmly believe that a good, decently formulated moisturizer can be safely and beneficially used on all areas of your face. If you have a chal-lenging skin problem, simply add a face oil blend or a serum suitable for this condition. The following products contain a lot of antioxidant and soothing agents that help regulate sebum production, relieve inflamma-tion, and prevent premature aging. You will find more about antiaging green skin care and green ways to handle acne later in this chapter.

## Green Product Guide: Moisturizers

In my opinion, it's virtually impossible to prepare an elegant, pleasant-to-use moisturizer at home unless you are a really gifted cosmetic chemist. To whip up a jar of day cream, you will need to do some exten-sive shopping, mostly online, and then spend about an hour steaming, double-boiling, blending, and whisking. I did it a few times, and while the outcome was perfectly natural, it just takes too much time, and the result-ing goop won't necessarily look like something you'd enjoy applying to your face daily. So instead of preparing a moisturizer from scratch, you can try to improve the existing green products with skin actives of your choice. The following are my recommended moisturizing products, rated from one to three leaves, with three being my favorite.

🍃 The emollient sunflower oil in **Burt's Bees Carrot Nutritive Day Crème** contains added linoleic acid. Other oils from wheat germ, avo-cado, grape seed, and carrot seed nourish skin and lock in moisture, while rosemary extract, vitamin E, and milk proteins calm the complexion. The only two drawbacks to this lightweight cream are the high content of potentially irritating balsam peru and an abundance of beta-carotene that may stain your collars or pillows. This cream can be mixed with many active ingredients, such as coenzyme Q10, green tea extract, and a pinch of alpha-lipoic acid (ALA).

🍃 **Weleda Iris Day Cream** is a basic day moisturizer that you can also use at night. Formulated with organic jojoba oil, beeswax, and bio-dynamic *Iris germanica* root extract, this flower-smelling lotion provides a great base for many active ingredients such as L-carnosine, green tea extract, hyaluronic acid, and most synthetic peptides for collagen synthesis.

🍃🍃 If you need a lightweight moisturizer to go under a heavy sunscreen, consider **Pangea Organics French Chamomile & Orange Blossom Facial Cream.** Originally formulated for oily skin, this featherlight serum is basically lavender tincture with organic plant oils, vegetable glycerin, and sugar emulsifiers, enriched with extracts of burdock, elderflower, witch hazel, and chamomile. Packed in a convenient pump bottle, it comes in a box stuffed with seeds that you can plant in your organic garden. This lotion blends well with such active ingredients as yeast beta glucans, copper peptide, Indian pennywort (*Centella asiatica*), and ellagic acid.

🍃🍃 **CARE by Stella McCartney 5 Benefits Moisturising Fluid** is a heavenly scented, lightly hydrating, firming, and healing fluid lotion. I use it during the summer, and it provides an excellent base for mineral foundations. Based on garden cornflower water, plant-derived fatty alcohols, sunflower seed, and soybean oils, this rich yet lightweight moisturizer delivers the goodness of sixteen (!) antioxidant and calming essential oils, as well as sodium hyaluronate. Packed in an airtight bottle, it requires no preservatives. This also means you won't be able to add any additional actives to the mix, but this cosmetic product is very good by itself.

🍃🍃🍃 **Moisturizers by Dr. Hauschka** are in a class of their own. They don't travel into the eyes (so you can use them around the eye area), they are just the right texture (feeling great under makeup), and they don't contain essential oils for added scent. I love using **Quince Day Cream** (the fashion industry favorite) in the summer, under mineral makeup for sun protection, **Rose Day Cream** in the winter and on my baby's bum, **Tinted Day Cream** all year around, when I feel like wearing just a hint of makeup, and **Moisturizing Lotion** anytime my skin misbehaves. These moisturizers come in handy (albeit smallish) tubes, so if you want to blend them with active ingredients, you'll need to transfer creams to a glass jar. Not sure if it's worth it: most Dr. Hauschka creams do not mix well with my favorite skin actives. Only **Rose Day Cream** works well with a scoop of **Philosophy Hope and a Prayer** topical vitamin C.

✐ ✐ ✐ **JASON Natural Cosmetics Pure 5,000 IU Vitamin E Oil** is a versatile moisturizer that will get you through many skin challenges. Surprisingly lightweight and fast penetrating, it is actually a blend of seven organic oils (sunflower, safflower, rice bran, apricot, peach kernel, avocado, and wheat germ oils)—even though the label states it's just five oils! It also contains emollient lecithin and a whopping 5,000 IU of vitamin E. This oil blends extremely well with such potent active ingredients as alpha lipoic acid (be gentle on this one!), lutein, lycopene, various carotenoids, and phytosterols.

## Green Beauty Oils

Most people shun oils as a beauty aid. Those with acne-prone skin want oil-free products because "oil clogs pores," and people with normal skin avoid oils for fear of tipping the scale of their skin balance toward the oily, acneic type. In fact, most pore-clogging ingredients aren't natural oils. They are mineral oil and animal fats. We now know that many high-quality moisturizers contain plain and essential oils because oils are wonderful at binding moisture to the skin and strengthening skin cell membranes.

Facial oil is the only moisturizer worth trying to cook at home. It will also serve you better than many commercially made creams and lotions. Beauty oil ingredients come cheap; you can twist and turn the formula to suit your skin's needs; you can make one oily serum for your blemishes and one for wrinkles; one for windy winter days when your cheeks turn beetroot pink and one to use after lazy summer afternoons on the beach. Just dab a few drops of oil of your choice and top it with your regular moisturizer, a heavy sunscreen that often leaves you no room for extra moisturizer, or leave the oil to work on your skin alone.

## Making Your Own Beauty Oils

Here are some topical oil-based treatments you may find useful. Preparing beauty oil is extremely easy. All you need is a glass pump bottle and a dropper. The formula usually consists of carrier oil and a few drops of essential oils. Pour the carrier oil into a bottle, add essential oils, drop by drop, shake well, and leave to synergize for one day. To use, apply a drop of oil to each fingertip. Rub fingers lightly against each other to warm the oils. Inhale the oils deeply. Press the fingertips gently against your skin and lightly spread in upward, gentle circular motions. Do not apply oils too close to the eye area.

## Glow-Reviving Oil

½ ounce avocado oil

1 drop neroli essential oil

1 drop clove essential oil

1 drop jasmine essential oil

½ teaspoon of nude golden mineral shimmer (try Aromaleigh Pure Hue Intense Multi-Purpose Powders in adobe or brocade)

**Yield: 4 ounces**

*This luxurious, fast-penetrating oil is versatile enough to use on the face, hands, and décolleté. Shake the bottle before use.*

1. Combine all the oils in a bottle and shake vigorously.

2. Add the mineral glimmer. Shake again to distribute the pigment. Shake before each use.

## Soothing Face Oil

1 tablespoon organic rose hip oil

1 tablespoon organic virgin olive oil

1 tablespoon organic aloe vera juice

2 drops calendula essential oil

1 drop chamomile oil

1 drop comfrey essential oil

**Yield: 5 ounces**

*This antioxidant oil blend comforts irritated, red, or hot skin, especially in wintertime or after prolonged sun exposure.*

Combine the oils in a pretty glass or china bottle and shake vigorously.

## Sun Protection Beauty Oil

1 tablespoon sesame oil

1 tablespoon carrot seed oil

1 tablespoon kukui seed oil

400 IU vitamin E

2 drops beta-carotene

2 drops vitamin D

**Yield:
4 ounces**

*This facial oil contains natural sun guards that will not replace a sunscreen but will boost its effectiveness and shield your skin from mild sunrays in wintertime. Many plants contain natural sun protection mechanisms, which are the best way to support the skin's own production of melanin.*

Combine the oils in a pretty glass or china bottle and shake vigorously.

## Green Eye Care

There's an old saying that the eyes are the mirrors of your soul. From a nutritionist's point of view, your eyes and the skin around them also mirror the health of your circulatory and digestive systems. Not only do our eyes reveal our natural radiance and allure, but also lack of sleep, water, and fiber in our diet, too much junk food, and too much sun exposure.

Just like our facial skin combines too many "skin types," the skin around the eyes has different areas that should be treated accordingly. The skin in the eye socket has very small pores, and it's the thinnest on our face. Blood vessels are only a fraction of an inch away from the surface of the skin, and constant movements of the eye require this skin to be pliable yet taut. The skin on the outer sides of the eyes, near your temples, is more similar to the facial skin on your cheeks and forehead, but it's prone to easy wrinkling because of the way we smile—and I hope you smile a lot!

Any eye treatment product should not be applied to the eye socket area. No matter what you choose to make your eyes look brighter and younger, keep the product at least one-quarter inch away from the lash line. You may apply a firming cream to your brow bone area, but make sure to keep it away from the eyelids.

There are a lot of skin care products aimed at the eye area: creams, lotions, serums, gels, patches, and masks. In your twenties, you don't need a special moisturizer for your eye area. If you use a natural, light-weight moisturizer and regularly shield your eyes with durable UV-coated sunglasses, then you can use your regular moisturizer under the eyes, making sure not to rub it into the eye sockets.

When I hear a recommendation that I should use a product that is specifically formulated for the eye area, I usually ask, "What's so different about it?" I usually hear that "these products are designed to be light enough for the eye area, yet still deliver a lot of moisture." A close examination of the ingredients list doesn't reveal any dramatic difference. For example, Kinerase Intensive Eye Cream contains the following ingredients: water, a blend of synthetic fatty acids and fatty alcohols that work as emollients (glyceryl stearate, laureth-23, isopropyl palmitate, stearic acid, cetyl alcohol, stearyl alcohol), penetration enhancers (propylene glycol, imidazolidinyl urea), slip agent dimethicone, preservatives (methylparaben, propylparaben), triethanolamine, and a few plant ingredients such as safflower seed oil, soya sterol, and aloe leaf juice. The cream also contains the powerful natural antioxidant N6-Furfuryladenine (kinetin) and a totally useless collagen and elastin that were proven ineffective as antiaging components many years ago.

Now let's take a look at Kinerase Cream, a favorite celebrity product that has a cult following. We see the same water, fatty alcohols as emollients, propylene glycol, silicone, safflower seed oil, soya sterol, aloe leaf juice, kinetin, and the same blend of preservatives. Not a single ingredient is different, except the concentration of the active ingredient, kinetin. The eye cream contains 0.125 percent, and the face cream contains 0.1 percent. The difference of 0.025 percent, or a microscopic 0.2 mg (worth a few cents when kinetin is bought in bulk) causes a double increase in price.

Many experts claim that using a rich facial cream around the eyes can cause milia, or small whiteheads that are similar in nature to acne but are not caused by inflammation. This happens because petrolatum-based, heavily scented, preservative-laden eye creams usually clog narrow pores in the eye area. If you don't use a cream with petrolatum, mineral oil, or paraffin in it, milia won't stand a chance.

Let me address another traditional "don't" of eye care: the one that says you should not apply a facial cream around the eyes if you wear contact lenses. I cannot imagine that a sensible woman would apply an eye cream at night without first removing her contact lenses or would start her morning beauty routine with her contact lenses on. Don't rub the eye cream into your eyes and keep it away from your eyelids, and your contact lenses will be safe.

It's true, however, that rich face moisturizers are prone to migrating into your eyes and causing irritation. To avoid this, use cream very sparingly and apply it a good one-quarter inch away from the lash line. There are many wonderful natural moisturizers that won't travel or migrate into the eye sockets. They will firm and moisturize, provided you use a small amount and keep it away from the lash line and inner corners of your eyes.

> There are many wonderful natural moisturizers that won't travel or migrate into the eye sockets. They will firm and moisturize, provided you use a small amount and keep it away from the lash line and inner corners of your eyes.

It's not that I am against eye creams. During my last twenty years of diligent use of eye creams, I've owned a few brilliant organic creations, and I regularly blend a jar of antioxidant-rich, depuffing, soothing concoction that I apply every night. For emergencies, I have a vial of light-weight gel-serum that I store in the fridge and apply in the mornings to reduce redness and puffiness resulting from entertaining my active toddler into the wee hours every other night.

So what makes a good green eye cream? First of all, let's see what makes a horrible eye cream: mineral oil, paraben or formaldehyde preservatives, artificial colors, synthetic fragrances, propylene glycol, triethanolamine, and petroleum-derived silicones. So, any cream that contains none of the above is worth considering.

Good green eye products should be based on water, beeswax, vegetable glycerin, or plant-derived emollients. Many natural eye creams contain vitamin E as a versatile antioxidant and vitamin C, which strengthens capillaries. Plant extracts helpful to the eye area include green tea, eyebright, aloe vera juice, cucumber, and chamomile extracts. A rich eye cream, Burt's Bees Beeswax & Royal Jelly Eye Crème, even contains magnesium-rich Epsom salts that are known for their ability to soothe any swelling or aches. Some vitamins are a no-no. Even though vitamin A is a good antiaging active, it can be too irritating for use around the eye area. Novel ingredients helpful in preserving the naturally youthful look of your eyes include antioxidant coenzyme Q10, various peptides that stimulate the formation of collagen, yeast, oat beta glucans,

Indian frankincense extract (*Boswellia serrata*), antioxidant proanthocyanidins from grape seed, moisture-boosting hyaluronic acid, and chrysin that virtually eliminates dark circles. You can read more about these ingredients in Chapter 5.

## Green Product Guide: Eye Care

Finding a very effective green eye cream is not an easy task. Most often, natural eye creams are hardly different from face creams but cost significantly more. You aren't likely to find peptide molecules, hyaluronic acid, epidermal growth factor, and coenzyme Q10, not to mention idebenone. That's why the best way to reap the benefits of these ingredients and stay green is to buy a relatively inexpensive eye product and add these ingredients yourself. Most of the products mentioned in the guide allow you to customize them. Just be careful to use active ingredients for use around the eyes very, very sparingly. The following are my recommended eye-care products, rated from one to three leaves, with three being my favorite.

🍃 **Organic Pharmacy Lip and Eye Cream** is a very nourishing, almost greasy eye cream, more suitable for use in the winter. Formulated with eyebright, antioxidant bilberry, and water-draining fennel, the cream does a perfect job moisturizing the eye area, but tends to stay on the surface and travel into the eyelashes, no matter how diligently you avoid applying it away from the lash line. Thanks to a DIY-friendly jar, you can adapt the formulation according to your needs.

🍃🍃 **REN Lipovector Peptide Anti-Wrinkle Eye Cream** provides deep moisturizing with proteins from wheat and plant collagen from yeast, while beta-carotene works against superficial lines. Almost scentless and very lightweight, this eye lotion works best for younger eyes or on top of an intensive eye serum. The airtight bottle doesn't allow any messing with the product.

🍃🍃 **Avalon Organics Revitalizing Eye Gel** can become your lifesaver if your nights involve more dancing, web surfing, or diaper changing than actual sleep. Keep it in the refrigerator for a morning boost of icy goodness. Loaded with calming lavender, depuffing green tea, soothing chamomile and licorice, antioxidant grape extract, moisturizing hyaluronic acid, and age-fighting peptides, this liquid gel penetrates almost instantly and can be reapplied without stickiness. I would have given it three leaves if not for the arnica extract (may be irritating) and phenoxyethanol (definitely not green).

🍃🍃🍃 **Lavere Ultimate Eye Care** cream is a godsend to those who need to deal with the double whammy of wrinkles and puffiness. Formulated with moisturizing collagen, rose hip and evening primrose oils, caffeine, grape seed, and ginseng extracts, this cream penetrates quickly and leaves the skin taut, not sticky. This cream cannot be modified with skin actives of your choice, but believe me, you really don't have to bother.

🍃🍃🍃 **Aubrey Organics Lumessence Rejuvenating Eye Crème with Liposomes** is a real gem. Packed with plant proteins and amino acids, deep-penetrating liposomes with vitamins and humectants, and more vitamins, the lightweight, nourishing, yet not greasy cream also contains a plethora of plant extracts and oils that form the basis of every decent eye cream: aloe vera, evening primrose oil, rose hip oil, white tea extract, and not one but two seaweeds (laminaria and carrageenan). The airtight bottle does not allow adding any more actives, but this cream is great as it is.

## Green Solutions for Dark Circles

Most green eye treatments moisturize and prevent wrinkles, but not many can handle the problem of under-eye puffiness and darkness. A mineral concealer may temporarily mask the problem, but the underlying issue will still exist.

There's a common notion that dark circles under the eyes form because of waste products accumulating around the eye area. This is not exactly true. The under-eye area is not a bladder or any type of bodily waste dump. Neither are dark circles caused by stress or fatigue. Dark circles are caused by a very complex physiological mechanism. Here's the skinny: fine, almost transparent skin under the eyes is meshed with capillaries, or tiny blood vessels. These capillaries are so narrow that red blood cells sometimes have to line up to get through. Sometimes red blood cells break through the walls of capillaries and leak into the surrounding skin. Special enzymes break down the red blood cells, which turn dark blue-black in color. So your dark under-eye circles are actually caused by leaky capillaries. It's the same mechanism that produces bruises when we are hit by something.

What can you do to prevent dark circles from forming? Actually, there isn't very much you can do. The thickness of the skin under the eyes and the leaking abilities of blood vessels are hereditary. People with darker skin have more visible dark circles because of the natural pigments in their skin. If you have deep-set eyes, natural shadows contribute to the dark circles under the eyes, making them more visible. Also, some medications that cause blood vessels to dilate may result in darkening circles around the eyes. Lack of sleep can make dark circles under the eyes more visible because fatigue contributes to poor circulation and your skin looks paler.

One thing you can do is get your blood moving. Try simple lymph drainage by dry brushing your body at least every other day. Use a soft, natural fiber brush with a long handle and a removable head with a strap, so that you are able to reach all areas of your body. Long sweeping strokes should start from the bottom of your feet upward, and from your hands toward your shoulders, and on the torso in an upward direction to help drain the lymph back toward your heart. Stroking away from your heart puts extra pressure on blood and lymph vessels and can make matters even worse. Now take a shower as usual.

Get a cucumber from the fridge, slice it one-quarter-inch thick, lie down, and place the slices on your eyes. Leave them on for at least five minutes. It's a good idea to set your alarm clock if you're doing this early in the morning. Cucumber has gentle whitening properties, and it's also cooling and moisturizing.

Try green tea bags soaked in water. The caffeine in green tea is a diuretic; that is, it helps the body lose excess water. When applied topically, it may shrink the puffiness and help boost circulation.

Couch potato remedy: slice a raw potato, and then place it on your eyes and relax on your couch. Potatoes contain catecholase, an enzyme that works like a skin lightener. Make sure to use raw, not cooked potato.

Add some relaxing cardio to your workout. Yoga can work wonders to dissolve under-eye circles. It takes a couple of months to see the results, but you may never need an under-eye concealer again.

Topical treatments may reduce dark eye circles. If darker skin under the eyes makes those unsightly circles more visible, try natural lightening agents, such as kojic, ferulic, and betulinic acids, bearberry (*Uva ursi*) extract, arbutine, niacinamide, vitamin C, and glucosamine. They will work gradually by training under-eye cells to produce less pigment and help make the pigmentation less visible. Natural skin lighteners are gentle but can take up to three months to bring noticeable results. Antioxidant products containing vitamin E are known to stimulate fibroblast activity in the dermal layer and help firm up the skin.

Some people swear by applying Preparation H with 0.25 percent phenylephrine. This well-known hemorrhoid ointment may help the capillaries constrict, causing dark circles to appear less visible. This is hardly a green treatment, but you may consider it as an emergency measure.

Sleep with your head elevated to prevent water from pooling around the eye area.

Dark circles under the eyes can also be the result of health issues, such as chronic allergies. Go to an allergist and get tested for allergies, especially to yeast, dairy, alcohol, and wheat. Cut back on caffeinated beverages, alcoholic beverages, diet sodas, and salt.

## Green Solutions for Wrinkles

If you are looking for a one-step organic treatment for wrinkles, then, sadly, you won't find one—not in this book and not anywhere else. Wrinkles are the result of hundreds of body processes, as well as our own actions. We can protect our skin from sun damage, quit smoking, and limit the use of toxic skin care. We can slow down free-radical damage, and we can eat well and supplement our bodies so our immune systems stay in peak condition. Unfortunately, we have little if no control over age-related processes, such as cell cessation and hormonal depletion, that result in reduced cell turnover, decreased fat and collagen content, and hormone loss. Environmental pollution also speeds up skin aging, and even if we move to less polluted areas, decades of living in toxic cities will eventually show up on our skin.

It would take another book to address every factor that makes our skin age from the green point of view; right now, let's find out what we can do to slow down skin aging using organic, natural cosmetic products. Every wrinkle takes decades to develop, so it's very unreasonable to hope that a smear of a cream will remove it completely and overnight. When you understand what can and what can't be done using cosmetic products, you'll be able to make informed choices and avoid spending money on products that are physically unable to live up to their claims.

What happens when we get wrinkles? Older skin has less fat in its dermis, which makes it look thinner and more transparent than younger skin. Facial muscles lose their shape and density, which causes facial features to sag and the skin to droop. Cell reproduction slows down, which shows up as an uneven skin structure and increased water loss. Skin cells lose vital elements such as hyaluronic acid, glycerin, and polysaccharides, which results in dryness and a parchmentlike look to the skin. The skin's support structures, collagen and elastin, deteriorate after decades of reckless sun exposure and hormonal changes, which results in sagging and wrinkles. Aging skin is more prone to allergic reactions, irritation, discoloration, and even acne because of the declining state of the immune system.

> Aging skin is more prone to allergic reactions, irritation, discoloration, and even acne because of the declining state of the immune system.

A proper skin care routine can deal with some of these factors—but not all of them. Popular wrinkle creams claim they can restore collagen and elastin, rejuvenate and repair skin cells, and even reprogram the DNA to produce younger, healthier skin. No matter how tempting it is to resolve all the issues of aging with one clever potion, it's impossible. Instead of wasting money on another "snake oil," let's see what we can actually do to delay the formation of wrinkles.

Protect the skin from environmental damage. Damage from the sun and free radicals resulting from pollution, an improper diet, and an overabundance of toxic chemicals in skin care products builds up in skin over time. This causes the DNA and RNA to stop skin cells from reproducing quickly, which slows skin cell turnover and thickens the layer of dead skin cells at the top layer of epidermis. Naturally derived or synthesized antioxidants, such as coenzyme Q10, idebenone, anthocyanidins and polyphenols from grapes, lycopene from tomatoes, superoxide dismutase, vitamins C and E, and alpha-lipoic acid, when added to skin care products, can slow down and even repair the damage done by free radicals.

*Protect the skin from sun damage.* Loss of elasticity due to the deterioration of collagen and elastin, and the formation of furrows, crow's feet, and brown spots on our face, necks, and hands, are largely due to sun damage that builds up over decades. Sun exposure causes damage by twisting cell DNA, which in turn shows up as abnormal cell growth, inadequate blood and lymph flow, and collagen loss. Unfortunately, sun damage is irreversible. Prevent further harm by applying a mineral-based sunscreen daily, ideally in two layers: by topping the moisturizer with sunscreen with mineral foundation.

*Exfoliate dead skin cells.* This has nothing to do with regular scrubs or peels. Exfoliation of mature skin should be more gentle and consistent. As the skin gets older, dry, misshapen cells linger on its surface longer, creating a flaky, uneven appearance and increasing water loss. When you remove dead skin cells, skin functions improve, and cells can perspire better and receive more moisture and nutrients. Exfoliation with retinoids (vitamin A acids), ascorbic acid, or plant enzymes should become part of your daily skin care routine.

*Moisturize, whiten, and heal.* While moisturizers do not prevent wrinkles, the dry top skin layer can form microscopic cracks that make the skin more irritable and prone to inflammation. Using moisturizers with emollients such as phospholipids and lecithin, humectants like glycerin and hyaluronic acid, and lipids from plant oils can help restore the skin's intercellular matrix, filling it with essential building blocks. Healing and soothing agents such as kinetin, sea kelp, Indian frankincense (better known as *Boswellia serrata*), licorice, propolis, green tea, chamomile, and vitamin B5 (niacinamide) help the skin recover from environmental assaults.

None of these ingredients is a panacea. Some newly synthesized peptides and proteins help reverse some of the damage done to the skin and restore some of its functions, but I don't want you to believe that even big guns, such as idebenone or plant-derived cytokine proteins (also known as epidermal growth factor), can permanently change the structure of your skin. Aging cannot be reversed, but it can be slowed down with smart and consistent chemical-free skin care, an organic diet, and an active, joyful lifestyle.

**the green beauty guide**

"Stay hydrated, attend the sauna, and exercise regularly to detox your skin and body, and avoid synthetic and toxic ingredients that cause health issues. The sun is very aging as well. Avoid excessive sun exposure. You cannot be too young to start protecting your skin with natural sunscreens. Every woman has beautiful features. You should try to enhance them through healthy exercise and healing sleep. 'You look healthy' or 'You look pretty' rather than 'Your makeup looks great' should be the ultimate compliment to aim for. And do not underestimate the beauty and appeal of a natural smile that reflects inner happiness and well-being."

—Ulrike Jacob,
Laveré Skin Care

## Green Solutions for Acne

Many believe that acne is simply an age-related rite of passage that does not need to be treated because you will outgrow it eventually. However, graduating from high school does not necessarily mean the end of acne drama. "Often, women are getting acne later in life," notes Susan West Kurz of Dr. Hauschka Skin Care, who insists there's more to acne than oily skin. "We try to look at the whole picture, consider a person's eating habits, lifestyle, and age. Acne could also be an allergy to a certain kind of protein. Sometimes, when people cannot digest something, even psychologically, it shows up on their skin. We have known hundreds of people who were treated for their acne with cortisone creams and Retin-A, but all these treatments address only symptoms, not the real cause. When you just treat the

> Sometimes, when people cannot digest something, even psychologically, it shows up on their skin.

symptoms, it's the same as putting your hand on the yellow flashing light on your car's dashboard. You try not to look at it instead of fixing the problem."

Instead of removing oil using concentrated foaming cleansers and drying lotions, holistic skin care experts rely on oily extracts of healing and antibacterial medicinal plants. "Your skin is responding to oil in a homeopathic way: if you put oil on the oily skin, it will help loosen impurities and refine the pores. It also sends a message to your skin that it is producing enough oil," says Susan West Kurz, "and your skin responds by slowing down its production of oil. So, if you overcome your prejudice against putting oil on oily skin, you will notice that your skin produces less oil. I remind people that you can't clean an oily substance with water because these two substances do not mix. People who remove oil from their skin often get dry, flaky skin on top and congested oily skin below. But if you put oil on a congested oily complexion, it will loosen impurities trapped in your skin and direct [the] metabolism to produce a healthy flow of sebum again. Oil also helps reduce the size of pores, because when your skin is blemished, your pores are enlarged. Oil flow is reestablished in a healthy way, and pores diminish, because elasticity returns to the skin. Oils are highly antioxidizing, and as your skin is healing from the blemishes, oil also helps prevent any kind of scarring and other problems associated with acne-prone skin."

If you have suffered with acne since your teenage years, past outbreaks have left lots of postacne brown spots and maybe even scars. To fade them and prevent new acne blemishes from arising, you should use a mild daily exfoliating product such as Santa Maria Novella Sulfur Soap or almond-based, anti-inflammatory Dr. Hauschka Cleansing Cream. Don't forget about sun protection, which will help prevent further postacne hyperpigmentation. Avoid inflammation by strengthening your skin's own defenses. Enrich your daily skin care regimen with antioxidants, vitamins, and anti-inflammatory substances.

There are many easy, natural, and inexpensive ways to treat acne. Because acne-prone skin is usually thicker and oilier, acne sufferers tend to overindulge in strong foaming, often abrasive, cleansers, caustic astringents, and oil-free moisturizers. This triple whammy leads to increased sensitivity, new breakouts, and faster skin aging due to a broken skin barrier, which results in increased moisture loss.

To successfully battle acne, you need a consistent and effective green skin care routine. Here are some general guidelines for taking care of acne-prone skin naturally:

*Cleanse gently.* Wash your face with a nonfoaming or lightly foaming water-soluble cleanser that does not sting or leave the skin feeling dry in the morning, and double-cleanse with a cleansing oil and a foaming cleanser at night. Cleanse only twice a day. Frequent or vigorous cleansing will increase irritation and inflammation but will not promote healing of your acne blemishes. You may replace the second cleanser with an exfoliating product containing alpha/beta hydroxy acid. Use scrubs only if you have no blemishes but want to fade postacne hyperpigmentation.

*Choose a toner* that contains witch hazel, tea tree oil, chamomile, aloe, cucumber, calendula, and fruit acids to gently exfoliate the skin. Plant-derived alcohols and clay can help quickly zap blemishes. To quickly soothe inflamed acne lesions and prepare your skin for a healthy night's sleep, apply milk of magnesia for a few minutes before going to bed. Use an unsweetened and unscented magnesium hydroxide solution—the common laxative and upset stomach treatment. Apply it with fingertips or a cotton ball, leave it to dry, and wash off with tepid water.

*Wear a daily moisturizer* with antioxidants and botanical anti-inflammatory agents such as chamomile, green tea, panthenol, provitamin B5, tocopherol (vitamin E), licorice, calendula, raspberry, rice and oats, seaweed (algae), evening primrose oil, arnica, and echinacea. Choose lightweight fluids and serums instead of oil-free moisturizers. One product to try is Suki Moisture Serum, which is formulated with organic chamomile, echinacea, and calendula in a lightweight oil base. It quickly soothes inflamed, fragile skin thanks to a high content of antioxidants, and it is suitable for sensitive, oily complexions that have trouble tolerating conventional oil-free lotions with benzoyl peroxide.

*Zap zits with topical treatments.* Tea tree oil is a traditional acne remedy that can be used directly or diluted with a toner or a mask. Apply a vitamin C powder directly onto blemishes. To treat larger areas affected with acne, mix 1 scoop of Philosophy Hope and a Prayer vitamin C with two or three drops of your favorite facial or body oil. The vitamin C will not dissolve completely, so this treatment is best left on overnight. Please note: this concoction may sting.

Make sure you wear sunscreen, especially in the summer and anytime you have active breakouts. Mineral sunscreen is perfect for acne-prone skin: you can wear it on top of your acne treatment of choice. Skipping sunscreen can result in dark postacne marks that are hard to get rid of.

## Making Your Own Acne Zappers

For problem skin, nothing beats tea tree oil. You can apply it directly on blemishes, dilute it in your favorite toner, and add a few drops to your masks and scrubs. Here are some quick and easy acne zappers that use the power of this green zit fighter.

### Sweet Tea Balm

1 tablespoon runny honey

1 tablespoon aloe vera juice (bottled or freshly squeezed from the plant)

10 drops tea tree oil

500 mg vitamin C (to act as a preservative)

*This all-purpose antibacterial healing concoction is inspired by the award-winning Harley Street Cosmetic Tea Tree Antibacterial Gel, but we won't be using any synthetic fillers!*

Combine all the ingredients in a shallow bowl and blend until smooth. Transfer into an empty lip balm jar. This blend can be stored in the fridge for up to six months and used on all sorts of blemishes and minor cuts.

Yield:
5 ounces

## Tea Tree Healing Oil

1 teaspoon apricot kernel oil

10 drops pure organic tea tree oil

3 drops chamomile essential oil

2 drops geranium essential oil

*This is a traditional recipe with an aromatherapeutic twist to it.*

Combine all the ingredients in a small pump bottle. Use twice daily on areas affected by acne. Avoid using during the first three months of pregnancy.

**Yield:
5 ounces**

## Spicy Tea Poultice

1 organic green tea bag

1 tablespoon fine sea salt

10 drops tea tree oil

5 drops chamomile essential oil

1 drop eucalyptus essential oil

1 elastic bandage, ideally one with a sticky edge all around

1 piece of sterile gauze

*A poultice is a soft, moist mass that is spread over an affected area and left to work its magic for an extended period of time. You can leave the poultice on overnight to see a noticeable improvement in your blemish size in the morning. This is a powerful emergency treatment that has to be used in skin crises only!*

1. Prepare a cupful of green tea. Remove the tea bag. Open the bag and scoop out the green tea mush. Blend it quickly with salt and essential oils.

2. Apply a dime-sized blob of the blend on the blemish. Cover with the gauze and secure it with a bandage.

3. Be prepared to see temporarily wrinkled skin around the almost invisible blemish in the morning. Wrinkles will go away in 10 minutes at most.

**Yield:
4 ounces**

chapter **10**

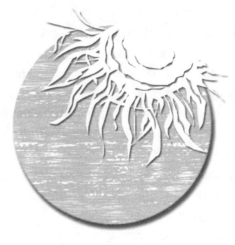

*green* **sun**
**protection**

**a**ll living beings have developed ways to protect themselves from harsh elements. It may be fur, a shell, feathers, or scales. Human skin protects itself by becoming thicker and darker.

The sun makes us look healthier and feel better. Just imagine what summer outdoors would be without the sun shining! As we bare our skin to soak up that sunny goodness, let's take a look at what is really happening to our skin as we tan.

Our skin has several built-in sun protection mechanisms. When exposed to the sun, the top skin layer thickens within four weeks to the equivalent of a weak sunsceen, approximately sun protection factor (SPF) 4. This type of protection takes time to develop and is too weak to completely shield us from the harmful effects of the sun's radiation.

Tanning is the skin's main way of protecting itself. In fact, it's an alarm signal pulled by our skin. Ultraviolet (UV) radiation stimulates skin cell melanocytes to produce more melanin pigment. Sun radiation causes the melanin to combine with oxygen, which creates the actual tan color in the skin. Melanin protects the body from absorbing an excess of solar radiation, which can be harmful. The more we expose ourselves to the sun, the more pigment is produced.

Apart from developing a nice golden tint, our skin undergoes less attractive changes. The sun's rays damage skin in several different ways. After sun exposure, our skin becomes thicker, drier, less pliable, and more prone to irritation. On a molecular level, UV radiation from the sun attacks keratin cells and fibroblasts, triggering a variety of molecular changes that cause a breakdown of collagen in the skin and a shutdown of new collagen synthesis. With decades of long sun exposure, the skin starts looking coarse and thick, and deep wrinkles form. In addition, too much exposure to UV radiation suppresses the body's immune system, triggering a complex cascade of changes on a cellular level, so you may develop increased sensitivity to sunlight and even react differently to immunizations. Scientists from the University of Münster in Germany found that ultraviolet radiation "can function as a complete carcinogen by inducing 'UV signature' DNA mutations and by suppressing protective cellular antitumoral immune responses." They found the precise mechanism by which frequent sun exposure damages skin: first, UV radiation damages skin cells' DNA, which results in the release of an immune-suppressing chemical called interleukin-10 (Beissert, Loser 2008). Even low levels of UV (type B) sun radiation can slow down the immune system of the skin for several weeks. This may explain why people often develop sun allergies and acne while on vacation.

## ABCs OF SUN

Ultraviolet radiation from the sun is a form of electromagnetic radiation. It is divided into three types: UVA, UVB, and UVC.

UVA radiation (320 to 400 nm wavelength) is weaker than UVA and UVC, but it is the most prevalent type of sun radiation. UVA radiation causes premature aging at a somewhat slower rate than the others, but this radiation causes melanoma, a very dangerous type of skin cancer. UVA is not blocked by many conventional sunscreens, but it can be effectively blocked by physical sunscreens and clothing.

UVB radiation (280 to 320 nm wavelength) has higher energy than UVA waves and is therefore more damaging and more carcinogenic. UVB rays burn our skin and cause instant damage. They also raise the risk for nonmelanoma skin cancers.

UVC radiation (200 to 280 nm wavelength) is successfully filtered by the ozone layer, although today, as the ozone layer is considerably thinner, scientists are concerned that dangerous, short wavelengths of sun radiation may be reaching Earth in higher amounts than in the past.

# Health Benefits of Tanning

The main source of vitamin D in humans is sun exposure to the skin. Research in Denmark in 2007 indicates that a lack of vitamin D may influence the development of autoimmune diseases such as inflammatory bowel disease, type 2 diabetes, multiple sclerosis, and rheumatoid arthritis (Heller et al. 2007).

Another recent study blames the prevalence of asthma and allergic diseases on a lack of vitamin D in human bodies (Litonjua, Weiss 2007; Shaheen 2008). Scientists from Brigham and Women's Hospital in Boston hypothesize that as people spend more time indoors, there is less exposure to sunlight, leading to decreased vitamin D production in the skin. Vitamin D deficiency, particularly in pregnant women, results in more asthma and allergies in children. Vitamin D has been linked to the immune system and lung development in babies, and epidemiologic studies show that higher vitamin D intake by pregnant mothers reduces asthma risk by as much as 40 percent in children (Litonjua, Weiss 2007).

While many studies avoid mentioning sunscreens when discussing lack of sun exposure, one 2007 study directly links heavy use of sunscreens to lack of vitamin D (Alpert, Shaikh 2007). Researchers from the University of Nevada—a state that receives a potent dose of sunshine every day!—aren't ecstatic about sunscreens. They say that since most sunscreens filter out UVB light, they are inhibiting vitamin D production. In their 2007 report, they note that long-term vitamin D deficiency leads to rickets, osteoporosis, type 1 diabetes, cancer, and multiple sclerosis. What's more, people with darker complexions have greater difficulty producing vitamin D because melanin acts as an effective natural sunscreen, requiring longer sun exposure to produce an adequate daily allotment of vitamin D.

But what about skin cancers, a dangerous consequence of inadequate sun protection? As we all know, skin cancers are associated with sun exposure—yet the same sunlight, through the production of vitamin D, may protect against some cancers. Scientists from Finland came to a shocking conclusion: patients with skin cancer have a lower risk of developing other cancers. Take a deep breath and please read on.

During a massive study of 416,134 cases of skin cancer and 3,776,501 cases of non-skin cancer as a first cancer, from both sunny countries

(Australia, Singapore, and Spain) and less sunny countries (Canada, Denmark, Finland, Iceland, Norway, Scotland, Slovenia, and Sweden), researchers found that all second solid primary cancers (except skin and lip) after skin melanoma were significantly lower for the sunny countries than in the less sunny countries (Tuohimaa et al. 2007). In sunny countries, the risk of a second primary cancer after nonmelanoma skin cancers was lower for most of the cancers except for lip, mouth, and non-Hodgkin's lymphoma. Scientists concluded that vitamin D production in the skin seems to decrease the risk of several solid cancers, especially stomach, colorectal, liver and gallbladder, pancreas, lung, female breast, prostate, bladder, and kidney cancers. The apparently protective effect of sun exposure against second primary cancer is more pronounced after nonmelanoma skin cancers than melanoma, which is consistent with earlier reports that nonmelanoma skin cancers reflect lifelong, cumulative sun exposure, whereas melanoma is related more to sunburn.

A smaller Australian study, conducted in 2007, found that recreational but not occupational sun exposure decreased risk, generally by 25 to 40 percent, of non-Hodgkin's lymphoma, one of the most mysterious types of cancer (Armstrong, Kricker 2007). Scientists believe that production of vitamin D from sun exposure offers us a protection mechanism against non-Hodgkin's lymphoma. A high dietary intake of vitamin D also reduces the risk of this cancer.

Does it mean we have to ditch sunscreens and embrace the sun in order to stave off the onset of multiple sclerosis and bone mass deficiency? Actually, we don't have to fry on a sunny beach for hours in order to keep healthy levels of vitamin D in our bodies, and of course we should *not* rely on artificial tanning beds as a source of vitamin D. While agreeing that UVB radiation does boost amounts of vitamin D, a recent article in the *Journal of the American Academy of Dermatology* stresses that therapeutically important changes in vitamin D can be achieved with minimal tanning (Armas et al. 2007). Sunbathing on a beach can generate 10,000 IUs of vitamin D or more in as little as fifteen minutes. Depending on skin pigmentation, valuable increases in vitamin D can be achieved by low doses of sun exposure that are enough to produce only a light tan.

There are other ways of maintaining healthy levels of vitamin D in our bodies. The biologically active vitamin D metabolite, also known as dihydroxyvitamin D3, is synthesized primarily in human skin, but there are newly available analogues of vitamin D that can also protect the immune system and various tissues against cancer and other diseases, including autoimmune and infectious diseases. A 2007 study suggested that such vitamin D analogues may be effective against acne (Reichrath 2007). Today, UV radiation is used to treat psoriasis and vitiligo.

## We Still Need Sun Protection!

It's impossible—and actually harmful—to avoid the sun completely. A light tan is more than enough to maintain healthy levels of vital vitamin D, but sun protection today is more important than ever. Sunburns are directly linked to a higher risk of developing the most disastrous skin cancer—melanoma—and it's much easier to get burned today than twenty years ago. When the tan was first made fashionable by Coco Chanel in the 1920s, the protective ozone layer was fairly intact, but the first study linking skin cancer to relentless sun exposure dates back to 1948. Fifty years ago, tanning was relatively safer than today. Now, huge gaps in the ozone layer, especially over large cities, allow more harmful short-wave sun radiation to wreak havoc on our vulnerable skin. Too much careless sun exposure can result in premature aging and uneven pigmentation, weakening of the skin's immune system, and most important, a higher risk of skin cancer.

*Valuable increases in vitamin D can be achieved by low doses of sun exposure.*

Sun exposure is indisputably linked to the development of melanoma, and blocking sun exposure is recommended by the American Academy of Dermatology, the Skin Cancer Foundation, the American Cancer Society, the Centers for Disease Control and Prevention and the Environmental Protection Agency. Melanoma is a malignant tumor of pigment-producing melanocyte cells; it is a relatively rare but deadly type of skin cancer.

According to the World Health Organization (WHO), melanoma kills about forty-eight thousand people worldwide every year. Blistering and peeling sunburns, especially those having occurred in childhood, are one of the main risk factors for melanoma, along with family history. People with fair complexions, red or blond hair, and birthmarks and moles are especially at risk.

Ultraviolet radiation is one of the main risk factors for melanoma. Yet, there's no need to go overboard and completely shun the sun, hiding inside and slathering cupfuls of sunscreen lotions every hour, as some ardent antisun experts recommend. Everything is good in moderation, and not a single sunscreen can completely shield you from skin aging or cancer.

# The Dark Secret About Sunscreens

It's a given fact that sunscreens prevent sunburn. However, there has never been epidemiological or laboratory evidence that most common sunscreens, including para-aminobenzoic acid (PABA), invented in 1922, prevent either melanoma or basal cell carcinoma in humans. All we know so far is that the same mechanism that causes sunburn may also trigger the formation of skin cancer. Sunburn by itself doesn't cause skin cancer, but it signals a harmful, excessive exposure to the sun.

Worldwide, the countries where chemical sunscreens have been recommended and adopted have experienced the greatest rise in skin cancers, with a simultaneous rise in death rates. In the United States, Canada, Australia, and the Scandinavian countries, melanoma rates have sky-rocketed, with the greatest increase occurring after the introduction of sunscreens at the end of the 1970s. According to the National Center for Health Statistics, death rates in the United States from melanoma doubled in women and tripled in men between the 1950s and the 1990s; yet melanoma remains a relatively rare type of cancer, killing twenty times fewer people than lung cancer (Miniño et al. 2007).

Could it be that sunscreens promote skin cancers instead of preventing them? Absolutely not, but there is something about sunscreens that needs careful attention. One explanation could be the ineffectiveness of sunscreens made in the 1980s and 1990s. Older formulations did not provide protection from all spectrums of the sun's radiation. Those sunscreens shielded more from burning UVB rays but did almost nothing about the more damaging UVA exposure. Both UVA and UVB types of sun radiation have been shown to mutate DNA and promote skin cancers in animals (Rass, Reichrath 2008). UVA also penetrates deeper and stimulates melanocytes at a much higher rate, yet for some reason UVA dangers were ignored. Slathered in sunscreen, people stayed in the sun longer without having proper protection, often over a period of ten or twenty years, before clinical symptoms of skin cancer appeared.

To understand why sun protective ingredients aren't able to actually protect us from skin cancer, let's first see if there's any difference between sunscreens and sunblocks. Sunscreens are a group of chemicals that get under our skin to absorb sun rays. They first need to get absorbed by skin so they can then absorb photons of sun radiation. Sunscreens usually contain benzophenones, such as oxybenzone, which protect against UVA, and salicylate and octyl methoxycinnamate, which protect against UVB. A major drawback of these sunscreen ingredients is that they break down after several hours of exposure to sunlight, which means you need to reapply them often, exposing yourself to a host of preservatives, penetration enhancers, petrochemicals, and artificial fragrances. Even when broad-spectrum sunscreens (ones that provide protection from both UVA and UVB sun radiation) were introduced in the early 1990s, they failed to completely shield us from harmful doses of sun radiation. High SPF factor gives us a false sense of security. The logic is simply deceptive: if a lotion with SPF15 allows you to stay in the scorching sun fifteen times longer, then lotion with SPF50 would give a whopping fifty times more protection. Right? Wrong.

Sunblocks are physically blocking sun rays. Also called mineral sunscreens, sunblocks include zinc oxide and titanium dioxide. They are highly effective in protecting against both UVA and UVB rays. They do not require any complex chemical cocktails to make them safe and effective, so they can be used in completely green and natural sun protective creams and lotions that are more suitable for children than deeply penetrating sunscreens. The only drawback is that sunblocks often appear white on the skin, however, the newest micronized forms of zinc oxide blend well into skin and appear to be invisible.

But let's go back to sunscreens since they are much more popular than sunblocks. So, what do we get with a conventional sunscreen—freshly scented, easily absorbed, packed in a convenient bottle? We get a nice skin moisturizer and relatively effective protection from UV radiation.

Instead of allowing our skin to accommodate the increased sun exposure by thickening the epidermis and increasing pigmentation, we switch off these biological mechanisms by slathering on even more sunscreen. At the same time, we turn off the skin's ability to produce vitamin D that may offer additional protection from various types of cancer, including melanoma. "Sunscreen users may compensate for their sunscreen use by staying out much longer in the sun, or may use sunscreen lotions inconsistently," noted Martin A. Weinstock, MD, PhD, director of the Photomedicine Unit of Brown Medical School Department of Dermatology, Rhode Island, noting that we may "require another decade or more of experience with sunscreen use" before we would know how sunscreen works against skin cancer.

Only a few epidemiological studies have examined the relationship of sunscreen use and skin cancer, yet two studies suggest that sunscreens may not be effective in preventing it. Researchers from the University of Southern California in San Diego found that the use of common sunscreen formulations that absorb UVB almost completely, but do not block UVA rays, may contribute to the risk of melanoma in people who live in southern regions (Gorham et al. 2007).

Another study focused on the use of sunscreens and the amount of skin hyperpigmentation in children. Dermatologists in Israel found that regular sunscreen use contributed to the risk of moles in children as young as seven years of age. Such moles can often evolve into melanoma, especially in people with fair skin and hair (Azizi et al. 2000). Scientists suggest that sometimes sunscreens can play a negative role in prevention of skin cancers because sunscreens suppress the natural warning signals of excessive sun exposure, while leaving the skin defenseless to the damaging UVA rays they do not block. Instead of cautious and sensible tanning, we heavily rely on SPF100 sunscreens and continue baking under the tropical sun for hours.

Another concern about sunscreens is their formulation. Most sunscreens appear to act as endocrine disruptors. During a 2001 study at the University of Zurich, some of the most popular sunscreens, including benzophenone, homosalate, methylbenzylidene camphor, methoxycinnamate, and octyl-dimethyl-para-aminobenzoic acid, showed estrogenic activity in animals (Schlumpf et al. 2001). Avid sunscreen proponents argue that animals in this study were fed sunscreens, and only a few received topical applications, so why should we worry? Humans don't eat sunscreens. Actually, sunscreen ingredients are able to penetrate the skin and enter our bloodstream. An earlier Swiss study has shown that benzophenone and methoxycinnamate can be found in dermis six hours after application (Chatelain et al. 2003), and a 2001 Australian study concluded that sunscreen chemicals are the most common cause of photoallergic contact dermatitis (Cook, Freeman 2001).

Let's not forget about our daily toxic burden due to an overabundance of carcinogenic chemicals in our food, cosmetics, and household products. Conventional sunscreen lotion is packed with petroleum-derived emollients, penetration enhancers, paraben and formaldehyde preservatives, and synthetic dyes and fragrances. Heat, rubbing, and perspiration drive these ingredients deeper into the skin. Generous use of toxic sunscreen and other skin care products could be another reason why the rates of cancers have skyrocketed in the past few years.

## On the Sunny Side

A decently formulated sunscreen is a very important step in your beauty regimen. As you already know, ultraviolet light provides us with vitamin D, but too much sun exposure can cause skin damage and melanoma. Different wavelengths of ultraviolet light penetrate the skin at different depths, causing varying levels of damage. Therefore, a good sunscreen should protect us from all types of the sun's rays, but should not be irritating or toxic, of course.

Spend a minute reading the ingredients label and avoid harsh chemical ingredients. These include para-aminobenzoic acid (PABA), benzophenones (benzophenone-3 and oxybenzone), cinnamates (octyl methoxycinnamate and methoxycinnamate), and salicylates (such as octyl salicylate).

Finding truly natural sun care products must be high on the organic shopper's priority list. This is easier said than done because many sunscreen products that are advertised as "natural" actually contain the same active chemical ingredients as mainstream brands. Chemical sunscreens, which absorb light, are popular because they are lightweight and penetrate quickly. However, their ability to trigger allergies and irritation is supercharged by sitting in the sun. Another downside of chemical ingredients is that they are not photostable and start breaking down when they have been exposed to the sun.

## What to Look for in a Sunscreen

To begin with, a good sunscreen should contain active ingredients that protect us from all types of sun radiation. Until now, most sunscreen products sold in the United States focused on blocking UVB rays. Newer substances, such as Mexoryl (also called ecamsule; chemical name terephthalylidene dicamphor sulfonic acid), provide efficient UVA protection, and they are more stable under the sun's rays. Sunscreens containing Mexoryl are widely used in Europe and Canada. In 2006, the U.S. Food and Drug Administration approved it for use in U.S. cosmetic products. Unfortunately, Mexoryl is exclusive to L'Oreal, and we have yet to see a truly green beauty product coming from under the French beauty giant's wing. Mexoryl is usually paired with potentially carcinogenic triethanolamine to keep the pH of the product in balance. To keep the formulation stable, large concentrations of paraben preservatives are also used.

Green beauty embraces mineral, physical sunblocks. Wearing a mineral sunscreen is like wearing thousands of tiny mirrors on the skin that reflect the sun's rays. They sit on top of the skin and are less irritating than sunscreens. Mineral sunscreens include zinc oxide and titanium oxide. Both minerals have a wider spectral range of activity than any synthetic sunscreen ingredients. While the entire range of UVA and UVB radiation is 280 to 400 nm, titanium dioxide's range of protection is 270 to 700 nm, and zinc dioxide shields from rays ranging from 290 to 700 nm.

Cosmetic chemists often combine mineral UV filters with DNA-repairing agents, offering better protection from photoaging. Throughout history, people have used avocado, olive, nut, and seed oils for skin protection. Natural oils contain essential fatty acids that can restore the pliability and elasticity to coarse, sun-drenched skin and thus partially offset harmful effects of excessive sun exposure, but they cannot reverse photoaging and protect you from skin cancer.

To avoid layering two products every morning, opt for a tinted moisturizer with built-in sunscreen. "SPF-containing tinted moisturizers have multiple benefits in one," says Karen Behnke, the founder of Juice Beauty. "They offer SPF15 or even SPF30 coverage, they are the ultimate moisturizers rich in antioxidants such as pomegranate juice, and they are mineral tinted for light coverage." Karen uses only organic juices in her formulations because organic juices are richer in antioxidants, and nutritional science supports her beliefs. In a 2004 study of organic and conventionally grown tomatoes, Alyson Mitchell, a food chemist at University of California at Davis, found that organic tomatoes had higher levels of vitamin C, while significantly higher levels of the cancer-protective flavonoids were found in organic broccoli.

Sunblocks should become part of multilayered sun protection that includes lightweight, tightly woven clothes made of cotton or linen, wide-brimmed hats, and an antioxidant-rich diet. Cover up more diligently if you have fair skin, red or blond hair, or lots of freckles.

## What About Tanning Oils?

Tanning oils or creams are slowly but steadily going out of fashion. In terms of sun protection, tanning oils are a joke. Favored by sun worshippers who prefer to coat their skin in some exotic oil instead of sunscreen because they like the softness and possible (more often, imaginary) anti-aging benefits, tanning oils rarely deliver on their promises. I believe that avid tanners like oils for their alluring glow on skin. "A tan protects me from the sun," my perennially tanned mom used to say, until last year, when she sheepishly asked me to choose a few strong sunscreens because she "developed a sun allergy." Most likely, her skin, exhausted by decades of relentless baking, just couldn't take any more. Now my mom gets her moles checked yearly and slathers on sunscreen diligently, rain or shine.

Often tanning oils contain beta-carotene, a naturally occurring form of vitamin A that offers antiaging benefits and in high doses adds a yellowish tint to the skin (and stains clothes and towels like crazy). Another popular additive to tanning oil is tyrosine, an amino acid found in large quantities in milk protein. Tyrosine is the precursor to the pigment melanin, and many makers of tanning oils, tanning accelerators, and tanning pills believe that tyrosine can stimulate melanocytes to produce more pigment. At this moment, there are no studies that can support this notion, and I believe that scientists can find much better ways to spend their grants than finding out whether or not tyrosine tanning oil helps some reckless tanners achieve their chocolate goals sooner.

## Sun in a Bottle: Not Too Safe Either

Self-tanning products have been around in one form or another since the invention of cosmetics. In 1960, Coppertone introduced its first sunless tanning product, Quick Tanning Lotion, which was so orange it instantly became a joke. Today's sunless tanning products produce much more realistic-looking results. Sunless spray tanning or self-tanning lotions and sprays can imitate a subtle bronze glow or a deep, dark tan. Self-tanners are the choice of many top models who are too blond and too smart to bake under the Riviera sun. Many fashion designers and stylists send their models to spray tanning booths or hire estheticians to rub self-tanners on their skin as they make final fittings before a big show.

But self-tanners aren't all that safe. Virtually all conventional and green self-tanners are made with dihydroxyacetone (DHA). Does that sound similar to acetone, that infamous, toxic nail polish remover? No wonder. They are cousins. When applied to the skin, dihydroxyacetone oxidizes and injects the top skin layer with a brownish color that sheds off in five to six days.

Sounds pretty safe, doesn't it? It's something like a long-wearing blusher for skin. But when I tried to impart some color into my pregnancy-stricken, milky-pale face with a perfectly natural DHA-based self-tanner from a well-known green German brand, I did some research aimed for pregnant women. The British hub for new mums at iVillage.co.uk revealed that dihydroxyacetone is not recommended for pregnant women because there were no studies that confirmed its safety. Concerned, I dug deeper, and here's what I found: dihydroxyacetone generates free radicals during UV exposure. A German study conducted in October 2007 found that DHA-treated skin was attacked by 180 percent more free radicals during sun exposure compared to untreated skin (Jung et al. 2007). In plain English, self-tanners actively promote skin aging. Needless to say, I passed on that self-tanner.

But what's a pale girl to do? Long live the bronzer. These pretty, shimmery powders yield immediate results and are easy to apply. When choosing a bronzing cream or a powder, steer clear of talc-based versions, for talc is not the safest cosmetic ingredient. Some studies link cosmetic use of talc to ovarian cancer, but the results are inconclusive (Langseth et al. 2008). Earlier, scientists voiced concerns that some cosmetic talcs may be contaminated with asbestos (Blount 1991). So if you prefer to err on the side of caution, look for titanium oxide–based bronzers that contain some mica and iron oxides for coloring. You can blend some mineral or cream bronzer with your body oil or SPF-rated sunscreen lotion and achieve a pretty glow that is healthy, too.

I know it's hard to ditch the idea that sun in a bottle is the safest way to get a tan. So here's a truly safe self-tanner recipe my mom honed as she started spending more and more time away from the sun and under an umbrella. This recipe takes more time than all the other recipes in this book combined (three months to soak the walnuts!), but the wait is worth the results. This oil contains iodine from walnut shells, so it may not be suitable for people with thyroid disorders.

## Golden Shimmer Nut Tanner

1 cup green walnut husks or young walnut shells

1 cup organic virgin olive oil

2 tea bags of organic green tea

2 tablespoons coconut butter

120 mg (3 capsules) vitamin E

10 drops beta-carotene

1 teaspoon Bare Escentuals Precious Diamond Face and Body Color

Yield: 4 ounces

1. Pour the oil over the walnut husks or shells, place in an airtight jar, and let stand in a warm place exposed to sunlight for about three months.

2. When the three months is up, pour the mixture into a small coffee press to divide the husks from the oil.

3. Meanwhile, steep the green tea in very hot water for 10 minutes. Cover the cup to prevent beneficial green tea antioxidants from escaping with the steam. When the tea is deep golden in color, remove the tea bags.

4. Melt coconut butter in a shallow stainless steel pan.

5. Add the pressed (deep brown) olive oil, steeped green tea, vitamin E, and beta-carotene. Briskly whisk to combine all the ingredients.

6. Now add the mineral shimmer, and your tanner is ready. Pour it into a nice pump bottle and apply sparingly. It won't stain your clothes or sheets, and the glow is unbelievable! The tint stays for up to four days, if you don't apply a body scrub.

# Smart Tanning (Yes, It Can Be Done)

For those who choose to tan, dermatologists recommend the following preventative measures.

*Choose a broad-spectrum mineral sunscreen.* Once in my lifetime, I had to face the fierce sun in southern France after a glycolic acid peel. While I usually rely on old-fashioned zinc oxide, to avoid uneven pigmentation I applied a layer cake of sunscreens: an organic zinc oxide baby sunscreen as a moisturizer and a Mexoryl-containing (yes, not quite organic, but water-soluble) product on top. This way, the sunscreens joined forces, and even though Mexoryl didn't penetrate my skin thanks to the highly occlusive, greasy baby sunscreen, my skin remained cool, blemish-free, and interestingly pale under the merciless July sun.

*Apply sunscreen generously.* To enjoy this process, pick a product that is a pleasure to use. Profit-oriented cosmetic manufacturers and dermatologists have routinely promoted a heavy application of chemical sunscreens for skin cancer prevention. This has not been proven by laboratory tests or epidemiological studies, yet common sense tells us that sun protection creams need to be applied frequently to make a difference. The sunblock must not disappear in the skin like a good foundation. A walnut-size blob may be enough to cover one arm; a hazelnut-size blob is sufficient for the face. If you are unsure of how much product to use or you plan to spend a lot of time in the open sun, use a product with minimum SPF30.

Reapply sunscreen every two to three hours and after swimming or sweating. When playing sports, and for babies splashing in the pool, the sunscreen should also be water-resistant. Waterproof sunscreen doesn't exist in nature. According to FDA, sunscreens are neither sweatproof nor waterproof. Most sunscreen formulations don't dissolve in water or sweat, but can be washed off or rubbed off during swimming and other sport activities. Thus, FDA insists that no sunscreen, green or synthetic, can be marketed as waterproof, and that cosmetic manufacturers can label their products only as water-resistant or sweat-resistant.

Famous brands of sunscreens claim to protect your skin from UVA and UVB radiation, but the actual products do little to protect against the longer waves of UVA rays. Sunscreen alone does not completely prevent skin cancers such as melanoma, because harmful types of sun rays can cause DNA damage without actually burning the skin. Not a single sunblock or sunscreen can completely shield you from the harmful effects of sun radiation. Protective clothing made of natural, breathable fabrics, wide-brimmed hats, beach parasols, and common sense are your most reliable allies against premature skin aging. Avoid sunbathing between 10 AM and 4 PM. Keep babies away from the sun during this time, too.

Remember that the sun's rays are stronger at higher elevations and near the equator. Here's a trick: check your shadow length. If your shadow is shorter than your actual height, the risk of sunburn is much higher. Be aware that reflective surfaces like snow and water can greatly increase the amount of UV radiation to which the skin is exposed.

According to the Skin Cancer Foundation, more than 1.5 million skin cancers are diagnosed in the U.S. each year. Don't become part of this sad statistic. Not a single sunscreen or sunblock, natural or chemical, allows you to bake in the sun for hours.

## Strengthen Your Skin's Defenses

We receive a major dose of sun radiation from our daily exposure to the sun, rather than at the beach where we are more likely to use sunscreens. Human skin has a built-in mechanism for sun protection, but an abundance of hormone-disrupting and toxic chemicals in the environment, a weak immune system, a less-than-perfect diet, and stress join forces to undermine our skin's natural ability to protect itself from the elements, including sun radiation. Here's how you can give your skin a helping hand.

If you choose to add just one natural antioxidant to your diet and skin care routine, make it green tea. Studies show that an antioxidant in green tea, a polyphenol called epigallocatechin gallate (EGCG), may prevent DNA damage from ultraviolet radiation (Morley et al. 2005). Human trials showed that green tea offered some protection from sun radiation even when volunteers drank it and then were exposed to twelve minutes of ultraviolet A radiation. Make sure you drink lots of iced green tea during the summer, and I believe that if you add a concentrated extract of epigallocatechin gallate to your sun protective moisturizer, the effect could be even greater. Powdered epigallocatechin gallate is available online.

Virtually all plants and animals protect themselves from the sun using vitamins C and E. A stable aqueous solution of 15 percent L-ascorbic acid (vitamin C) and 1 percent alpha-tocopherol (vitamin E) can provide significant protection against sunburn by warding off free radicals. Scientists say that either L-ascorbic acid or 1 percent alpha-tocopherol alone is also protective, but a combination works much better (Lin et al. 2003). Consistent use for at least four days produced even better protection from photoaging. Many sunscreen products contain vitamins C and E in their formulations.

One of nature's most potent sun protectors is edelweiss. This precious flower protects itself from the intense sun at the tops of mountains thanks to carotenoids and vitamin E, which help this summer-flowering alpine herb survive exposure to intense UV radiation. "Edelweiss is useful in protecting human skin, too," says Roger Barsby of Weleda. "Active compounds in the plant alleviate irritation and help prevent premature aging and wrinkling, as well as protect blood vessels and so impeding fine thread veins. Edelweiss extract contains powerful free-radical scavengers, which bind the free radicals and render them ineffective." Weleda's sunscreens contain organic edelweiss extract blended with carrot and light sesame oil, which are also valued for their UV-filtering properties.

As effective as vitamins C and E already are, their performance really shines when ferulic acid, another powerful plant antioxidant, steps in. When ferulic acid works in synergy with vitamins C and E, the skin receives eight times more protection from sunburns and skin cancer. This antioxidant formulation also greatly reduces damage of skin cell DNA (Lin et al. 2005).

Carotenoids are natural pigments that protect us from sun radiation by scavenging free radicals. Studies show that a carotenoid-rich diet is very efficient in sun protection, and eating foods rich in lutein, zeaxanthin, alpha-carotene, beta-carotene, and lycopene can significantly lower your chances of getting a sunburn (Stahl, Sies 2005). A 2004 German study found that treatment with carotenoids is needed for a period of at least ten weeks, and increased consumption of carotenoids in tomatoes, spinach, broccoli, zucchini, and, of course, carrots, may contribute to lifelong protection against UV-induced damage (Sies, Stahl 2004). Pure lutein and beta-carotene are also available as food supplements.

# Green Product Guide: Sunscreens

Exposure to sunlight has always been a natural part of life, and even though the ozone layer is diminishing, there is no reason to avoid sunshine. Just be careful and use a natural mineral sunscreen. Common sense tells us that too much of anything is unhealthy, so use your judgment when outdoors. The following are my recommended sunscreens, rated from one to three leaves, with three being my favorite.

🍃 **Lavera SPF30 Baby and Child Sun Spray** can be used by the whole family. Fine zinc oxide and titanium dioxide do not leave a whitish cast on skin, and the smell is fresh and summery but not too noticeable. Fatty acids from certified organic ingredients moisturize and ensure even application. The spray bottle allows adding antioxidants such as green tea extract, vitamin E, and a few drops of eucalyptus oil for bug repelling purposes. The only drawback is the presence of alumina in the formulation: I have mixed feelings about aluminum in any form in my skin care products.

🍃🍃 **Juice Organics SPF30 Light Tint Moisturizer** is the only product I need on a summer morning. A formula with titanium dioxide sits on my skin nicely, while a load of antioxidant plant extracts (white grape, pomegranate, aloe, apple, cucumber, green tea) join forces with serious skin soothers and plumpers like vitamin C, E, and B5; allantoin; and hyaluronic acid. It contains no paraben preservatives or synthetic dyes, but does have essential oil fragrance, which may be irritating to sensitive skin.

🍃🍃🍃 **Dr. Hauschka Sunscreen Cream SPF30** is an extremely green and versatile product, and the only sunscreen we use in our family. And as with any family member, we have learned how to live with its shortcomings. Shortcomings? Any mineral sunscreen may leave a whitish cast if you apply it thickly or frequently. Newer, micronized zinc sunscreens are not as heavy and may not leave a white film. Any mineral may cause you to break out (if you can't stand zinc oxide, try titanium oxide, and vice versa). Spread it well and top it off with mineral foundation powder to set it up.

## Final Thought

There's just one reliable formula for sunscreen, and I found it in *Alive* magazine. All the rest are variations, and mine is no exception. You can easily tailor it to your skin's needs: greasier skins should use sweet almond oil alone; sensitive types will be better off with a drop of chamomile oil instead. Please note that chamomile is mildly lightening, so use with caution. Mature, drier skins would benefit from a drop or three of rose hip or evening primrose oil in addition to sweet almond oil.

## Skin-feeding Sunscreen

3 ounces sesame oil

2 ounces sweet almond oil

½ ounce pure beeswax

4 ounces distilled water

2 tablespoons zinc oxide

*Optional:*

  5 drops rose hip oil

  5 drops chamomile essential oil

  5 drops evening primrose oil

**Yield:** 4 ounces

1. Melt the sesame and sweet almond oils and beeswax in a double boiler over medium heat.

2. Remove from the heat, add the water, and blend with a stick blender until uniform.

3. Allow the mixture to cool. Add the zinc oxide and other essential oils of your choice, if using. Blend some more.

4. Transfer the mixture into a glass jar. You can store this sunscreen cream for up to six months.

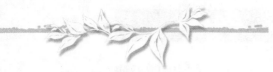

"Natural beauty to me is loving acceptance and celebration of who you are as an individual. When you have that loving acceptance and celebrate your life, it leads to sustainable choices that support yourself, the community, and the earth. Natural beauty is a woman going in her own unique, beautiful way."

—Susan West Kurtz,
President of Hauschka Skincare

I think it's unhealthy to treat the sun as an enemy. The sun has always been with us and is involved in delicate, complex mechanisms in our bodies. By artificially blocking the sun, we may be shutting down more than vitamin D production. It's just not natural.

All of nature's gifts can become poisonous when overdone. Take red wine. If you drink one small glass a day, red wine provides cancer-fighting chemicals and may protect against heart disease. If you drink a bottle of red wine a day, you are damaging your liver and increasing your risk of certain cancers. Another example is olive oil. When you pour a tablespoon over your green salad, you are reaping the goodness of antioxidants and skin-benefiting fatty acids. But when you load everything with oil, you will likely soon gain weight, become obese, and suffer the dreadful health consequences that come with excess weight, from diabetes to cancer. Moderation is the key, whether you are dealing with red wine, olive oil, or the sun.

*chapter* **11**

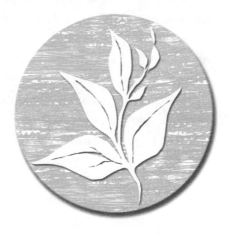

*green* **body**
**care**

Call it body discrimination, but not all areas of our skin receive the same attention. Smooth, dewy skin epitomizes youth, beauty, and health, yet many of us concentrate our efforts on the skin from the neck up. We would happily spend ten minutes washing, scrubbing, and nurturing our face and styling our hair, but all we do for the major portion of our skin—that is, the skin covering our arms, legs, and torso—is slapping on some moisturizer, with some occasional scrubbing with a loofah or exfoliating shower cream.

To truly pamper yourself, you should give as much thought to your body care as you do to your face. There is absolutely no excuse for you to neglect any part of your body: in health food stores, drugstores, and glittering counters of department stores, not to mention online, you will find a scrub, toner, and lotion for every nook and cranny. But how much thought do we put into buying them? Do we buy them for real results, or are we swayed by the airbrushed advertising? As you read the next few pages, you will learn how to choose the best products to use during a shower, a soothing and relaxing bath, cellulite massage treatments, hair removal, and nail care sessions, and they should be part of your green beauty routine.

Body care products are perhaps the most populated area of the green beauty industry. On a good day in Whole Foods Market or in your local health food store, you will find shower gels and soaps in every imaginable scent, and endless varieties of body lotions, scrubs, and massage oils. These days, many spas are offering toluene- and formaldehyde-free manicures and organic wax hair removals. Many conventional cosmetic manufacturers are reformulating their body products, removing sodium laureth/lauryl sulfates, ethoxylated ingredients, and synthetic fragrances. Sadly, the makers of many "natural" beauty products too often cut corners by adding chemical junk to their products. We gladly buy them to soak, scrub, moisturize, fight unsightly dimples, and wash away our emotional woes. So how do you make informed decisions and buy green beauty products that truly deliver results? Read on!

# Green Shower

Body cleansers, no matter if they are packed in an elegant glass bottle or a minimalist tube made of corn, all function in a very simple way. They cleanse the skin using surfactants, chemicals that lift up the oil, dead skin cells, and daily body grime, and then mix with water and wash away. Some cleansers leave a faint layer of oil on the skin. Some have antibacterial properties. Some contain vitamins, amino acids, fruit acids, plant extracts, and exfoliating granules. All these ingredients may offer excellent benefits in a face or body lotion, but they have little chance to make any difference when used in a body wash. They are simply washed off too quickly. All you want to pay for in a body wash, green or not, is a surfactant mix and some gentle emollients. Save your money for a decent body moisturizer, and let the body wash do its job, which is cleansing your body.

A green cleanser should use plant-derived cleansing agents, derived from olives, coconuts, or sugar beets without the use of sulfates. Many so-called natural shower gels still use sodium myreth sulfate and lauramide MEA (JASON Organics), sodium laureth sulfate (Bain de-luxe, Korres Natural Products), sodium lauryl sulfate, cocoamide MEA, paraben preservatives (Kiss My Face), or polyethylene glycols and tromethamine (Nature's Gate Organics) and therefore cannot be recommended due to their contamination with the carcinogen 1,4-Dioxane (refer to Chapter 2). To "offset" the use of toxic and irritating detergents, many "organic" manufacturers stuff their shower gels with plant extracts, which are of little use because they are quickly washed off.

# Green Cleansing 101

All cleansing products, whether they are meant for use on the face, body, or hair, are based on one of three types of cleansing agents: detergents, soaps, or saponins.

*Detergents* are the most ubiquitous type of cleansers. Essentially, all soaps work as detergents because they all allow oil and water to mix so that oily grime can be removed during rinsing. But in the cosmetic industry, detergents refer to anionic and nonionic surfactants: one side of a molecule prefers water (hydrophilic) and another side prefers oils and fats (hydrophobic). The hydrophilic side attaches to water molecules, and the hydrophobic side attaches to oil molecules, allowing them to be washed away. Detergents include *nonionic surfactants* like polyethylene glycol esters (PEGs), *anionic surfactants* ammonium laureth or lauryl sulfate and sodium laureth or lauryl sulfate, and gentler yet still derived from petrochemicals *amphoteric* surfactants such as cocoamidopropyl betaine and lauryl glucoside.

Natural plant *soaps* are made by saponifying olive, jojoba, or coconut oils with an alkali (potassium hydroxide, sodium hydroxide, wood ashes, or the ashes of other plants). Soaps are classified as anionic surfactants. While there are many wonderfully informative books on soap making, I've never ventured into cooking my own soap at home because I prefer the convenience of certified organic, ready-made castile soap base. For my own cosmetic products, I use liquid soap made of certified organic olive oil.

*Saponins* are plant glycosides that derive their name from their soap-like properties. They occur in a great many plant species, including soap-wort (*Saponaria officinalis*), soap lily (*Chlorogalum pomeridianum*), and soap berry tree (*Sapindus mukorossi*), whose dried nuts make a wonderful all-natural laundry detergent.

Personally, I feel that my skin is cleanest after bar soap. Your bar cleanser shouldn't be the typical, heavy-scented, animal tallow–based bar soap that is blasted by all beauty experts. Plant-based, naturally scented bar soaps are very effective body cleansers. On the downside, soap bars tend to get slushy when left in a shower for long, so if you buy a good olive bar soap or receive a fancy box of exotic soaps as a gift, keep them out of steamy showers and treat them to a nice soap dish. I once spent untold money on an elegant plastic designer container for a soap (okay, it was Chanel) and then used it for my humble organic glycerin bar. Finding a really good soap dish with a lid is not that easy, but you can find a real jewel on Ebay or in a local thrift store.

## Green Product Guide: Shower Gels

Trying to concoct a shower gel at the kitchen sink is just not worth the effort. Here are some really good body cleansers to consider. As always, those with three leaves are my favorite.

☞ **Tom's of Maine Natural Moisturizing Body Wash** is one of the few truly green products from this mainstay of health food stores. This basic, no-nonsense body cleanser is very gentle and soothing and not overly moisturizing—just right for summertime use. The light scent makes this shower gel a good choice if you are sensitive to essential oil fragrances. It is reasonably priced, too.

☞ **Dr. Hauschka Rose Body Wash** is a rich, creamy shower gel with a relaxing, sensual aroma of jasmine, lilac, and rose. It's very good for use in wintertime thanks to its highly emollient base of nonsulfate surfactants, jojoba oil, shea butter, and soothing propolis. However, it may not be suitable for sensitive skins because of the high content of essential oils, and the price is a little steep for a tube that is usually finished in ten days.

☞ ☞ ☞ **Pangea Organics shower gels** are some of the few body cleansers out there that are true to their organic claims. Formulated with saponified organic oils, aloe vera, vegetable glycerin, and a dozen plant extracts, including lavender, calendula, gotu cola, linden flower, and red clover, these thick, rich shower gels last a really long time, helping you save money by buying less.

☞ ☞ ☞ If you want to start your green beauty routine with just one natural product, make it a generously sized bottle of **Dr. Bronner's 18-in-1 Pure-Castile Hemp Baby Mild Soap**. Very concentrated, very natural (nothing but water, coconut soap, olive oil, hemp, and vitamin E with some citric acid as a preservative), this cleanser can be used in tons of different ways: when diluted, it makes a good gentle shampoo, body wash, mouth rinse, diaper soak, baby laundry detergent, and even a baby bath.

## Green and White: Basics of Natural Tooth Care

If you decided to go organic because you care about your health, you may decide to put natural tooth care products close to the top of your list. Some parts of the body, including the gums, are more absorbent than others, making it easier for chemicals to pass into the bloodstream, which is another reason your tooth care should be as healthy, natural, and chemical-free as the food you eat.

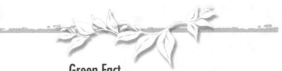

## Green Fact

Many natural toothpastes are made of ingredients that are good enough to eat, which, if you're using it in your mouth, makes perfect sense, since we swallow nearly a whole tube of toothpaste in one year.

While claiming to create healthier, brighter smiles, many types of toothpaste are a long way from pure and natural. Here are some chemicals you should avoid in your tooth care products.

Fluoride. Many experts claim fluoride helps fight decay, yet this chemical has also been linked to many adverse effects, including cancer. Fluoride was found to actually increase teeth and bone decay by causing a condition called dental fluorosis, says a study done by the School of Public Health of the University of Michigan (Heller et al. 1997). A 2008 study by French researchers confirms the findings and explains that elevated fluoride intake causes fluorosis by triggering DNA changes (Wurtz et al. 2008). Scientists of Harvard School of Dental Medicine found "an association between fluoride exposure in drinking water during childhood and the incidence of osteosarcoma among males" (Bassin et al. 2006). Polish scientists in February 2008 found that fluoride greatly diminished the protective abilities of kidneys in animals (Blaszczyk et al. 2008). It seems that fluoride also has an adverse impact on our hormonal system. Scientists at the National Center for Toxicological Research reported a close correlation between decreasing fertility rates in women and increasing fluoride levels (Freni 1994). Last but not least, fluoride appears to increase the lead content in our bodies. In 2007, U.S. researchers found that children living in communities with fluoridated water have elevated blood lead, which may be explained by corrosion of lead-containing plumbing by fluoride chemicals in water (Coplan et al. 2007). I think that just one of the above reasons is enough to reconsider the use of a fluoride-loaded toothpaste and adopting a less sugary diet to avoid tooth decay.

Sodium Laureth Sulfate. Many so-called natural types of toothpaste still use this harsh detergent to make the product foam lavishly. However, we already know that sulfate-based detergents are strong irritants and should never be ingested, even in small amounts.

Hydrogen Peroxide. This potent bleach in the form of carbamide peroxide is frequently used in whitening gels and strips in concentrations of up to 6 percent. This popular whitening agent is not currently thought to cause mouth cancer in humans, but toxicologists from São Paulo State

University in Brazil concluded in 2006 that "dental bleaching agents may be a factor that increases the level of DNA damage" in vitro (Ribeiro et al. 2006). To date, science knows that while carbamide peroxide removes surface stains, it attacks both organic and mineral components of dentin, causing irreversible changes in the mineral components of teeth. Besides, it can be toxic when eaten or accidentally swallowed. The National Poisons Information Service in the United Kingdom says that swallowing of hydrogen peroxide in concentrations similar to those during professional tooth whitening "may cause irritation of the gastrointestinal tract with nausea, vomiting. . . . Painful gastric distension and belching may be caused by the liberation of large volumes of oxygen in the stomach" (Watt et al. 2004). Stomach troubles were also recorded in a study when animals swallowed a commercially available 6 percent hydrogen peroxide whitener (Redmond et al. 1997). So if you choose to brighten up your smile a bit, do it under a doctor's supervision and make sure not to swallow any of the bleach.

Saccharin (sodium saccharin). This artificial sweetener is used in toothpastes to make them more palatable. Yet studies dating back to the 1970s have linked saccharin to cancer in animals (Bryan et al. 1970). Results of these studies were labeled as irrelevant to humans. Debates about the safety of saccharin are still ongoing, and science has not yet provided clear enough evidence of a lack of association between saccharin and cancer in people. One of the recent human studies on saccharin involved the whole state of Lucknow, India, where children have such a sweet tooth they ate up to three times the recommended amounts of saccharin in candies, ice cream, and desserts. After observation of children between six and ten years of age, scientists found that they "may be susceptible to the toxic effects of saccharin, including bladder distention, elevated urine osmolality and bladder cancer" (Tripathi et al. 2006). That same year, a study done by oncologists of University of Leicester in the United Kingdom showed that saccharin, along with acesulfame K in carbonated drinks, triggers overactive bladder symptoms (Dasgupta et al. 2006). Yes, that doesn't scare quite the same as bladder cancer, but if there are other options available, why risk it? Who knows what will studies show in five years?

My advice remains simple: don't be fooled by the word "natural" on the toothpaste's label. Many popular "natural" types of toothpaste contain FD&C dyes, propylene glycol, aluminum, and other potential contaminants that we discussed in Chapter 2, "Beauty and the Toxic Beast."

So, do green toothpastes exist? And if they do, do they taste awful, foam even worse, and feel like chalk in the mouth? Not really. To gently polish away stains, green toothpastes use silica, baking soda, and mineral calcium carbonate. To leave the mouth fresh, nothing beats good old peppermint. To soothe gums, green toothpastes use sea salt, aloe vera, and chamomile.

To make green toothpastes even sweeter, xylitol, a "tooth friendly" sugar replacement, is added. Unlike most artificial sweeteners, xylitol can be extracted from corn, birch, raspberries, and plums, and studies show that it not only strengthens teeth enamel, but also wards off yeast and bacteria (Edgar 1998). To ease symptoms of canker sores, many toothpastes are now sodium laureth sulfate-free, with added licorice and aloe. Other excellent green soothers for canker sores include cloves and myrrh, available in toothpastes by Green People and Tom's of Maine.

Finding pure, nontoxic toothpaste is easier than you think. JASON Natural Cosmetics PowerSmile is a brilliant whitening toothpaste without any synthetic junk in it, and Dr. Hauschka Lemon & Salt Toothpaste is suitable for sensitive teeth or bleeding gums—there's no menthol or peppermint in it. Would you like to whiten those choppers but hate to swallow bleach? Try rubbing your teeth with strawberries (rinse off quickly to avoid enamel decay!) or brush them with a baking soda and salt mixture. Some people believe that gargling with diluted hydrogen peroxide helps to bleach teeth, but be extra careful not to overdo it. As we learned earlier, swallowing even weak solution of hydrogen peroxide can seriously irritate your stomach.

## Green Bath Time

Taking a bath is probably the most indulgent beauty treatment. A tranquil, carefully prepared bath can do wonders for your mood and your skin's health. I denied myself long bath soaks during my whole pregnancy, and what a torture it was! I loved being pregnant, but the bath ban was very hard to tolerate.

Physiologically, the relaxing effects of soaking in water are easy to understand: warm water suspends your weight, making you feel lighter, and thus helping to relax the muscles. As your blood vessels dilate from

  **the green beauty guide**

the warmth, your blood pressure drops. Warm water can relax sore and tired joints and release tension. The warm cocoon feels like a womb, making you feel safe and secure. While showers can be called the skin's fast food, a warm bath is definitely on top of the skin's comfort foods.

The less expensive your bath product is, the better. One-half cup of olive, sweet almond, or grape seed oil is much better for your skin than a glittering, bubbling bath bomb made of skin-drying chemicals and synthetic fragrances. Rose and orange water, Epsom salt, apple cider vinegar, whole-fat milk, lemon and orange juices, green tea bags—all these kitchen staples can be put to use.

## Green Bath Aromatherapy

It couldn't be easier to go green when you bathe. Instead of detergent-based bath foams, switch to plain milk, salts, and fragrant oils. Oils will protect skin from dehydration, because long, hot soaks in the bath or showers can strip natural moisturizing oils from your skin. You can buy premixed bath oil blends based on pure vegetable oils and essential oils. Make sure to check the label for preservatives and avoid mineral oil, which will wrap your skin in a waterproof film and obstruct your skin's perspiration.

**Green Tip**

Carefully concocted oil compositions may help improve your mood while nourishing your skin as you soak.

By carefully blending gentle essential oils, you can supercharge your bathing ritual. You can create wonderfully inexpensive and 100 percent green bath salts by adding blends of essential oils to Epsom or Dead Sea salts, which are especially good if you have psoriasis or seborrhea.

Sometimes essential oils in your bath can do more harm than good to your skin. The strong fragrance components can easily irritate your skin, especially in the vaginal area, so your carefully planned bath experience may end with itching and soreness. Among the safer essential oils used in bath oils and milks are lavender, sandalwood, chamomile, spruce, and rose, while citrus oils, as well as jasmine, bergamot, and sage have more irritation potential. Plant extracts and infusions can be used instead of oils.

Here are some classic recipes for delightful bath treatments with a green twist. Enjoy them, treat your family to them, and pack them in pretty jars to give to friends. I recommend storing bath salts in clay spice jars or clear glass jars with spring lids. Plastic is more practical, but many types of plastic can release chemicals, especially when in contact with the volatile compounds in essential oils.

*Please note:* Whenever you use essential oils, keep them out of the reach of children. Most essential oils are poisonous if ingested, even in small quantities.

## Cleopatra Milk Bath

1 cup organic reconstituted or condensed milk

2 tablespoons honey

2 drops vanilla extract

1 drop chamomile essential oil

1 drop lavender essential oil

**Yield: 4 ounces**

*You can use whole milk straight from the carton in this recipe, and any baby formula works as well.*

Blend the ingredients well and use immediately to create a soothing, deeply moisturizing balmy bath.

## Green Tibet Bath Salt

1 cup grape seed oil

1 cup green tea

1 tablespoon baking soda

½ cup Epsom salt

1 drop lavender essential oil

1 drop frankincense essential oil

**Yield: 5 ounces**

*This bath salt recipe reminds me of a famous Tibetan green tea traditionally prepared with salt, butter, and baking soda. It will invigorate your senses and stimulate blood circulation. This bath salt will also soften the water.*

Mix all the ingredients in a bowl and store in your favorite jar. Add half-cup of the infusion to the running bathwater. To keep the essential oils from evaporating too quickly, you can add the bath salts just before getting into the tub. Sitting on undissolved bath salts can be uncomfortable (though nicely exfoliating for your bum), so make sure the salts have dissolved well before entering.

## Stress-Relieving Fruity Bath

1 cup virgin olive oil

1 drop rose essential oil

1 drop lavender essential oil

1 drop vetiver essential oil

2 drops mandarin essential oil

5 organic unwaxed oranges, cut into quarters

**Yield: 4 ounces**

1. Add the essential oils to the olive oil and pour the mixture under running water into the bathtub so that the oils spread evenly without forming greasy puddles.

2. Add the oranges and let them float around. As you bathe, squeeze the oranges lightly and wipe your face with their juices.

## Babassu Milk Bath Ritual

(courtesy of Anne Dolbeau, founder of Inara)

2 teaspoons full-fat milk powder or buttermilk powder

2 teaspoons sea salt

1 tablespoon (15 ml) of your favorite massage oil or any lightweight unscented oil of your choice

**Yield: 4 ounces**

Combine ingredients in a bowl and whisk. Be sure you use enough oil so that you thoroughly moisten the salt and the buttermilk or milk powder. Start your bath and pour the mixture directly into the running water. Get your bath to the desired temperature and enjoy!

## Making Your Own Herbal Bath Blends

Dried herbs, flower petals, and herbal teas make wonderful additions to your bath. You can use many herbs from your garden or buy them already dried from health food stores and online.

You can harvest your own leafy herbs in midsummer, just before they flower. After flowering starts, the oils in the leaves are not as potent. You'll want to harvest flowers when they are at their peak, in the middle of a dry day. Do not collect flowers when the air is damp or if they are covered in morning dew. To avoid damaging the petals, remove whole flowers with some of the stalk; discard any damaged petals. Put them in an open container; they may sweat and rot in a closed container.

To air-dry herbs and flowers, be guided by the plant. Lavender and sage may be used whole, with only roots and dry leaves removed; rose petals need to be carefully peeled off; sage, lemon balm (melissa), and thyme may be used with stems and all the leaves on the stalk, removing only roots; with chamomile and marigold, only florets can be used. Prepare the herbs, flowers, and petals by wiping off any moisture on the stems with paper towels. If drying flowers on stems, make bunches of five to ten stems, and secure them with an elastic band. Hang the bunches upside down in a dark, well-ventilated place at a temperature of about 68°F (20°C ) until they are dry. Dry whole florets and petals on an unbleached tissue paper or cotton towel in a cool, dry place away from direct sunlight. The drying time will vary from days to weeks. Store dried herbs and flowers in dark, airtight, clearly labeled glass jars.

You can also dry herbs in a conventional oven on low heat (no more than 200°F [100°C /Gas 1/2]), or even in a microwave oven. I do not recommend microwaving food, but you aren't going to eat bath blends, are you? To use a microwave oven, wrap chopped herbs loosely in a paper towel and cook them on high for a minute at a time. Place a cup of water in the microwave; herbs do not contain much moisture.

To prepare an herbal bath blend, crush the stems or chop the leaves and florets (such as those given in the recipes that follow) and mix thoroughly in a small bowl. To use, place the mixture in an unbleached muslin or organic cotton drawstring bag. These are easily found at herbal body care shops or online, and come in many different sizes. A good size to use for herbal bath mixtures is 3 inches by 4 inches (or 3 inches by 5 inches). In Chapter 13, you can also learn how to prepare herbal bath pouches for your baby. You can also boil an herbal blend in a small enamel pan, sieve off the herbs, and pour the mix into your bathwater.

## Winter Soothing Bath Blend

¼ cup dried chamomile flowers

1 cup dried lavender blossoms

1 cup dried fennel seeds

1 cup dried rose petals

**Yield: 4 ounces**

*This blend soothes dry, wind-blasted skin and aching muscles better than a Swedish massage session! Oat bran nourishes the skin, while rose petals add a warm, luxurious touch.*

The best way to use an herbal blend is to put it into a small, unbleached muslin (or organic cotton) bag and tie it with a ribbon or string. Just put the bag under running water as you prepare your bath. When you are done bathing, remove the bag, let it dry, then discard the contents and rinse the bag. It's ready to be used again!

## Bath Full of Joy Blend

1 cup dried lemongrass

2 cups dried lemon peel

¼ cup dried peppermint leaves

¼ cup loose green tea

¼ cup bay leaves

**Yield: 4 ounces**

*This bath blend has a very long shelf life. It also makes a great holiday stocking stuffer. Buy a handful of fabric drawstring gift bags (they are fabulously inexpensive!) and fill them with this fragrant blend. You can also use this blend as potpourri to add a fresh aroma to your lingerie drawers or wardrobe.*

## Skin Rejoice Bath Blend

1 cup Dead Sea salt

1 cup cornmeal

1 cup dried rose petals

½ cup hops flowers

½ cup dried chamomile flowers

½ cup dried calendula (marigold) flowers

**Yield: 4 ounces**

*This versatile bath blend can be used to soothe itchy skin, sunburns, and rashes. I used this blend to bathe my newborn daughter when she had a bit of a rash (I skipped the rose petals, though), and it seemed to work really well.*

# Green Scrubs and Peels

Skin exfoliation is very beneficial, no matter if you rub a creamy scrub, use mild acids, or simply brush your body with a loofah. Exfoliation helps unclog pores and improve circulation so that moisturizers and bath ingredients can penetrate better. It's good to dry brush (see Chapter 9) or briskly scrub your body before a therapeutic herbal bath. Keep in mind, though, that no scrub or peel can remove a single dimple from your thighs. Cellulite doesn't respond to physical exfoliation, although scrubbing can definitely help skin look smoother. Avoid scrubbing over blemishes, rashes, sunburn, or other skin irritations.

There are many wonderfully green products that effectively get rid of dead skin cells. Body scrubs are usually more coarse and thicker than facial scrubs because body skin can tolerate more aggressive friction. Good green scrubs contain plant waxes, oils, butters, and glycerin, and they exfoliate with crushed plant kernels, salt, sugar, nutshells, or seaweed. They usually contain ample amounts of essential oils, which may not benefit those of us who have sensitive skin. Topical products with alpha hydroxy acid (AHA) and salicylic acid may be an excellent option for the face, but I found that it's quite hard to control the application in a steamy shower.

I've tried dozens of body scrubs, from very expensive to very basic ones, and I believe that the only way to get a really good scrub is to cook it at home. Luckily, making a great body polish is easy, costs mere pennies, and all the ingredients are usually already in your kitchen.

## Making Your Own Body Polish

Here are some of my favorite body polish recipes. Most of them use sugar and other kitchen staples, so it is only natural to base them on our favorite dessert recipes. Use them, share them, make them in batches, and sell them, but please make sure to send me a thank-you note!

## Key Lime Body Scrub

2 small key limes

1 cup condensed milk

1 free-range egg yolk

1 cup brown sugar, preferably muscovado

**Yield: 4 ounces**

*This gentle AHA-based exfoliant makes a great whitening mask if left on to work for a few minutes. This scrub can be used on your face, too. Store it in the refrigerator for up to one week. If you plan to make a large batch of this Florida state-pie scrub, skip the egg yolk and add three drops of grapefruit seed extract.*

1. Squeeze the juice out of the limes and mix with the milk and egg yolk. Blend until thick.

2. Add sugar, but make sure it doesn't dissolve completely. Apply in circular motions using light pressure. As the sugar dissolves on your skin, it will become thinner, so there's little risk of scrubbing too hard.

## Oatmeal Cookie Scrub

½ cup baking soda (sodium bicarbonate)

½ cup steel-cut oat flakes

½ cup raw brown sugar

1 cup goat milk

½ cup jojoba or grape seed oil

**Yield: 4 ounces**

*This soft scrub combines two types of exfoliating granules: oil-absorbing oat flakes and mildly exfoliating baking soda.*

Blend all the ingredients well and store in the refrigerator in an airtight container for up to one week.

## Zesty Apple Rub

½ cup apple cider vinegar

½ cup fine Dead Sea salt or plain sea salt

½ cup almond meal

3 tablespoons applesauce

2 drops rosemary essential oil

1 drop lemon essential oil

3 drops grapefruit seed essential oil

**Yield: 5 ounces**

*This is a strong exfoliant. Save the original version for your feet, elbows, and knees, but if you dilute the mix with some honey or aloe vera juice, you can use it to exfoliate the rest of your body.*

Blend all the ingredients in a china bowl. Wet yourself thoroughly in the shower. Rub the scrub over your body using your hands. Rub in gentle circles, moving from your extremities toward your chest. Rinse the salt off thoroughly. You can store the scrub in the refrigerator in an airtight container for up to one month.

# Green Body Oils

The skin on our bodies has a surface area of around 1.5 to 2.0 square meters. This means that our exposure to harmful chemicals from a body cream will be much higher than from an eye serum. Luckily for us, there are many perfectly green, ready-made body moisturizers available at reasonable prices. Weleda, Dr. Hauschka, Avalon Organics, Burt's Bees, Lavera, and REN make wonderful body lotions, and Lavanila and Jo Wood Organics make luxurious aromatherapeutic fragrant body mists and oils for the moments when you feel like spoiling yourself.

Pure plant oils are the ultimate skin moisturizers. Some people shun oils because they believe they make skin oilier and leave a greasy film on the skin, while lotions penetrate, or "soak" into the skin. The main difference between lotions and oils is the texture, not the way they moisturize. Lotions are oil-in-water emulsions, and when the water and alcohol evaporate, oil, possibly beeswax, and some plant extracts are left on the skin's surface. With body oils, you are not wasting your money on water and alcohol. You get pure oil that can be applied lightly or heavily, depending on your preferences. There's also "dry oil," a lightweight oil blend that is sprayed on the skin to leave minimal greasy residue. Many cosmetic brands make "dry oil" by blending olive or jojoba oil with silicones. Dry oil sprays are incredibly versatile: you can apply them to damp skin after a shower or bath, you can spray them on your hair when it feels frizzy or dry, and you can also lightly spray it on your face for a dewy glow.

To prepare your own dry oil and moisturizing oil blends, you will need pure plant oils such as jojoba, almond, or grape seed, and a selection of your favorite essential oils. If you have sensitive skin or nose, skip stronger essential oils and add a subtle fragrance with one or two drops of chamomile or lavender oils. Most plant oils have fresh, earthy aromas of their own.

Many oil blends don't need preservatives to stay uncontaminated, but some require a bit of a help from essential oils or antioxidant vitamins. Jojoba and coconut oils, which are technically liquid plant waxes, have a longer shelf life, but most oils have to be used up within a year. Besides, many oils originate many thousand miles away from you and may well have spent months in transit before finally arriving at your bathroom or kitchen counter. This is a good reason to buy smaller sizes of organic oils regularly. If stored properly, in a cool, dark place, or at least in dark glass bottles, most body oil blends have a safe shelf life of six to twelve months. By adding ester of vitamin C and vitamin E, as well as grapefruit and tea tree oils, you can extend shelf life, but not dramatically.

## Sweet and Spicy Body Oil

1 ounce sweet almond oil

1 ounce apricot kernel oil

1 ounce grape seed oil

2 drops clary sage essential oil

2 drops mandarin essential oil

2 drops chamomile essential oil

1 drop ylang-ylang essential oil

1 drop lavender essential oil

**Yield: 4 ounces**

Pour the premeasured amounts of oils into a glass bottle and shake vigorously to blend.

## Sun Glow Dry Oil

½ ounce (15 ml) jojoba oil

½ ounce (15 ml) coconut oil

3 drops vanilla extract

2 drops sandalwood essential oil

800 IU vitamin E

1 teaspoon mineral shimmer

**Yield: 5 ounces**

*This is a green cross between my once-favorites NARS Body Glow and Stila Sun Shimmer Dry Oil. It adds a gorgeous natural-looking tint with a hint of shimmer. Lightweight plant oils do not form a greasy film, and they spread evenly. Ideally, you should make this oil with just a teaspoon Bare Escentuals Bare Minerals Glimmer in Tan Lines or True Gold. However, you can substitute any less-expensive mineral shimmering powder in shades of gold or sand. Be creative and blend mineral powders as you like, but don't use light pink or beige shimmers, even if you have pale skin. Opt for golden corals and pinks instead.*

Combine all the oils in a spray bottle. Carefully pour in the mineral pigment. Shake well before each use.

# Green Solutions for Cellulite

The first time I started to question the potentially toxic impact of cosmetics on my body was after massaging my skin with a fabulous, highly perfumed "anticellulite" lotion. After five minutes of massaging my tummy with a special rolling head, the lotion had soaked in. Where did it go? The water and alcohol must have evaporated, but what about the rest? If it's dissolving my cellulite, where does the fat go? Into my bloodstream? Into my lymph? Does it mean I will have fat cells in my blood? All these were uncomfortable and probably dumb questions. I knew I would never learn exactly what had entered my bloodstream and, hopefully, had been filtered out by my liver.

We know it as orange peel syndrome, cottage cheese skin, and the mattress phenomenon. Medical names for cellulite include *adiposis edematosa, dermopanniculosis deformans, status protrusus cutis,* and *gynoid lipodystrophy*. Don't confuse relatively harmless cellulite with the infectious disease cellulitis, when inflammation damages the underlying connective tissues of the skin.

Doctors are not entirely clear on what causes cellulite. Some say that cellulite is caused by weakened supportive collagen and elastin tissue and protruding fat cells. Others blame hormones, rapid weight loss, excessive water retention, and sluggish lymph flow. All we know is that cellulite plagues both the toned buttocks of supermodels and flabby tummies of new moms. Cellulite can appear on the upper arms, the back of the neck, and around the knees.

Like acne, cellulite is not an isolated cosmetic problem. It sends us a message that our body systems are not functioning properly, possibly due to hormonal shifts or toxin buildup. In any case, cellulite has to be addressed from inside and outside at the same time. Massaging creams will not make much of a difference at all.

I have to admit that a few years ago there wasn't a single cellulite cream in stores that I hadn't tried. Cooling, warming, tightening, smoothing, exfoliating, massaging lotions, even Nicoderm-like patches—I used them all diligently, with little to no result. I am a witness that there is no cure in a bottle for cellulite. At the same time, rigorous dieting and weekly detox alone won't get rid of cellulite either. Cellulite is not made of toxins or fat accumulating under skin, so flushing fat without paying attention to the efficiency of blood flow and lymph circulation won't get you anywhere.

After spending untold money on cellulite creams and spa procedures, I have put together a natural, green plan that is easy to follow and involves no hormone-disrupting chemicals.

*Improve lymph flow.* The fluid between your cells is filtered by the lymphatic system, and when the body gets congested, this process doesn't work well. As a result, the lymph system gets overloaded with toxins. To improve lymph flow, perform a dry skin brushing every day or at least every other day. You can also invest in roller massagers with wooden or metal heads that physically propel fluids in cellulite-affected areas. Contrast showers (alternating cold and warm water as you shower) do wonders for blood flow—you will see a healthy glow on your face immediately!

*Improve bowel function.* I noticed that many women who get cellulite also tend to have constipation. This is a clear sign of congestion and poor removal of waste products from the body. By adopting a toxin-free, organic diet and making regular Green Beauty Detox a habit (see Chapter 16), you will reduce the toxin load on your elimination system and help your cells exchange nutrients, clear toxins, and burn fat more efficiently.

*Avoid water retention.* Alcohol, saturated fats, and excessive amounts of salt all increase the swelling of skin tissue surrounding fat cells. Wearing tight clothes and sitting or standing in the same position for long periods of time have also been shown to contribute to cellulite. Drinking proper amounts of water (the proverbial eight glasses a day) helps fight excessive water pressure in the skin. You drink more, but you pee more too.

*Burn the fat.* Enlarged fat cells make the connective tissue weaken and eventually burst under pressure, creating an uneven, bumpy texture. Exercising and eating a healthy diet will reduce the fat buildup under your skin, as well as improve blood and lymph flow. Yoga and Pilates are especially good at promoting healthy fluid exchange in your skin.

*Try health supplements.* There are many health supplements that are believed to have an effect on cellulite. These include coenzyme Q10, amino acid l-carnitine, and gotu kola *(Centella Asiatica)*, which improve connective tissue activity, and Indian chestnut, ginkgo biloba, and rutin, which boost microcirculation. None of them have proved to be a miracle cellulite pill, but you may find them useful as part of a holistic cellulite plan. Consult your doctor before adding any health supplements to your diet.

*Use a body oil.* Improve the skin's elasticity and strengthen its cells with a nutritious, tightening body oil that can be combined with a massage. Here's a recipe that worked well on my stubborn wobbly bits.

## Green Skin Toning Oil

1 ounce evening primrose oil

½ ounce rose hip oil

15,000 IU vitamin E (from capsules)

5 mg horse chestnut extract

5 drops grapefruit essential oil

3 drops ylang-ylang essential oil

**Yield: 4 ounces**

*This potent blend of moisturizers and nutrients allows the skin to breathe and helps heal any stretch marks you may have on your tummy and thighs.*

Premix horse chestnut extract with a teaspoon of any of the oils to completely dissolve it. Combine all oils and other ingredients in a glass bottle and shake vigorously. Use it twice daily.

None of these steps will make a difference in your fight against dimpled skin if used separately from the rest. Just like acne, cellulite cannot be cured with a single magic potion. It requires consistent efforts that benefit your whole body. I usually begin my anticellulite regimen in February, allowing twenty-eight days for the skin renewal cycle to complete. Since cellulite has to be attacked both from inside and outside, I start with a gentle detox and continue drinking the skin-cleansing, fat-melting cocktail Green Detox Drink (see recipe in Chapter 16) during the whole month. Every day I dry brush my whole body and massage my thighs, arms, and belly with my own Green Skin Toning Oil or Weleda Birch Cellulite Oil, using a simple wood rolling massager. In total, I spend four intensive hours in February keeping

"Here's my beauty secret: use organic skin care; eat mostly organic foods, such as whole grains, vegetables, fruits, and organic salmon; exercise aerobically; practice yoga or strength training; get plenty of sleep; and drink lots of water."

—Karen Behnke,
founder of Juice Beauty

cellulite at bay, with five-minute daily upkeep during the rest of the year. And so far, I haven't had to bring any heavy artillery, such as Endermologie or a similarly expensive procedure, into play.

## Green Hair Removal

Most women prefer to shave their unwanted hair, but there are many other options that will leave you silky smooth. You can safely tweeze, wax, or sugar wax any area, as long as you are not prone to bruises. You cannot wax legs if you have varicose veins, though.

No matter how tempting it is to freeze unwanted hairs in their tracks, avoid any topical hair-removal creams or lotions that claim to slow hair growth. Chemicals in cream hair removers, such as potassium thioglycolate, potassium hydroxide, lithium silicates, urea, and some essential oils, can be easily absorbed by your skin. The safety of these chemicals has never been studied on humans.

Waxing, the ancient method of hair removal, has been used for centuries. Waxing pulls hair out by its roots, so the results last from four to eight weeks, and the new hair grows in soft and fine—or may not grow back at all!

Commercially available waxing kits almost always contain some sort of chemicals—preservatives, thickeners, emulsifiers, and such—that are able to penetrate the skin, especially when heated, and we clearly don't want that. Instead, we can prepare our own organic body wax to work on our legs, arms, and even bikini line. With a bit of practice, as you develop a lighter touch, you can use the blend on your face, too.

Waxing can be painful when done for the first time, so practice on your arms and lower leg before applying wax to underarms or the bikini line. Don't attempt a Brazilian wax—complete hair removal from the bikini area—at home. Try waxing the bikini line first before considering a Brazilian. Going to a salon for a professional wax is also recommended before you attempt to duplicate the hair-removal procedure at

**Green Tip**

Waxing can be painful when done for the first time, so practice on your arms and lower leg before applying wax to underarms or the bikini line.

home. Try to find a place that offers natural sugar wax so you are not treated with unwanted chemicals. Before waxing, you will need to brace yourself and allow at least one-eighth inch of hair to grow out.

Here's what you will need for your green home wax:

15–20 cotton strips, 2-inch wide for legs and arms, and ½-inch wide for facial hair and bikini line. You can cut these from a piece of fabric or purchase a roll from a beauty supply store.

Cornstarch-based baby powder

Flat wooden sticks or Popsicle sticks (avoid metal or plastic)

Two saucepans: one small and deep, one wide and shallow

Green Sugar Wax (recipe follows)

Grape seed, jojoba, avocado, or other body oil

Cotton cloth for cleanups (not cotton balls!)

Green Soothing Spray (recipe follows)

Making your own natural wax is easy and inexpensive. Make a smaller batch for the first waxing session. You can always make more wax when you need it. The recipe yields enough wax to treat two lower legs or two arms and a bikini line. I do not recommend reusing leftovers as they rarely reheat evenly.

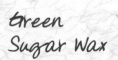

## Green Sugar Wax

2 cups organic brown sugar (any type)

½ cup filtered water

½ cup steeped chamomile tea

2 tablespoons freshly squeezed lemon juice

Yield:
4 ounces

1. Half-fill a wide, shallow saucepan with water, bring to a boil, and then turn heat to low. Mix all the ingredients in a small, deep saucepan and bring to a boil over medium heat, stirring constantly.

2. When the sugar mixture ("wax") boils, place the small saucepan into the wide, shallow saucepan and leave it on low heat. The wax should remain liquid and golden in color, not stiff and brown, so stir constantly. To prevent the mixture from becoming too dark, avoid stirring too briskly, so that the sugar mixture doesn't stick to the sides of a pan. When the wax bubbles gently and looks thin enough to pour, add 1 cup of boiling water from the shallow pan, stir thoroughly, and remove from the heat.

3. When the wax has reached the consistency of fresh honey, transfer it to a glass bowl and allow it to cool down before using. Never put the freshly prepared wax on your body! You may burn yourself badly.

4. While the wax is cooling, pour hot water into a wide, shallow bowl to use as a water bath to keep your wax warm and pliable.

  **the green beauty guide**

Make sure you have all the waxing supplies—baby powder, cotton strips, wooden sticks, and oil—within easy reach.

Coat the area that you plan to wax—your arm or lower leg—with baby powder. This is essential to keep the skin protected from wax sticking to it and causing redness and bruising, especially now, as your blood flow to the area will increase. Check the temperature of the wax. It should be warm to the touch, not hot. Using a wooden stick, apply a thin coat of wax in quick gliding strokes in the direction of the hair growth: from inside to outside on your arm, from knee to foot on your leg. You need to dip your stick in the wax about 2 inches deep—this way, you will be applying a thin coat that will stick to the cotton strip at once. Cover an area the width of your cotton strips and 4 inches long for legs, 1 inch long for face and bikini line.

Now apply a cotton strip to the area covered with sticky wax, also in the direction of hair growth. Press gently and rub to make sure the strip sticks without bulging. Take a deep breath, then lift the strip by the lower end and pull quickly! Here you go—your skin is smooth and hairless. Repeat the procedure until you've covered all desired areas. Use the strip until it is completely covered with hair and can't pick up any more wax. After that, get a new strip. Meanwhile, keep the wax warm and fluid by adding some hot water to the water bath. When done, remove any remaining wax smudges with baby oil and soothe the skin with a freshly made soothing spray.

## Green Soothing Spray

½ cup freshly steeped organic green tea

1 cup freshly steeped chamomile tea

2 tablespoons fresh aloe vera juice

1 teaspoon calendula extract

5 drops peppermint essential oil

½ teaspoon willow bark extract

**Yield: 4 ounces**

*Green tea and chamomile are known herbal anti-inflammatories, while aloe vera and calendula (marigold) are known for their soothing, healing properties. Peppermint oil is optional, but it can cool the raw, freshly waxed area in no time! Willow bark extract is a source of natural salicylic acid, which prevents ingrown hair.*

Blend all the ingredients in a spray bottle, shake well, and keep in the refrigerator until ready to use.

The first time is the most painful waxing experience. Start with waxing simple areas, such as the lower legs, forearms and upper arms, eyebrows, chin, and upper lip. After a few sessions, the hair will get weaker, and waxing will be much easier. Plus, you will build up some tolerance and will become handier at applying the wax and ripping out the hair. When you gain experience, you can move to the underarms and bikini line. Just remember the rule: always apply wax in the direction of the hair growth and pull the cotton strip in the opposite direction, not forgetting to soothe and moisturize your skin after you are done waxing!

## Making Your Own Hand and Foot Treatments

Many of these recipes work just as well as ready-made treatments, but I hope you never wish to delete spa services from your list of priorities. No matter how down-to-earth you strive to be, there is nothing quite like having someone else give your feet a massage!

## Green Cuticle Softener

¹/₃ ounce soy wax

2 teaspoons sweet almond oil

10 drops beta-carotene

1,000 IU vitamin E

2 teaspoons lemon juice

¼ teaspoon sodium hydroxide (available at most home improvement stores)

**Yield: 4 ounces**

*This blend was inspired by my all-time favorite, Burt's Bees Lemon Butter Cuticle Creme, but with added mild cuticle dissolvers. One batch will last you at least six months.*

Warm the soy wax in a pan and add the oil and other ingredients. Thoroughly blend and transfer to a pump bottle.

## Green Cuticle Oil

½ ounce rape seed oil

½ ounce sweet almond oil

3 drops lavender essential oil

3 drops chamomile
  essential oil

3 drops tea tree
  essential oil

**Yield:
4 ounces**

*This makes a three-month supply of moisturizing and mildly antiseptic oil. It can be massaged into nails morning and night to prevent them from peeling and breaking.*

Simply blend all ingredients in a pump bottle. You can use an old bottle from eye or face serum, but make sure to wash and rinse it well to prevent any leftover product from messing up your efforts.

## Hand Rescue Cream

½ ounce beeswax

Juice of one freshly squeezed
  lemon

1 tablespoon sweet almond oil

5 drops lemon essential oil

2 drops lavender essential oil

**Yield:
5 ounces**

*There are some wonderful all-natural hand creams on the market. Weleda, Jurlique, Logona, Dr. Hauschka, Suki Naturals and many more make excellent, entirely natural creams and balms, but here is an inexpensive alternative that will do the same job minus the price tag.*

1. Melt beeswax in a pan.
2. Add the lemon juice and oils and stir with a wooden spoon until blended.
3. Transfer to a jar. Shake occasionally until the cream is cooled and uniform.

## Manicure in a Jar

½ cup organic brown sugar

½ cup grape seed oil

5 drops vanilla extract

2 drops lavender
  essential oil

1 drop sandalwood
  essential oil

**Yield:
4 ounces**

*This is my personal hand savior when I need my hands to look freshly manicured in two minutes.*

Combine the ingredients in a small bowl and transfer to a wide-necked jar so you can dip your fingers into the mix. Do just that: one by one, dip your fingertips into the jar, massaging the sugary mixture gently into cuticles and knuckles, wave hands gently to please your senses (the scent is lovely!), and briskly immerse your hands in warm water to remove excess oil. Dry your hands and apply Hand Rescue Cream.

## QUICK TIP FOR STRONG NAILS AND SOFT HANDS

Soaking your nails daily in almond or olive oil strengthens the nails better than any conventional nail hardener. Simply soak for five minutes, wipe your hands clean, and massage in the remaining oil until it disappears into the skin. For the same results, but with the added benefit of soothing, mix a teaspoon of honey with two teaspoons of almond or olive oil, and massage into the hands after gardening or other strenuous activities. When burning an organic soy candle, use the melted oil for a deeply penetrating "paraffin" treatment, but be careful not to spill the hot oil, and do not poke your fingers into the candle while it's still burning! For ultimate hand softening, apply deep moisturizing oil, such as jojoba or grape seed, put on a pair of organic cotton gloves, and sleep in them. It works best if you're sleeping alone!

## Green Feet Fizzy

1 cup baking soda

½ cup cornstarch

¼ cup Epsom salt

½ cup citric acid

½ cup purified water

5 drops peppermint
essential oil

5 drops tea tree
essential oil

*This is a green duplicate of LUSH Bath Bombs but without any preservatives or synthetic perfumes. You can also use your favorite essential oils to make as many different bath soaks as you want.*

Mix all the ingredients in a china bowl. Stuff the mixture into ice cube trays or form small balls and let dry. For a foot soak, use one apricot-size cube. For bubbly bath, use three cubes. Store the tablets in a plastic container with a lid or in a decorative bottle or jar.

Yield:
4 ounces

  **the green beauty guide**

## Green Feet Reviving Spray

1 cup purified water

½ cup witch hazel

½ ounce white clay (kaolin)

5 drops peppermint essential oil

5 drops tea tree essential oil

**Yield: 5 ounces**

Combine the ingredients in a spray bottle and store in the refrigerator. Shake well before use.

## Green Wax Hand and Foot Treatment

7 ounces soybean wax

½ ounce sweet almond or jojoba oil

5 drops rose essential oil

**Yield: 4 ounces**

*Remember how good it feels to wrap your hands in warm, pliable wax and let nutrients penetrate the skin as it gets softer? You can treat your hands to this decadent procedure at home using completely natural ingredients instead of petrochemicals.*

1. Melt wax in a microwave oven according to the instructions on the package. Add the jojoba or sweet almond oil and rose essential oil. Remove from heat and pour mixture into a shallow glass container with a lid. Let cool about five minutes.

2. When the wax mixture is still hot but not burning, apply a thick coating of jojoba oil or heavy all-natural hand balm to your hands, and dip them into the wax bath. Leave your hands in the wax for at least five minutes, then remove hands from the container and peel off the hardened wax. Save the remaining wax for the next time.

## What to Eat for Healthy Nails

A common cause of brittle nails is thought to be iron deficiency. Too little vitamin A, zinc, and calcium also cause nail discolorations, dryness, and brittleness, while an inadequate intake of vitamin B2 may cause the slow growth of nails.

So what should we eat to keep our nails strong? Vitamin A is contained in raw and dried apricots, carrots, papaya, mango, watermelons, egg yolk, tuna, and salmon. Zinc is contained in Brazil nuts, walnuts, hazelnuts, and coconuts, as well as in currants, figs, and salmon. Calcium in its natural form is contained in dairy products, broccoli, raisins, oranges, kiwis, and mandarins, while dried plums, dried figs, tamarind, and egg yolk are especially rich in biotin, a natural form of vitamin B2.

## The Nail Polish Dilemma

To color or not to color? This is a burning question. If you want to be truly green, not just greenwashed, you must ditch your toxic nail polishes completely. Yes, even that pretty shimmery pink. I know it cost you a fortune, but it seems like nail polishes are real toxic bombs loaded with more carcinogens than any other beauty product I have reviewed so far.

A truly nontoxic nail polish doesn't exist in nature. While many brands remove some of the harmful ingredients, the nail polishes become less toxic but not completely harmless. Let's discuss nail polishes in more detail.

The most abundant toxin in conventional nail polish is solvent formaldehyde and formaldehyde resin. Formaldehyde is a proven carcinogen, according to the U.S. Environmental Protection Agency. In 2006, the International Agency for Research on Cancer categorized formaldehyde as a substance carcinogenic to humans. Formaldehyde was linked to nasopharyngeal cancer and leukemia (Bosetti et al. 2008), as well as severe allergic reactions (Sainio et al. 1997) in European studies, but the link is strongly disputed in the U.S. Today, the use of formaldehyde in cosmetics is strictly limited in the European Union and Japan, but last time I checked, this chemical was found in the majority of nail polishes and other nail products sold in the U.S.

Small amounts of formaldehyde can be absorbed through skin and the nail bed, but the worst thing is that you also inhale formaldehyde when someone else does your manicure or pedicure. Many manicurists today wear protective masks that give them some sort of air filtration. But too many times I have seen a very pregnant lady practically bathing in a cloud of formaldehyde as she was having her nails painted bright red. To me, women who have their nails painted during pregnancy are no better than pregnant smokers or drinkers.

To make the polish cover the nail smoothly, the pretty goo also contains plasticizer dibutyl phthalate, a known hormone disruptor. Little is known about health effects of phthalates, but about one thing science is pretty certain: phthalates are linked to the worsening state of the male reproductive system, including sexual dysfunctions, decreasing sperm count, low production of testosterone, as well as various abnormalities in male reproductive organs (Lottrup et al. 2006). Recent epidemiological evidence shows that boys born to women exposed to phthalates during pregnancy "have an increased incidence of cryptorchidism (*absence of one or both testes from the scrotum*), hypospadias (*a birth defect of the urethra that involves an abnormally placed urinary openining*), testicular cancer and spermatogenic dysfunction," say Chinese pathologists who studied the effects of phthalate exposure in 2007 (Chen et al. 2007). Researchers from Denmark found that contamination of human breast milk with phthalates "has direct influence on the postnatal surge of reproductive hormones in newborn boys" (Main et al. 2006). Many cosmetic companies agreed to remove phthalates from their nail products. For example, most L'Oreal, Estée Lauder, Milani, Lumene, and Revlon nail polishes today do not contain formaldehyde or dibutyl phthalate. Yet there are many, many more popular nail products that proudly display phthalates in the ingredients list.

The rest of the ingredients of your average nail polish are not that safe, either. Solvent acetone smells ghastly, but its hidden effects are even worse: in 2008, scientists of Brookhaven National Laboratory in New York found that animals who inhaled acetone were slower and less agile (Lee et al. 2008). Reports about acetone intoxication date back to the 1990s (Kechijian 1991), and recently Hong Kong researchers found that there's more to acetone than its ability to irritate skin and make rats high: acetone is often contaminated with another toxin, formaldehyde (Huang et al. 2007). It's another reason to use nonacetone nail polish remover—if you decide to use nail polish after all you now know.

Are there any natural, nontoxic nail polishes available? Yes, but don't expect them to be as pretty and long-lasting as their synthetic counterparts. They would still contain nitrocellulose, ethyl acetate, and isopropyl alcohol, but at least there would be no formaldehyde, toluene, or phthalates. HoneyBee Gardens, No Miss, Sante, and Suncoat make natural-looking polishes that come in a sophisticated palette of colors. Safer conventional nail products include top coats by Revlon, Estée Lauder, and Mary Kay that give your nails a natural groomed look without formaldehyde, toluene, phthalates, or FD&C dyes.

But if you are pregnant or are trying to be completely green in your beauty routine, consider avoiding nail polishes altogether. Until science comes up with something truly nontoxic, the only option to keep our tips and toes groomed is buffing and lots of cuticle oil. When you are having a manicure or a pedicure, ask the manicurist to buff your nails with a special buffing pad and buy your own buffer for use at home. Apply a coat of nourishing cuticle oil every night and regularly exfoliate your cuticles with a homemade sugar scrub. I stopped wearing nail polish three years ago, and my nails today look healthier than ever.

*chapter* **12**

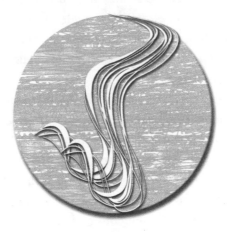

*green* **hair**
**care**

The human hair is stronger than nylon, aluminum, or copper fiber of the same size, yet it often behaves as a fussy, ill-tempered toddler after too much chocolate. The manes of many of us seem to live lives of their own, and it's now our turn to teach our locks the benefits of green living.

Our hair has structure similar to skin, but unlike skin, all the layers of hair follicles are dead. Outside, the hair is composed of thick, horny cells known as cuticle. These cells are made of keratin, a protein held together by amino acids, most importantly cysteine and methionine. Keratin fibers shield *medulla*, an inner layer of cells containing fat granules, oxygen, and pigments. One end of the hair reaches the sky, or at least peaks some place where our hairstyle allows it; another end roots in the skin. There, a small onion-shaped hair papilla is producing new keratin cells while being continuously nourished by blood vessels. Each follicle can only grow about twenty hairs in a person's lifetime. Separate sebum glands running along the hair follicle provide shine and protection to the new cuticle cells of the hair. This is why it's vitally important to feed your hair with sufficient amounts of good proteins and essential fatty acids.

The average human head has about 100,000 hair follicles, and blonds definitely have more fun, at least when it comes to hair. Scientists meticulously calculated that people with blond hair have almost 50 percent more hairs than those with red or dark hair. But, no matter what the color is, our hair, this incredible living fabric, requires much gentler handling than most couture textiles. That's why the words "natural" and "organic" that so commonly adorn bottles and tubes of various hair treatments often mean very little. Follow this guide to truly natural hair products.

## Green Cleansing for Hair

Well-groomed, shiny, and resilient hair is a surefire way to boost attractiveness and self-confidence. We eagerly wash, moisturize, condition, straighten, and add volume and shine to our locks. Since the scalp is the most absorbent part of our body, choosing genuinely green hair care should certainly become a shopping priority.

Shampoo is the most frequently used hair product. Water and detergent make up almost all of a conventional shampoo's formulation, featured at the beginning of ingredients labels, with moisturizing emollients and plant extracts often adding up to no more than 1 percent. But let's not be deceived by the word "organic" on the label. The amount of organic aloe vera extract in a shampoo may be very minuscule—sometimes less than 1 percent! What truly matters for the health of our hair is the bulk of the shampoo, namely, the quality of the detergent and the amount of emollients. Both have to be of plant origin, derived without the use of toxic chemical processes.

We love the idea of herbs and botanical ingredients nurturing our hair back to health, but while many mainstream herbal shampoos brazenly claim to be natural and organic, most contain tiny amounts of beneficial botanical ingredients, with the bulk of the product consisting of harsh detergents, preservatives, and petroleum-derived silicones.

The quality of a detergent—that foam-producing ingredient that dissolves oil and grime—is the most important thing to consider when choosing a shampoo. The very nature of the detergent action of shampoo interferes with the scalp's natural barrier function and makes it even easier for chemicals to penetrate. Most often you will find sodium lauryl sulfate and its milder brother, sodium laureth sulfate, on the label. Both have been questioned as cancer-causing ingredients, although a research panel organized and sponsored by the cosmetic industry declared them safe for use. Also, steer clear of cocoamide diethanolamine (DEA) and ammonium laureth sulfate, which often make up to one-third of an average shampoo bottle. Any ethoxylated compounds are a major no-no in a truly organic beauty product.

Even shampoos that claim to be organic can contain harsh cleansing agents. This is one of those rare cases when buying products in a health food store doesn't always help, because most otherwise green and ethical brands still use detergents from the sulfate family as well as ammonium laureth sulfate or cocoamide DEA/MEA. Sometimes keen marketers add a clause "derived from coconut" following the dubious ingredient, but the fact that sodium laureth sulfate has coconut as its distant relative doesn't make this detergent any safer. For dangers of ethoxylated ingredients and

The quality of a detergent—that foam-producing ingredient that dissolves oil and grime—is the most important thing to consider when choosing a shampoo.

particularly detergents, refer to Chapter 2, particularly the section on 1,4-Dioxane.

Close label reading reveals that, instead of sodium laureth sulfate, some natural brands use other sulfate family members, such as sodium myreth sulfate. Needless to say, such ingredients do not contribute to the health of your hair and scalp, and they cannot be recommended for use in truly green products.

There aren't many green cleansing agents available. Many natural brands favor cocamidopropyl betaine, derived from coconut using petrochemicals, and petroleum-derived olefin sulfonate. One of the greenest, lauryl glucoside, is a soapy blend of coconut oil, corn starch, and sugar, but it isn't used frequently because of its higher price. It's necessary to remember that most organic beauty manufacturers are in the business to make money, and they are often prone to cut corners and replace quality ingredients with cheaper alternatives after the product has been launched successfully.

Humectants and emollients in shampoos are nice additions, but they make little difference because they are washed off so quickly. Still, vegetable glycerin, aloe extract, jojoba oil, honey, and lecithin make shampoo more nourishing as they fill in the pores of a hair shaft and keep the hair surface smooth. They also soothe and moisturize the scalp. Since human hair is made of dead protein, it's impossible to infuse it with proteins—but milk, wheat, soy, rice, and oat extracts do make hair softer and more resilient. Some plants, such as calendula, yarrow, and burdock, work as mild astringents and can soothe scalp irritation, while citrus oils, apple cider vinegar, and rosemary seal the hair cuticle and help create a brilliant shine. Many organic brands offer concentrated shampoos with little added water. This is economical, since you only need a drop of shampoo to make a nice lather, and this also eliminates the need for strong preservatives. Grapefruit seed oil, vitamins A, C, and E, benzoin extract, and wheat germ act as natural preservatives in these shampoos.

How often should you shampoo? It depends on the state of your hair. If your hair is fine and dry, daily shampooing, even with the mildest product, can increase dryness. If you spend a lot of time in the sun, or if you wear lots of styling products, shampooing daily is recommended. Look at the condition of your hair and act accordingly! Yet be aware that frequent washes in hard water can make your hair brittle and prone to split ends. "Women use way too much shampoo," notes John Masters, the

the green beauty guide

pioneer of professional organic hair care and colors. "Besides, they use too much pressure when they wash their hair. Daily shampooing is not essential. You have to learn to be gentle to your hair."

## Green Product Guide: Shampoos

I would love to say that making your own shampoo is easy, but it isn't. It certainly can be done, but it's nearly impossible to create an effective and pleasant-to-use shampoo at home. Instead, look for the following all-natural shampoos that keep their formulations true to their green claims.

**Burt's Bees More Moisture Raspberry & Brazil Nut Shampoo** smells heavenly and cleanses well with a soapy, all-natural surfactant. Rich in natural omega-3 essential fatty acids, honey, soy protein, and a dozen plant oils, this preservative-free hair wash is not too moisturizing, which is great for summertime use or if your hair is on the oily side.

**Kiss My Face Whenever Shampoo** is a true miracle in a bottle. Gentle enough for daily use on sensitive scalps, this shampoo is bursting with flower waters, wheat protein, and plant extracts and infusions, including rosemary, chamomile, nettle, olive leaf, calendula, sage, green tea, and lavender. Based on mild (albeit petroleum-derived) surfactants, this shampoo has no added fragrance and relies on natural preservatives such as vitamin E, lime oil, citric acid, and potassium sorbate.

**John Masters Organics Zinc & Sage Shampoo with Conditioner** is a must for anyone whose scalp has been sensitized by harsh weather conditions or chemicals. Naturally derived, mild synthetic surfactants are thoroughly cleansing to hair and scalp, while nurturing the scalp with hyaluronic, linoleic, and linolenic acids, and reducing irritation with zinc and sulfur. Rosemary, nettle, horsetail, and lavender are very beneficial for hair, while carefully blended essential oils perform an aromatherapy session each time you shampoo.

If you are looking for the ultimate green shampoo that will be faithful when your hair is dry and then suddenly oily, head to your local health food store for a bottle of **Aubrey Organics Honeysuckle Rose Moisturizing Shampoo**. Based on coconut and corn soaps, rich in organic soy protein, aloe vera, and organic rose hip oil, this humbly scented, concentrated shampoo contains virtually every plant extract ever recommended for healthy hair, such as fennel, hops, ginseng, horsetail, coltsfoot, and magnolia, to name just a few. As always with Aubrey Organics, there are no added fragrances or synthetic preservatives.

## Making Your Own Hair Conditioners

"Our sense of true beauty begins with self-knowledge and self-acceptance, and it grows as we learn to adopt images of beauty that are real, alive, and strong. We should work with nature, not against her, and enhance our individuality, our own beauty in a way that promotes our health and respects our intelligence. Get to know your beauty and become empowered with information because, as I grew to understand more and more about this industry, my eyes were opened. I feel it's my duty to educate others and help everyone to become as knowledgeable as I am now. Take matters into your own hands because there really isn't anyone looking out for you better than you can."

—Suki Kramer, Creator of Suki Naturals

Remember all those magic shampoos that promised to instantly revitalize your hair? Let me remind you once again: your hair is made of dead keratin molecules and cannot be revived from the outside. You cannot feed it or improve its structure by applying minerals or vitamins or chemicals on its surface. All you can do is to temporarily smooth and stiffen the hair shaft so it looks shiny and more manageable. By coating hair follicles in silicones, plant oils, or waxes, you can make brushing and styling easier, too.

There are several types of conditioners available today. The most popular type is a rinse-off conditioner, which is applied after the shampoo, left on to penetrate a minute or two, and then rinsed off. There are also leave-in conditioners that you apply before brushing your wet hair and you don't rinse out. Finally, there are deep rinse-off conditioners that you apply once a week or whenever you feel your hair needs a quick fix of nutrients or a boost in shine.

Oily hair benefits most from rinse-off conditioners; dry hair needs a weekly deep hot oil treatment in addition to a moisturizing conditioner used after every wash. Colored, permed, or sun-bleached hair benefits from leave-on conditioners with essential oils, amino acids, and plant proteins. Those lucky few whose hair behaves well but whose scalp sometimes feels itchy can benefit from conditioners and rinses with aloe vera, zinc, and plant-derived silicones. By all means avoid propylene glycol, cetrimonium chloride, mineral oil, petroleum-derived silicones, and hydrolyzed animal protein, found in practically all conventional conditioners.

Making a quick and perfectly green conditioner is extremely easy. As with face masks, you usually already have all the ingredients in your kitchen cupboard. If not, they are readily available in health food stores and online. While there are excellent, lovely scented conditioners for every possible hair dilemma, your own conditioner will come at a fraction of the price, and you can custom-tailor the blend to suit your needs.

"Any of my conditioners can be recreated at home," says John Masters, who started blending his own shampoos and conditioners from his kitchen to use on clients in his home salon back in the 1980s. "Olive and jojoba oil make ultimate hair conditioners. Always use organic extra virgin olive oil on your hair for deep conditioning and massage. It can solve so many problems!" Another praised natural hair conditioner is avocado, rich in omega-3 oils and proteins, which you can mash and put directly on your hair. "Essential oils of lavender, rosemary, cedarwood, ylang-ylang, palmarosa, and geranium are all beneficial for the hair," adds Masters.

## Green Solutions for Oily Hair

If your hair tends to be greasy and you need to wash it every day, you need to rebalance the oil production in your scalp. Use a mild shampoo, or better yet, an organic baby shampoo, which is generally more oil-stripping than adult shampoos, and apply an oil-balancing hot oil treatment once a week. (Don't be scared, extra oil won't make your scalp oilier!) The next recipe also works well against dandruff because dandruff and oily scalp march hand in hand in many people.

If your hair is oily, look for shampoos with natural astringents such as sage, tea tree, juniper, and lemon.

Apple cider vinegar is a traditional, time-tested treatment for oily hair. You can use vinegar if you have dandruff, too, even if you think your hair is dry. Splash some vinegar in the palm of your hand and run it through your hair with your head tilted back. Massage the vinegar into the scalp. The odor may seem strong, but some people find it uplifting, and it will be gone after shampooing. After just one application, your hair will be more bouncy and shiny. With daily applications, you will soon be receiving compliments about your hair!

Honeydew melon makes an express hair treatment for oily hair. Simply mash or blend a quarter of an organic melon, then massage the puree into your scalp. Cover with a clean towel and relax for ten minutes, then shampoo and rinse out.

Neutral henna is an excellent toner for oily scalps that are prone to dandruff. Prepare a quick hair mask with neutral (uncolored) henna, aloe vera juice, and lemon juice, blended in equal proportions, and then massage it into your hair and scalp. Leave it on for a few minutes. This mask can lighten your hair color a little bit, so you may want to replace lemon juice with organic apple cider vinegar.

## Sweet and Sour Oily Hair Conditioner

1 cup jojoba oil

½ cup lemon juice

2 teaspoons brown sugar

5 drops rosemary essential oil

5 drops sage essential oil

5 drops tea tree essential oil

**Yield:**
**4 ounces**

*Brown sugar works as a mild soothing agent. For dark hair, you may substitute apple cider vinegar for the lemon juice because it can be mildly bleaching. But if you do want to lighten your hair a little bit, go ahead and use lemon juice!*

1. Combine all ingredients in a glass container and shake well to dissolve the sugar.

2. Apply the blend to dry, unwashed hair, starting at the roots and massaging the oil into the scalp. Rub the oil into the hair in a downward motion away from the scalp to seal the hair cuticle. Scalp massage encourages the penetration of active essential oils and helps prevent pore clogging with dry sebum and dead skin cells.

3. Comb the hair through. Follow with a mild shampoo. Massage the shampoo into hair, slowly adding water as the oil dissolves. Lather as usual and rinse.

## Green Solutions for Dry, Damaged Hair

Coloring, highlighting, perming, straightening, air-conditioning in the summer, heating during the winter, too little sleep, too many chemicals in your shampoo—all of these can dry out hair and make the scalp itchy and flaky. This should not be mistaken for dandruff, which is usually accompanied by a greasy scalp.

While conventional conditioners simply coat the hair and scalp in silicones and mineral oil, providing instant results that are gone before the end of the day, natural solutions work slowly but the effect remains longer.

Shampoo your hair with plain egg. It may sound ridiculous and feels even worse, but the effect is completely worth it. Eggs won't lather and will try to sneak through your fingers. Be prepared to waste a few eggs down the drain until you master the technique. The trick is to carefully separate the yolk and use it on your hair; save the egg white for a tightening, nourishing mask or a quick salt scrub for your face. If you prefer your shampoo to lather, make a simple egg shampoo by blending one egg yolk with one tablespoon (or two squirts) of castile soap. Blend them briskly in the palm of your hand and rub into your hair immediately.

In ready-made shampoos for dry hair, look for ingredients such as jojoba oil, aloe vera, cucumber and licorice extracts, milk and soy proteins, vegetable glycerin, and panthenol (vitamin B5). Some of the best shampoos for dry hair include John Masters Honey & Hibiscus Hair Reconstructing Shampoo, Lavera Rose Milk Repair Shampoo for Dry Hair, Aubrey Organics Honeysuckle Rose Moisturizing Shampoo, and Avalon Organics Lavender Nourishing Shampoo.

Keep plain jojoba oil in your shower and massage a handful of oil into your scalp at least once a week. You may also add a few drops of jojoba oil to your shampoo as you work it through your hair, but make sure to rinse thoroughly. Desert Essence sells a generously sized bottle of organic jojoba oil (Desert Essence Jojoba Oil for Hair, Skin & Scalp) that you can use as a facial cleanser and a nutritious mask for dry hair.

Diet matters, too. In the winter, when many people suffer from drier hair and scalp, introduce more oily fruits and vegetables, such as avocado and broccoli, in your diet. "Your lifestyle has a synergistic effect

**Green Tip**

Pure plant oil is the best conditioner for dry hair.

on your health and appearance," says John Masters. "A diet rich in organic raw fruits and vegetables is extremely beneficial for the condition of your hair. Olive, avocado, and fish oils will help keep hair healthy and shiny."

Here's a recipe for a nutritious preshampoo conditioner that infuses your hair and scalp with much-needed moisture.

## Mediterranean Garden Preshampoo Hair Butter

3 tablespoons organic virgin olive oil

2 tablespoons avocado oil

2 tablespoons whole-wheat flour

1 teaspoon organic spirulina extract

10,000 IU vitamin E

2 drops lavender essential oil

2 drops bergamot essential oil

2 drops chamomile essential oil

**Yield:**
4 ounces

*Use daily before shampooing for maximum results. This hair mask will last for one week of daily treatments.*

1. Blend all ingredients in a small bowl, making sure the essential oils spread evenly.

2. Massage one tablespoon of the treatment into wet hair and scalp, concentrating on split ends and areas of itchiness. Leave on for ten minutes for intensive conditioning.

3. Rinse thoroughly and shampoo as usual.

Use a leave-in conditioner that doubles as a styling aid. Look for soothing and calming ingredients such as aloe vera gel, oat and soy proteins, panthenol, cysteine, and other amino acids. Too much oil in your leave-in conditioner can weigh your hair down, so save oils for a conditioning mask or an oil massage.

If you can pull off a "bedroom hair" look, or disheveled, carelessly pinned or twisted hair, go for it. For corporate types, it's still possible to skip every other shampooing by adopting chic ponytails on long hair. If you have short hair, you can refresh your look by dabbing a bit of cornstarch into the scalp followed by blow-drying on a low setting.

Air-dry your hair whenever you can. Frequent blow-drying can damage the hair, causing split ends. If you must blow-dry, make sure that your hair is thoroughly towel dried first. I have found that organic cotton towels absorb more moisture than conventional ones, perhaps because the fibers aren't damaged by chlorine bleaching.

If you are going into the swimming pool or ocean, soak your hair in fresh water first and seal the cuticles with a light mist of jojoba oil so your hair won't be exposed to moisture-drenching salt or toxic chlorine.

Always remember to wear a hat in the sun or windy, cold weather. Hats prevent damage from UV radiation and dehydration from wind and frost.

### Green Tip

If your hair is fragile, make it a rule to shampoo half as often as you are used to.

## Sultry Shine Liquid Hair Mask

1 apple, peeled and cored

3 tablespoons neutral henna

½ cup light beer

1 tablespoon baking soda

1 drop lemon essential oil (optional)

1 drop hops essential oil (optional)

**Yield: 4 ounces**

*Apples provide vitamins, and the malic acid gently exfoliates scalp and hair follicles. Beer also is a time-tested shine booster. For best results, use flat beer with no bubbles.*

1. Puree the apple in a blender. Add the henna, beer, and baking soda and mix thoroughly. Add the essential oils, if using.

2. Apply the mask on freshly cleansed hair, leave on for five minutes, and rinse off with tepid water. You can store this mask in a glass jar in the refrigerator for up to three days.

## Green Solutions for Boosting Shine

Silicone serums are not the only solutions for vibrant, shiny hair. You can achieve far better and long-lasting results without the greasiness of petrochemicals if you try one of the following recipes.

To bring out the natural shine, start with your shampoo. If you have less than two ounces of shampoo left in the bottle, try adding a teaspoon of baking soda, which removes any residue from your hair without stripping too much natural moisture. If you are happy with the result, buy a bottle of inexpensive organic shampoo (aim for a basic formula without bells and whistles) and add 1 teaspoon of baking soda per 2 ounces of shampoo. Shake well and sit for about an hour before using. Don't expect soda crystals to dissolve completely. You will get a softening, mildly scrubbing scalp cleanser that you can use once a week to keep your scalp healthy and itch-free.

The simplest rinse to boost shine is apple cider vinegar. Dilute one-half cup of organic vinegar in one cup of water and use it as a final rinse after a thorough shampooing. Lemon juice mixed with water in the same proportion can also be used as a last rinse to give your hair a shiny and bouncy look. But beware: both mixtures should be applied carefully, with your head tilted back, so they do not get into your eyes!

If you have dark hair and would rather not experiment with bleaching lemon juice, try bringing up extra shine with coffee. Brew a cup of strong organic coffee, let it cool, and use it as a hair rinse.

Finally, the simplest recipe for shiny hair: after shampooing, just rinse your hair with cool water to close the hair cuticles. Don't use cold water, though: this can restrict blood vessels too much, resulting in a headache.

## Green Solutions for Increased Hair Volume

Our hair may look limp and lifeless for many reasons. We may use the wrong styling products that weigh down our hair instead of holding it up. We may use conventional conditioners loaded with silicones and quaterniums (synthetic polymers) that coat the hair with a shiny film. The shine will wear off by midday, leaving limp, greasy locks behind. Whatever the reason, we can easily correct it by some of the following methods.

First, ditch your conditioner with mineral oil, quaterniums, polyquaterniums, stearalkonium chloride, and similar industrial-strength hair softeners. Check the ingredients label, since these ingredients may hide between plant extracts and infusions. Try wonderfully natural volumizing conditioners such as Burt's Bees Very Volumizing Conditioner, Avalon Organics Biotin B-Complex Thickening Conditioner, or Aubrey Organics Ginseng Biotin Energizing Scalp Tonic, which is marketed for men but makes an excellent leave-on volume-boosting conditioner for anyone. Among the volume-boosting ingredients to look for are panthenol, hops, coltsfoot, nettle, and horsetail extracts, and the amino acids cysteine and methionine (the building blocks of hair follicles). Make sure these ingredients are near the beginning on the ingredients list of the conditioner.

Second, determine whether the lack of body in your hair is due to excessive oil production or to a lack of natural sebum. If your hair feels like straw by midday, most likely you have dry hair, and you'll want to follow the recommendations in the section on solutions for dry, damaged hair. If your hair feels like a bowl of spaghetti, then your hair is on the oily side, and adopting some steps from the solutions for oily hair section will certainly help.

If you have a few minutes of spare time and a head of limp, lifeless locks to deal with, try blending up a quick volumizing conditioner at home. Here's what you will need.

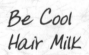

## Be Cool Hair Milk

½ cup witch hazel

⅓ ounce vodka, cognac, or brandy

3 drops peppermint essential oil

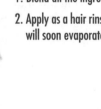

*Yield:*
4 ounces

1. Blend all the ingredients in a stainless steel shaker. Don't try to sniff!
2. Apply as a hair rinse, keep on for a few minutes, and rinse off. The smell will soon evaporate, leaving a faint herbal scent.

To boost circulation and make your hair follicles strong and perky, you will find a weekly scalp massage a blessing. For an invigorating rub, pour two drops of lavender oil and two drops of rosemary oil onto your fingertips, rub them together to warm up the oils, and then massage in strong circular motions. Massaging with essential oils boosts the blood flow to the scalp and encourages strong hair growth.

## Natural Hair Styling

Take a look at the label of your average hair styling spray, and what do you see? Petroleum-derived polymers diluted with alcohol and propylene glycol, spiffed up with synthetic fragrances and minuscule doses of plant extracts. Most bestselling hair sprays, from expensive René Furterer to affordable Thicker Fuller Hair, contain hydrofluorocarbon, a cooling liquid used in air conditioners and freezers that contributes to global warming and is a target of the Kyoto Protocol, an international agreement that aims to reduce greenhouse gases that cause global climate change. As of today, 136 countries, including Canada and European Union, but not the U.S., have ratified the Kyoto Protocol agreeing to keep greenhouse emissions at certain levels. The United States is the world's largest single emitter of carbon dioxide, according to the latest official energy statistics from the U.S. government (Energy Information Administration 2007).

But sometimes energy is what our hair is lacking. What's a limp-locked yet health-conscious girl (or guy) to do? Start with correctly chosen hair conditioner, recommends John Masters. "When you condition your scalp, your hair will gain so much volume you didn't realize you had," he says. "As you improve the circulation, your hair raises naturally, creating lasting volume." Another trick is to regularly remove product buildup, which leaves hair lighter and bouncier.

A sea salt spray adds instant texture and volume. John Masters prepares his with sea salt and essential oils, and he says you can easily recreate this bestselling (and very expensive) product at home. Just mix a tablespoon of fine sea salt in a cup of water and add a drop or two of your favorite essential oil. Peppermint, jasmine, and neroli work wonders for boosting circulation in the scalp while keeping hair deliciously scented.

A word about a common styling product ingredient, PVM/MA copolymer. Chemically known as polyvinylmethyl ether maleic acid, this petroleum derivative is frequently used in toothpastes and so-called "natural" hair products. In fact, there's nothing green or natural about PVM/MA copolymer, but there are many things that concern me. This synthetic resin is formed from vinyl methyl ether. The U.S. Personal Care Products Council, formerly the Cosmetic, Toiletry and Fragrance Association, insists that PVM/MA copolymer is safe for use. However, the U.S. consumer safety organization Environmental Working Group found that this chemical has never been assessed for human safety. Personally, I would rather not use anything that has undergone ethoxylation, especially if vinyl, a highly questionable compound, is present. I found a very disturbing study by scientists of the University of Wisconsin Medical School in 1997 that clearly shows that vinyl ethers form "mutagenic and tumorigenic metabolites" in animals (Park et al. 1997). As science begins to look closely at the toxic potential of various polymers, including vinyl, I would rather err on the side of caution and stick—pun intended—to botanical hair spray ingredients. Luckily, as technology moves on, green alternatives to petroleum-derived plastics become available.

Want shine and definition? The usual shine booster is pure silicone, a petroleum-derived clear liquid that works pretty much the same way Vaseline does on your skin. "Silicones provide an instant effect, but they do more damage in the long run," says John Masters. "Hair reprograms itself and stops producing natural emollients. As a result, the hair shaft becomes dull and lifeless, and you need to use more and more silicones to keep up the shine." Instead, use plant-based styling products that contain gum arabic and sugars for definition. Good green choices include B5 Design Gel by Aubrey Organics, Kiss My Face Upper Management Natural Styling Gel, and Lavera Volume & Shine Extra Strong Hold Styling Mousse. Trick of the trade: because organic styling sprays are much harder to find than organic styling gels, pour some gel into a spray bottle and dilute with water and grain alcohol or witch hazel. Here's what I use for my homemade styling spray: 1 ounce of B5 Design Gel by Aubrey Organic mixed with 2 ounces of purified water (avoid using mineral water because it may leave unsightly residue) and 1 ounce of organic grain alcohol (vodka). Combine all ingredients in a spray bottle, add a couple of drops of your favorite essential oil for a truly luxurious green experience, and shake well.

# Green Hair Coloring

If you take to heart only one piece of advice from this book, make it this one: do not color your hair with the toxic brew of chemicals sold in every drugstore and used in every salon. What makes the following information extremely important is not only the good condition of your hair. Synthetic hair dyes directly affect our health. We are talking serious health risks here.

To the dismay of cosmetic manufacturers and hairstylists worldwide, it eventually became clear that synthetic hair dyes were dramatically increasing the risks of some of the deadliest cancers. It was found that permanent hair dyes contain ingredients that are not only irritating—they are proven carcinogens (Bolt, Golka 2007; Miligi et al. 2005).

Two out of three women today color their hair. They color their hair every five weeks on average. The process of dyeing hair at home is so familiar that we don't even look at the instructions. We assume we know everything about hair colors, because our grandmother, and mother, and sister, and celebrity stylist—everybody—is doing it, so we guess it's just fine. *It's not.*

How does chemical hair color work? First of all, we have to blend a tube of coloring solution with a mixture of hydrogen peroxide and ammonia. Most permanent hair colors first remove the original color of the hair and then deposit a new color. Ammonia opens the hair cuticle to allow for the penetration of hydrogen peroxide, and it also increases the penetration of this potent bleach. No matter which shade you choose, a dark mahogany or light ash blond, every time you color your hair, hydrogen peroxide removes the original color and then the new color is deposited. Peroxide breaks chemical bonds in hair, releasing sulfur. When the color is gone, a new permanent color is injected into the hair shaft. After we have washed off the excess color, we use a silicone-based conditioner to close and seal the cuticle.

Here's what is happening to our body as we apply the hair color. Hydrogen peroxide, sulfur, and ammonia, well-known respiratory tract irritants, fill our lungs. Pigment-forming chemicals, known as aromatic amines, particularly phenylenediamines and aminophenols, are known to penetrate the skin and enter the bloodstream. We usually apply the coloring solution directly to the scalp, nearest the root, and most of us also stain our forehead, neck, and ears. The scalp is where the blood supply is the richest in the entire human body. This rich blood supply carries carcinogenic components right into the bloodstream, spreading them across the body, accumulating toxins in lymph tissue, and dumping them into the bladder.

No wonder bladder cancer, non-Hodgkin's lymphoma, and bone marrow cancers have a higher incidence in hair care professionals who work with hair dyes daily for long periods of time (Bolt, Golka 2007). In 2008, scientists of Yale University, reporting in the *American Journal of Epidemiology,* observed that "increased risk of non-Hodgkins lymphoma associated with hair-dye use was observed among women who began using hair dye before 1980" (Zhang et al. 2008). In 1995, the *European Journal of Cancer Prevention* found that hairstylists and colorists also have a higher risk of developing breast cancer (La Vecchia, Tavani 1995). But, while hairstylists are usually exposed to the fumes of hair dyes (mind you, they are wearing gloves!), the carcinogenic cocktail of chemicals is applied directly to our skin, exposing us to significantly higher amounts of toxins. In one study, the risk increased with more prolonged exposure to darker, more concentrated, permanent dyes (Miligi et al. 2005).

Many experts still prefer to insist that hair dyes may not be harmful at all. Most often, these experts have strong ties to the cosmetic industry or perform research that was paid for by cosmetic corporations. For example, in 2008, an industrial consultancy firm Exponent performed *a study of studies* on hair dyes and made a verdict that hair dyes are safe: "No association was found between any personal use of hair dye and bladder cancer among women" (Kelsh et al. 2008). To achieve these conclusions, scientists "compared, updated, and expanded the analyses of two previous meta-analyses" on hair dyes. No independent, scientifically sound research was done to support the optimism about hair dyes.

Writing about hair dyes is very painful for me. My mother continues dyeing her hair every two weeks despite all my pleas to stop or at least to switch to safer, less chemical dyes. Until five years ago, I couldn't be without the darkest brown dyed hair, heavily styled with petrochemically laden foams and sprays. So instead of crying wolf, let's see what real science has said recently about the troubling relationship between hair dyes and cancer.

A large population-based case-control study at the Centre for Study and Cancer Prevention, Florence, Italy, in 2005 found an association between the use of hair dyes and non-Hodgkin's lymphoma, leukemia, multiple myeloma, and Hodgkin's disease (Miligi et al. 2005). Women who used black hair dye colors were at an increased risk of developing leukemia, in particular chronic lymphocytic leukemia. Another 2007 study in Germany found that human bladder cancers, induced by aromatic amines, can often hide for more than twenty years, which means that hair colors could make their deadly impact many years later (Bolt, Golka 2007).

A Spanish study in 2007 analyzed 2,302 incident cases of lymphoid neoplasms from all over Europe in 1998–2003 (de Sanjosé et al. 2006). Use of hair dyes was reported by 74 percent of women and 7 percent of men. The lymphoma risk among dye users was increased by 19 percent in comparison with no use and by 26 percent among those people who used hair dyes twelve or more times per year. The lymphoma risk was significantly higher among people who had started coloring their hair before 1980 and people who had used hair dyes only before 1980.

Researchers at Roswell Park Cancer Institute in Buffalo, New York, in 2007 found that hair dyes, along with tobacco exposure and a diet rich in meat, increase a woman's risk of breast cancer (Ambrosone et al. 2007).

A small study in Nebraska in 2005 found that among women newly diagnosed with brain cancer, a 1.7-fold increased risk of glioma was observed for women who had ever used hair coloring products and a 2.4-fold risk for those who had used permanent hair coloring products (Heineman et al. 2005). For women with the most aggressive form of glioma, the risk increased after twenty-one or more years of permanent hair coloring use.

What's worse, women using hair dyes not only up their own risk of getting brain cancer, they may be passing this risk on to their children. A 2005 study conducted by scientists at the University of North Carolina linked maternal hair dye use and the elevated risk of childhood cancer, including neuroblastoma (McCall et al. 2005). Doctors analyzed children with neuroblastoma diagnosed between 1992 and 1994 at hospitals in the United States and Canada. They found that use of any hair dye in the month before and/or during pregnancy was associated with a moderately increased risk of neuroblastoma. Use of temporary (nonpermanent dyes, marketed as "low ammonia") hair colors was more strongly associated with neuroblastoma than use of permanent hair dyes.

For some reason that is beyond the scope of this book, cosmetic manufacturers consistently ignore these findings, launching new brands of at-home coloring kits. Would someone buy a hair coloring kit if it contained a warning "Caution: May Cause Cancer," similar to those on tobacco products? Many young people start coloring their hair as early as twelve years old, and I was shocked to see a toddler girl with intricately placed pink and golden highlights in her freshly colored black hair. It turned out her mom was a student of hairdressing, and she used her two-year-old daughter as a training model! These children and teenagers are accumulating a toxic load at an incredibly fast rate. The first calls to remove carcinogens from hair dyes and adopt appropriate labeling of hair-coloring products to reduce the risk of cancer were voiced as far back as 1994, yet nothing has been done so far in this direction.

## Dyes That Kill

So how do you know if your hair color is slowly killing you? There is only one way to tell. You have to take a thorough look at the ingredients list printed on the box. The list is usually printed in all-capitalized letters, making it incredibly hard to read, and there's a good reason for this. You will see that cancer-causing ingredients are found in all conventional hair dyes currently on sale in the United States, Canada, and the United Kingdom.

The next time you feel like changing your hair color, check the ingredients label on the box for one of the following chemicals:

phenylenediamine
aminophenol
ethanolamine
hydroquinone
2,4-diaminophenoxyethanol

If even one of these ingredients is present, you should not purchase the hair dye.

The following ingredients in hair colors have been shown to cause nausea when inhaled, dermatitis, and/or breathing difficulties: p-phenylenediamine, resorcinol, 2-methylresorcinol, toluene (4-amino-2-hydroxytoluene), ammonium hydroxide, sodium metabisulfite, tetrasodium pyrophosphate, nonoxynol-4, nonoxynol-9, phosphoric acid, 1-naphthol, etidronic acid. The list can go on and on, but these are the most popular ingredients found in the majority of hair dyes currently on the market.

There is no such thing as a safe chemical hair color. Basic home hair coloring kits sold at drugstores and expensive highlighting jobs at upscale hair salons are equally damaging to your health. Your hair may look glossy and pretty, but the damage to your bladder, breasts, lungs, and immune and endocrine systems is irreversible.

## Are There Any Alternatives?

Consider green hair dyes. While they don't always have the broad color palette and can be messy to apply, their damage rarely goes further than stained towels. Most often, natural hair dyes are based on henna with the addition of mineral pigments. They do not contain carcinogenic chemicals, ammonia, or peroxide.

Some so-called herbal hair dyes, such as Herbatint, are not much different from conventional coloring kits sold in groceries and drugstores. The last time I checked, some of the most popular "herbal" dyes contained p-phenylenediamine, p-aminophenol, resorcinol, ethanolamine, and tetrasodium EDTA, to name just a few offenders. The only thing green about these hair dyes is the color of the boxes. Don't be fooled by natural-sounding names. Always check what goes in the product, and don't be seduced by "green" claims until you verify yourself that they have any substance.

There are several plants that can be used as natural coloring agents. Henna is the oldest and most popular one. It was used in ancient Egypt, most notably by Queen Cleopatra, and today henna remains an important beauty tool in the Middle East and India. There are three types of henna: red henna (*Lawsonia inermis, Lawsonia alba,* and *Lawsonia spinosa*), neutral henna (*Lyzifus spina christi*), and black henna (*Indigofera tinctora*). To achieve color variations, all three types of henna can be blended together, with the addition of indigo and iron oxides. The active ingredient in henna, lawsone, has the chemical name 2-dihydroxy-1,4-naphtaqiunone (not directly related to hydroquinone or 1-naphthalene), which makes henna a stable, yet semipermanent hair dye. It will nourish your hair and bring out beautiful golden highlights in dark hair.

Henna is the only colorant to have been safety-approved by the FDA. Unfortunately, it doesn't always produce the expected hair shade. If your hair has been previously dyed with conventional hair dyes, henna is not recommended. Wait for a few months to let the chemical color wash out, and then perform a strand test with henna, similar to a patch test. Blend a small amount of henna according to package instructions and apply it on one lock of hair, preferably behind the ear.

Many women use henna not for color but for other benefits, such as increased volume, scalp irritation relief, and improved manageability of hair. To reap the benefits of henna without dyeing your hair, you can use shampoos and conditioners with neutral henna. This plant extract will not change your hair color.

Among the better hair dyes with henna, I would choose Light Mountain Natural (nonbrassy shades that flatter all skin tones, including Chestnut, Medium Brown, and Dark Brown) and Aubrey Organics Color Me Natural, which is both perfectly permanent and natural.

## Green Color Maintenance

A switch to green, all-natural hair color requires courage, especially if you are used to changing your hair shade at a single whim of fashion. There are plenty of color-boosting shampoos, conditioners, gels, and sprays that help protect your natural new hair color. They contain plant extracts that play up color tones and prevent color from fading. For lighter hair colors, choose treatment shampoos and masks with lemon, chamomile, sunflower, and calendula. Redheads must include products with henna (neutral or golden) in their hair care regimen. Dark hair colors benefit from black walnut, black tea, coffee, and licorice root in their conditioners.

Sadly, most "natural" hair color preserving lines—including ShiKai Color Enhancing line, Nature's Gate Organics In Living Color, and Aveda Color Conserve and Color Enhancing shampoos and conditioners—are formulated with paraben preservatives, polyquaterniums, disodium EDTA, and urea. Some of the safe green products for colored hair include Kiss My Face Miss Treated Organic Hair Care Shampoo, Aubrey Organics White Camellia Ultra-Smoothing Shampoo, and amazing Colorcare Henna Hair Shampoo for dark hair by Logona. Colored hair conditioners are more scarce. From all that I tried (and I tried a lot), Real Purity Native Earth Moisturizing Hair Rinse and Dr. Hauschka Jojoba and Marshmallow Conditioner are the best. For deep treatment, a dry mask Zen Hair and Scalp Detox Spa Therapy by Morocco Method is simply unrivalled.

For added hair health, use the following all-natural home treatments weekly to maintain the shade of your hair.

## Chamomile Rinse for Blond Hair

6 tea bags chamomile tea

½ cup plain yogurt

5 drops lemon essential oil

*This rinse will bring beautiful highlights to naturally fair hair or revive your existing highlights for a sunny, summery look.*

1. Boil 1 cup of water and steep the tea bags for fifteen minutes.
2. Add yogurt and lemon oil to the chamomile tea and mix thoroughly.
3. Apply the mixture to dry hair, working through to the ends. Cover with a non-PVC plastic shower cap and relax for twenty minutes. Shampoo your hair as usual.

Alternatively, you can add 1 cup of dry chamomile flowers to 3 cups of boiling water and simmer on low heat for fifteen minutes to prepare a concentrated chamomile infusion. You can add a pinch of vitamin C to act as a mild preservative and store it in a spray bottle in the refrigerator for up to one month. You can use this infusion as a leave-on conditioner: simply spray evenly on freshly washed hair and air dry or blow dry as usual.

**Yield:**
4 ounces

## Chocolate Brunette Hair Rinse

2 cups purified water
(do not use mineral water)

5 tablespoons dark roast ground coffee

1 ounce black chocolate

*This rinse will not ruin your highlights but instead will make your brown color deeper and more vibrant. Do not use a coffeemaker to prepare the rinse, as the concentration of coffee won't be strong enough.*

1. Boil the ground coffee in two cups of water in a shallow pan for 10 minutes.
2. Add the chocolate while the coffee is hot. Let the mixture cool and carefully soak your hair with the flavorful blend. Beware of the spills!
3. Cover with a non-PVC plastic shower cap, wait for 10 minutes, rinse off, and shampoo as usual.

**Yield:**
4 ounces

## Red Hair
## Shine Enhancer

½ cup beet juice

½ cup carrot juice

½ cup lemon juice

**Yield:
4 ounces**

*Word of caution: Do not use this blend if you have high-lights. Use only if your hair is relatively uniform in color.*

1. Mix all ingredients together and pour over clean, slightly damp hair. Cover with a non-PVC plastic shower cap.

2. Slowly heat the cap with a hot towel, a hair dryer on medium heat, or just by sitting in the sun for one hour. If using a hair dryer, aim for ten minutes of gentle heating—no need to burn the cap with the blast of hot air! Once you are done heating, rinse and shampoo as usual.

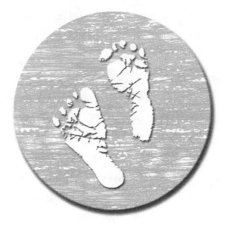

*green* **baby care**

how many times have you walked through the baby section of a drugstore cooing over all those cute, adorable, teddy-bear adorned bottles and tubes? There's everything your baby (or any baby in your life) will possibly need: moisturizers, bath gels, body washes, powders, diaper creams, and even sunscreens. They smell like little pink roses and feel much softer and gentler than adult versions. We automatically assume that the creators of these cute-as-pie concoctions have gone to great lengths to formulate completely safe, gentle, and soothing products for all those little behinds and toes. Well, don't assume anything.

We all know that a baby's skin is much thinner and more delicate than an adult's. As a result, it can absorb anything applied to it at a much faster rate. Babies scratch themselves more easily, they are more prone to irritations and rashes, and even a loose cloth tag left inside a onesie can leave scary red wounds that look worse than they are and heal by the next morning. Babies are soft, helpless, vulnerable human beings, and their skin cannot yet protect them from the dangers of the outside world.

Despite this obvious, commonsense information, virtually all conventional baby products you find on grocery and drugstore shelves are filled to the brim with ingredients that are anything but safe for a baby's health. Fragrances, penetration enhancers, sulfate detergents, preservatives, and synthetic dyes are not safe for babies. Neither are they for any adult. Yet these ingredients are contained in baby products at high concentrations. I know this may sound harsh, but the truth about baby products is that they are often worse for human health than adult ones. Ninety-nine percent of products marketed for delicate, fragile skin are nothing but bottled irritations, chapping, diaper rash, and watery eyes. Here is a quick checklist of things you should by all means avoid in your baby products:

*I know this may sound harsh, but the truth about baby products is that they are often worse for human health than adult products.*

*Propylene glycol.* This penetration enhancer and emulsifier can cause intense burning in the vaginal and perianal area. In 1998, a premature infant went into a coma after absorbing too much propylene glycol from topical applications when this chemical was used as a solvent in antiseptic dressings (Peleg et al. 1998). I certainly hope that your average drugstore baby wipe doesn't contain enough propylene glycol to send your baby into a coma, but the irritating, allergenic qualities of propylene glycol are well-known and well-documented.

Mineral oil. Also known as liquid petrolatum, mineral oil is praised for its lubricating action and low price. Mineral oil is a by-product of petroleum distillation, and its production is quite toxic, involving sulfuric acid, absorbents, solvents, and alkalis. It only takes a drop of synthetic fragrance to transform mineral oil into baby oil. In baby products, mineral oil is also used in lotions, diaper rash creams, and baby wipes. While it's considered to be nongenotoxic and generally nonirritating, mineral oil forms an airtight film on the skin's surface, preventing it from normal functioning. And there's another bothering fact about mineral oil. Researchers from the Innsbruck Medical University say that mineral paraffins appear to be the largest contaminant of our bodies, "widely amounting to 1g per person and reaching 10 g in extreme cases" (Concin et al. 2008). They found mineral oil in breast milk and fat tissue in new moms, and since mineral oil is frequently used to protect nipples between breastfeedings, babies ingest this petrochemical from the very first days of their lives.

Triethanolamine (TEA) is a popular emollient and acidity adjuster. We have already learned that this irritating chemical may be contaminated with the potent carcinogen 1,4-Dioxane. Why take chances? There are lots of green baby lotions and creams that do not contain triethanolamine or any member of the TEA/DEA/MEA family.

Paraben and other preservatives. A baby's hormonal system is not yet mature, and hormone disruptors can cause irreparable damage to the developing endocrine system. There have been no studies confirming the safety of paraben preservatives for babies. Why should your little bundle of joy participate in this gigantic experiment with an unknown outcome?

Fragrance. Conventional baby products are usually highly fragranced. These powdery scents are more appealing to moms than to babies, and manufacturers are in no hurry to remove the scents, simply because fragranced products usually sell better than unscented ones. Any synthetic fragrance, as we already know, is nothing but an irritation.

*Synthetic color.* Most baby products have a cute pink or yellow tint in them. Babies do not care about the color of their diaper cream or baby wash! All they want is zero irritation. More often than not, the color in baby baths, washes, and lotions is achieved by adding synthetic colorants, such as D&C Yellow 10 (Quinoline Yellow) or D&C Orange 4 (Acid Orange 7), considered to be potentially genotoxic substances.

Want to add more color to your baby's bath? Steep some herbal tea with berries, such as strawberries or raspberries for at least 10 minutes and pour it into the bath—believe me, everyone will be happier.

*Other toxic synthetic junk.* Other chemicals to avoid include fabric softeners such as cetrimonium chloride in baby hair detanglers, formaldehyde-releasing preservatives disodium EDTA and DMDM hydantoin in baby wipes and creams, and petroleum-derived silicones in diaper creams.

*Irritating plant extracts and essential oils.* These include peppermint, eucalyptus, ylang-ylang, sage, bergamot, and citrus oils. You may use eucalyptus in a vaporizer during colds, though.

It's vitally important to avoid all baby products that contain any of the above ingredients. Just a quick glance at the ingredients list will provide you with more information than any cute packaging or adorable scent. Which is more important to you—the cute little baby on the label or your own little pink darling who depends on your ability to discern between safe and unsafe products?

## Green Bath for Your Baby

Babies love to be bathed. Bathing relaxes them and may soothe any minor skin irritation, especially if you keep bath time less than ten minutes. And the smell of a baby right out of the bath . . . mmm, it's so yummy!

You don't need special cleansers for a baby's face, hands, hair, and behind. One gentle plant-based cleanser is more than enough. The best green cleansers are based on corn, palm, or coconut-derived surfactants that are prepared without the use of sulfates. These include decyl polyglucose, coco-glycoside, olivoil glutinate, sodium cocoyl glutamate, and the less green cocamidopropyl betaine. Aloe vera, calendula, chamomile, and olive leaf extracts are soothing and healing. They are usually well tolerated by all babies, even newborns.

To bathe a newborn, you don't really need anything other than warm water. Many doctors recommend bathing babies in plain water until they are six months old. We tried it, and our baby came out clean and good smelling. Newborns do not get sweaty or dirty except in the diaper area or if they spit up. You will need a foaming cleanser or a mild soap for cleaning the diaper area, though organic baby oil or organic virgin olive oil usually work just fine. If the water in your area is particularly hard, you can alternate water-only baths with foam or herbal baths. And use a mild cleanser to wash soiled cloth diapers.

## Green Product Guide: Baby Washes

**California Baby Calming Shampoo & Bodywash** is a no-nonsense, pure, and unscented all-purpose body wash and a shampoo that can also double as a facial cleanser for moms. Formulated with aloe vera, sugar-derived surfactants, and softening vitamin E and glycerin, this cleanser is very concentrated, so a little squirt goes a long way. Unlike many products by California Baby, this cleanser contains no paraben preservatives, so feel safe using it on your little green darling.

**Weleda Baby Calendula Shampoo & Body Wash** is a gentle, moisturizing, all-purpose body wash and shampoo with emollient sesame and sweet almond oils and soothing calendula extract. Rinses off clean and doesn't seem to irritate the baby's eyes.

**Dr. Bronner's 18-in-1 Hemp Pure-Castile Soap (Baby Mild)** is probably the most economical organic product available on the market. Just a dash of soap in warm water makes sudsy yet nonirritating bubbles, and you can also use it for baby laundry and to soak cloth diapers. Unscented, vegan, and organic—a truly ingenious product!

## Green Product Guide: Baby Washes

You can quickly create a baby herbal bath blend or bath oil using just a few basic ingredients. Please note that any essential oil may pose the threat of irritation to your baby's skin. Always perform a patch test if you are concerned about allergic reactions, especially if you have a family history of skin allergies. Dilute a drop of the essential oil in two tablespoons of virgin olive oil and apply a dot on the back of your baby's arm (the oil won't end up in her mouth). Leave the oil on overnight and check for any signs of redness in the morning. If no reaction occurs, the oil is likely to be well-tolerated. If you see any kind of redness, do not use the oil on your baby. You may use the scented batch of oil to massage your skin, though! Always use half the amount of essential oil that you would use in an adult product.

Although many baby products are formulated with lavender, I prefer to err on the side of caution with this aromatic herb. Suspected endocrine-disrupting abilities of lavender are currently being researched. However, lavender has been used in traditional medicine for centuries, and its ability to promote sleep is well-proven. Remember, it's easy to go overboard with lavender. When used in excessive amounts, this fragrant flower can stimulate instead of promote sleep.

## Skin-Clearing Herbal Bath

4 cups of purified water
½ cup dried birch leaves
½ cup marigold flowers
½ cup dried sage leaves

**Yield: 4 ounces**

*This is a traditional Russian recipe that we used to soothe redness and mild rash in our baby when she was one week old.*

1. Boil all ingredients for fifteen minutes in 4 cups of purified water.
2. Strain and discard the herbs and flowers.
3. Use two cups for one bath and store the remaining two cups of the infusion in the refrigerator. It must be used within two days.

## Soothing Milk Bath

⅛ cup organic milk powder

5 drops chamomile essential oil

2 drops rose essential oil

*This blend was inspired by the popular (and quite expensive) Burt's Bees Baby Bee Buttermilk Bath Soak, but we skipped an unknown "fragrance" and used well-diluted chamomile oil instead.*

1. Mix the essential oils with three tablespoons of milk powder and blend thoroughly so that the oil completely disappears into the powder. Mix this in with the remaining milk powder.

2. To use, dissolve two to three tablespoons in a warm bath. Let your baby relax in the milky water for ten minutes.

Yield:
4 ounces

## Baby Oatmeal Bath Pouches

2 cups organic oatmeal

2 cups organic milk powder

½ cup organic lavender flowers

½ cup dried calendula or chamomile flowers

2 drops chamomile essential oil

*You can use muslin or pieces of organic cotton to make reusable bath pouches. Cut 4-inch by 8-inch fabric rectangles and sew three sides together. Use fabric ribbons to tie the top. This recipe makes enough for twenty pouches.*

Blend all the ingredients thoroughly and fill the prepared pouches. To use, immerse one pouch in the bathwater and rub it over the baby's skin like a washcloth.

Yield:
4 ounces

## Making Your Own Baby Wipes

I had an upsetting experience with baby wipes, which I discussed in Chapter 2, "Beauty and the Toxic Beast." There are many truly green baby wipes available, including TenderCare Flushable Wipes, Seventh Generation Unscented Baby Wipes, and Tushies Baby Wipes, but I now prefer to make my own. It's cheaper, and I know exactly what goes into them.

## Green Baby Wipe Solution

1 cup purified water

½ cup witch hazel

5 drops calendula extract

5 drops aloe vera extract

3 drops tea tree essential oil

5,000 IU vitamin E
  (as a preservative)

**Yield:
4 ounces**

*Some DIY fans prefer to make baby wipes from a roll of paper towels cut in half, but I found that any really worn-out cotton T-shirt cut in squares works just fine. Start with twenty squares (a day's supply) and see how it goes. If you decide to modify the formulation, you won't waste too much fabric. Added bonus: fabric wipes are super-eco-friendly, as you can wash them with the rest of baby's laundry or diapers.*

1. Blend all the ingredients in a bottle. Shake well to dissolve vitamin E.
2. Place paper or fabric squares measuring approximately 4x4 inches in airtight, waterproof container and pour the solution over them. The fabric should be completely saturated, and some fluid should remain at the bottom. You can use an empty box from refillable baby wipes such as Tushies (when you have used up the wipes). Alternatively, any ceramic, glass, or polypropylene (plastic #5) food storage container would be suitable, too. You can find such containers in most discount stores and online.
3. Put the lid back on the box and turn it upside down so the solution is absorbed.

## Green Baby Massage

A baby massage is a greatly underestimated nonmedication solution for many baby ailments. Massage therapy has been consistently shown to increase weight gain and decrease stress in preterm babies (Lahat et al. 2007), and various studies show that baby massage helps ease colic, soothe stomach disorders, and help with sleep (Underdown et al. 2006). A study in Finland showed that 93 percent of participating parents reported that colic symptoms decreased during the three-week baby massage therapy (Huhtala et al. 2000). Baby massage is great for moms, too—by gently stroking and rubbing her little bundle of joy, a mom can alleviate symptoms of postnatal depression, British researchers reported in July 2008 (O Higgins et al. 2008).

You can easily perform a baby massage at home without attending courses or buying instructional videos. Choose a moment when your baby is content and relaxed, ideally after a bath but before the evening feeding. Put the baby on a clean receiving blanket and pour some massage oil on your hands. Rub them to warm the oil.

A baby massage flows from the head to the toes. Work with soft and gentle touches on the head, face, shoulders, arms, chest, stomach, and legs. Learn how much pressure you can use by closing your eyes and pressing on your eyelids. That's it! Unlike adult massages that penetrate to the muscles, baby massages shouldn't go any deeper than the skin. Use your fingertips to massage hands, feet, and face, and use the palm of your hand to massage the stomach area, legs, and arms. There is not one "right" way to massage your baby. Listen to your heart and be gentle. Don't worry: baby will love whatever you do!

Among some things to avoid are the following: Make sure not to massage the genital areas; do not put any pressure on the baby's knees or elbows; do not massage baby's face with any massage oils that contain essential oils; do not press too hard on the baby's neck or stomach. Do not force your baby to lie on her stomach; if she wants to turn over, use this opportunity to massage her back. Keep the massage oil away from your baby.

Here's a soothing, nourishing baby oil blend that you can also use to moisturize dry areas and for general cleanups after poops or spit-ups.

Virtually any unscented organic plant oil can be used to moisturize a baby's skin. Avocado, grape seed, and virgin olive oils are among the best. Just pour the necessary amount into a pretty glass bottle with a pump top and use as needed. I know that glass bottles may break when dropped, but this is still a better option than contaminating the baby product with chemicals leaching from plastic bottles.

You can easily perform a baby massage at home without attending courses or buying instructional videos.

## Soothing Baby Massage Oil

½ cup grape seed oil

½ cup wheat germ oil

*Optional:*

3 drops lavender essential oil

  *or*

2 drops rose essential oil

  *or*

3 drops calendula herbal oil
(available at Mountain
Rose Herbs)

Combine all ingredients in a glass bottle with a flip-top cap. Shake well to allow oils to blend uniformly.

**Yield:
4 ounces**

## Natural Diaper Area Care

There's a saying by Canadian social reformer and educator Martin McLuhan: "Diaper backward spells repaid." One thing is pretty certain—a wise choice of diaper care products can be repaid with quieter nights and happier daytime play.

Almost all babies develop at least one bout of diaper rash before they are potty-trained. There's no way around it. Frequent diaper changes, water rinsing instead of baby wipes when practical, a regular application of lightweight baby oils, and use of all-natural baby wipes can help control, if not completely prevent, diaper rash.

Sometimes diaper rash can be caused by the very diapers you use. Cloth diapers are more prone to cause skin irritations, perhaps because the moisture is not quickly wiped off the skin, as it is by disposable diapers.

Unlike many other green moms, I am not a firm believer in cloth diapers. (I already envision skeptical frowns.) Before my baby was born, I stocked an ample supply of soft, fluffy cloth diapers, woolen pants, and waterproof pads, none of which came cheap. After a month of daily diaper washes, our water and electricity bills skyrocketed! The almost constant diaper rash despite frequent changes and use of only natural detergents (Dr. Bronner's soap and plain unscented soap flakes, not Fairy liquid!) was also a decisive factor. We switched to biodegradable, chlorine-free disposables made of corn, and my daughter hasn't had a single episode of diaper rash since. With a monthly cost of $40 (instead of the $100-plus that advocates of cloth diapering claim the disposable diapers cost) and substantially lower environmental impact, I am happy to use disposable diapers with biodegradable liners and pack them in compostable diaper sacks. Even if you choose to use cloth diapers, keep a pack of larger-sized disposable diapers (not training pants) for diaper rash emergencies. If keeping an emergency supply of disposable diapers, always go one size up because babies grow so fast, and she may outgrow the diapers you've stocked if you use them only occasionally.

To soothe a baby's diaper rash, always wash the diaper area with water instead of cleaning with wipes, even if you've made your own completely green ones. Pat the area dry and apply a barrier cream with zinc oxide, calendula, aloe, or chamomile.

It's worth spending an extra five minutes to whip up a simple baby balm if no natural diaper products are available nearby.

## Happy Bum Flower Balm

½ cup shea butter
(if possible, organic)

½ cup coconut butter
(if possible, organic)

1 teaspoon zinc oxide

5 drops rose essential oil

2 drops sage essential oil

2,000 IU vitamin E

5 drops colloidal silver

Yield:
4 ounces

*When your baby is teething, you may want to use the cream more frequently, as babies are prone to diaper rash before their new teeth sprout.*

1. Heat the shea butter and coconut oil in a shallow pan, but do not boil.

2. Gradually add the rest of the ingredients. Add zinc oxide while the mixture is still liquid. Remove from heat and stir until the mixture starts to cool, about 3 minutes. Add the essential oils after the mixture cools a bit so that their properties don't disperse in the heat as quickly. Gradually add vitamin E and the colloidal silver. Stir well.

3. Transfer into a glass jar and use as often as necessary when you notice redness in the diaper area.

# Green Little Bunz Baby Powder

½ cup baking soda

½ cup kaolin (white clay)

1 tablespoon zinc oxide

5 drops chamomile essential oil

5 drops rose essential oil

**Yield:
5 ounces**

*Sometimes it's unclear whether your baby has diaper rash or a yeast infection. Cornstarch, a popular ingredient in natural baby powders, can worsen yeast rash by forming yeast-feeding wet clumps in skin folds. This powder avoids cornstarch.*

1. Combine baking soda, kaolin, and zinc oxide in a sifter.

2. Add oils one drop at a time while sifting. Sift a second time to mix the oil thoroughly.

3. Make a paper funnel and pour mixture into a shaker bottle. If your baby develops redness that doesn't go away after treatment with diaper rash cream, change the tactic and use the powder for one day instead.

*chapter* **14**

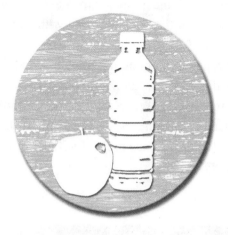

*green* **mineral**
**makeup**

**W**e all want to look good naturally. In a perfect world, we could face anyone barefaced and confident, but most of us need a helping hand from makeup.

Makeup is one area where many people compromise, opting for ease of application, staying power, and color selection instead of natural ingredients. When was the last time you checked the ingredients of that "vinyl shine" lip-gloss? Something tells me never. After all, we apply paint to such small areas of the skin compared with our bodies that we believe a little makeup isn't really going to hurt—or is it?

While the jury is still out, troubling research is published every day: lead is found in lipsticks, aluminum lurks in eye shadows, coal tar dyes give color to mascara. While things have certainly improved since the time of Queen Elizabeth I, when her distinguishing white makeup gave her lead poisoning, women are still willing to use toxic makeup for the sake of beauty.

## Color Me Healthy

Consider the ingredients list of an average bottle of liquid foundation. Water is at the beginning, followed by silicones, talc, glycerin, paraffin, synthetic wax, aluminum starch, propylene glycol, more mineral oil, more silicones, sodium laureth sulfate, synthetic fragrance, and some FDA-approved pigments. In some foundations, paraffin and mineral oil are listed several times! All of these ingredients have been shown to block skin pores and cause irritation in human or animal studies. Let's not forget about the potent blend of preservatives contained in any foundation, fluid or powder. These usually include formaldehyde-releasing butylated hydroxytoluene (BHT) and disodium EDTA, triethanolamine, and the strong contact allergen iodopropynyl butylcarbamate. The only natural ingredients occurring in conventional foundations are usually limited to panthenol, menthol, camphor, beeswax, and beta-carotene. Remove all the irritants, potential and proven toxins, and fragrance, and what are we left with? A pinch of mineral pigments.

No wonder mineral makeup, which is nothing more than finely powdered minerals, is becoming the makeup of choice of health-conscious models, celebrities, and makeup artists. Thanks to the latest technologies, minerals can be milled so finely that they stick to the skin's surface without any need for additional binding and slip agents such as silicones, and since mineral powder contains no water, there's no need to use preservatives either.

The bulk of a mineral makeup powder is composed of titanium oxide, a naturally occurring white mineral that can be found in its purest form in white beach sand. Titanium oxide can make up one-quarter of a jar of mineral foundation, serving as a base color and a physical sunscreen. Another key ingredient is zinc oxide, occurring in nature as the opaque white mineral zincite. Zinc serves an important role in skin health, protecting it from inflammation caused by bacteria and oxidative damage. It can even speed up wound healing! Other mineral makeup ingredients include iron oxides and mica.

There has been a lot of debate regarding the safety of bismuth oxychloride, which is found in many popular mineral makeup products. There have been claims that bismuth oxychloride can cause cancer, but authors of such articles and blog posts often confuse bismuth salts (not scary) with pure bismuth (can be quite toxic). It's the same with titanium and titanium oxide. No one is using pure metal titanium in mineral makeup, and no one is using pure bismuth! According to recent studies published by the Carcinogenic Potency Project at the University of California, tests on animals did not reveal any carcinogenic activity caused by bismuth oxychloride, and studies on animals back in 1975 also failed to find any carcinogenicity of this mineral (Preussmann, Ivankovic 1975). While bismuth oxychloride sounds similar to bismuth chloride, it's not the same chemical. Bismuth chloride is obtained by treating bismuth with hydrochloric acid and is indeed highly toxic. Bismuth oxychloride, a naturally occurring mineral salt that produces a subtle shimmer in mineral makeup products, has excellent antibacterial properties, and no study has ever shown any carcinogenic potential concerning this mineral.

Another dispute over the safety of mineral makeup concerns its physical qualities. Smoothness and long-lasting coverage in mineral makeup is achieved by pulverizing or "micronizing" minerals into microscopic or even nanoparticle size, but some researchers say that such wonderful qualities of mineral makeup come at a price. Experts from the Environmental Working Group claim that some nanoparticles can have very different, and even toxic, properties than the same chemical in a nonmicronized state.

Scientists are still trying to come to a definitive answer regarding the potential harm of zinc oxide and titanium oxide nanoparticles. The only recent research referring to the irritation potential of zinc and titanium oxide nanoparticles is a 2007 Scottish study showing that zinc chloride in nanoparticle form can irritate the lungs (Wilson et al. 2007). However, be advised that zinc oxide and zinc chloride are two different chemicals. Also in 2007, scientists at Boise State University in Idaho confirmed that while zinc oxide nanoparticles had clear antibacterial action, they had minimal effects on human cells (Reddy et al. 2007). Similar findings—that zinc oxide nanoparticles can kill both gram-negative and gram-positive bacteria without harming human cells—have also been reported by researchers of the University of South Dakota in February 2008 (Jones et al. 2008). If you prefer to err on the side of caution, stick to pressed mineral powder and fluid mineral foundations that do not require buffing in with a fluffy brush.

Iron oxide pigments and mica create most color variations in mineral makeup. Most of the iron oxide pigments used in cosmetics are approved by the FDA. When used in extremely high concentrations—for example, during tattooing and permanent pigmentation of eyebrows and lashes—iron oxides can cause irritation, but in mineral makeup the concentration is far lower. If you have a family history of allergies, you will be better off with plant-based kohl eyeliners instead of dark mineral eye shadows.

## Mineral Foundations: Not All Alike

Your foundation is going to sit on your face all day long, so going mineral helps you avoid unnecessary synthetic fillers and preservatives contained in a conventional foundation. Cleverly formulated mineral foundations will also help protect your face from sun exposure and excessive sebum production.

Invented thirty years ago, mineral foundations are quickly becoming the hottest-selling mineral makeup product. They come in powder and cream forms, packed in sifter jars and pump bottles. Those who love and use mineral makeup praise the dewy, natural, long-lasting glow and ability to layer the powder over problem areas without added bulk. Most important, pure formulations without synthetic bulk are safer and better for sensitive and acne- or rosacea-prone skin, especially after cosmetic surgeries. Fans of chemical skin care complain that mineral makeup is complicated to apply, drying, not portable, and accentuates wrinkles.

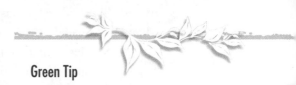

**Green Tip**

If you are going to buy just one green makeup product, make it a mineral foundation.

Makeup sensitivity is often the result of synthetic dyes, fragrances, and preservatives. While mineral makeup is made of generally the same color ingredients that have been used in synthetic makeup for ages, it's the absence of classic irritants like fragrances, silicone binders, penetration enhancers, synthetic dyes, and preservatives that give mineral makeup its special health and beauty properties.

Another big advantage of mineral makeup is its built-in sun protection. With an average SPF rating of fifteen, Bare Minerals has the Skin Cancer Foundation seal of approval as a sunscreen. Jane Iredale claims similar protective effects due to high contents of the physical sunscreens titanium dioxide and zinc oxide. But keep in mind that mineral makeup alone will not give you all the sun protection you need. You aren't likely to cover your ears and neck with mineral foundation, and even on the face the layer can be too sheer to provide reliable protection. Prime your skin before applying mineral foundation with moisturizer or sunscreen cream with an SPF of fifteen or higher.

## What Makes a Good Mineral Foundation?

As always, don't be fooled by the "all natural" or "all-mineral formula" on the label. Mineral makeup can still contain paraben preservatives and other fillers. Since there is no set regulation for what constitutes a "mineral" makeup, any product containing some minerals as a primary ingredient can be marketed as such—even if it contains a whole lot of synthetic ingredients. It's the same thing with "organic": any cosmetic product can be labeled organic if it contains just a pinch of organic aloe vera.

Here are some greener mineral brands that do not use synthetic additives, preservatives, or colorants in their products: Purely Cosmetics, Jane

Iredale, Sheer Cover, Laura Mercier, Youngblood, and BeLeeVe. Bare Minerals has excellent additive-free mineral foundations, but some of their mineral powders still contain paraben preservatives. If you prefer to use a mineral foundation without bismuth oxychloride, here are some brands you may find useful: Kathleen Meow Cosmetics, Perfect Earth Mineral Foundations, and Sheer Cover. All these brands are available online only.

When chosen wisely, foundation is virtually revolutionary in its benefits to your skin. Gone are the days when natural foundations came in ghastly color palettes that were often too pink or too orange to match real people's skin tones. Green foundations today are actually good for your skin, formulated with ingredients that make your skin healthier.

## Choosing the Right Green Foundation

Of all the makeup products, foundation is the hardest to buy. You want your color to be sheer, but you want the coverage to be good enough to cover imperfections. You want your texture silky, with a slight dewy glow, but not shiny. You want your foundation to diffuse little wrinkles, but you don't want it to be heavy and greasy. So many demands . . . and luckily, more than enough choices.

With mineral foundations, your only concern should be the ideal match for your skin tone. You can adjust the coverage and the texture later, using the right primers and mists.

Each of us has a skin tone that is based on yellow or pink. Here's how you can determine whether you have a pink undertone or a yellow undertone, which is crucial in choosing the right color. You have yellow undertones if your eyes are brown or hazel and you look best in gold jewelry and clothes that are orange, bronze, cream, or brown. You have pink undertones if your eyes are cool hazel, blue, green, or blue-gray, and you look best in silver jewelry and clothes that are violet, plum, pale blue, or pure white. Many cosmetic brands list colors for pink undertones as "neutral," while yellow undertones are often labeled as "golden."

Still unsure? If shopping in a department store, ask for a small sample in a clean jar. If shopping online, buy a small sample. Decent retailers are always happy to accommodate a cautious customer, because when you make informed buying decisions, you are less likely to return a product.

Mineral foundations today come in powder and fluid form. Powders are more versatile but less portable. Fluid mineral foundations are less common. Jane Iredale and Miessence make the best ones I have found so far. Fluid mineral foundations are a much better choice for aging skin. In addition to mineral pigments, they contain emollients, humectants, and plant antioxidants, which means that fluid foundations can double as moisturizers. Fluid mineral foundations can be "sealed" with powder mineral foundation, especially if you need to hide birthmarks, acne scars, or brown spots. In the summer you can also use Dr. Hauschka Toned Day Cream, which provides quite a substantial layer of natural-looking glowing tint. You can top the tinted moisturizer with a subtle layer of a mineral powder foundation to obtain some sun protection, but don't rely on the sun-protective qualities of mineral foundation! It cannot be your sole sunscreen. The tinted moisturizer, ideally with SPF rating fifteen or higher underneath the mineral powder, will provide moisture and prevent the powder from getting cakey and accentuating fine lines and wrinkles.

If your skin feels oilier in the summer, you can try the excellent Suki-color Tinted Active Moisturizer that contains vitamin C, retinol, organic plant extracts, and willow bark, an antioxidant rich in salicylic acid. I found that the coverage is quite sufficient when applied with fingertips, but for lighter coverage you can mix the foundation with a few drops of your regular moisturizer.

Shopping for the right color is no walk in the park. Here are some tips that you will find useful.

*Always test the color in the middle of your cheek* where you can see it. Many sales consultants want you to test the foundation at your neck so the color "will not leave a visible line." I find this practice useless. People first see your face, not your neck. The foundation must match your facial skin tone. Plus, it's virtually impossible to see your neck clearly in a mirror. For the same reason, don't test for color on your hand unless you are trying to camouflage some scars on your hands. Always test where you will actually apply the foundation and ignore all attempts to smear your neck or hand. Mineral foundations allow for seamless blendability, so the visible line at your chin should be the least of your worries.

### Green Tip

When you find a color that looks good indoors under florescent lights, *take a small mirror and walk outside* to check the color in natural light. Many colors will prove themselves too shimmery or too bronzy for everyday use.

Choosing the right foundation color can be tough for women with darker skin tones. That's why many women with dark complexions faithfully stick to their foundations and are reluctant to trade them for mineral versions, no matter how pure they are. Fortunately, most mineral makeup producers have broadened their color spectrum to suit every skin tone. Bare Escentuals carries excellent warm and neutral shades ranging from golden caramel to darkest espresso brown. The darkest shades can be found in Cover FX Powder FX Mineral Powder Foundation, which unfortunately is loaded with talc, silicones, and other additives. Dark-toned mineral foundations must contain a bit of a golden shimmer to avoid that unattractive ashy effect on dark and olive skin. A dry complexion can make dark skin look grayish. Make sure you wear a good moisturizer underneath your foundation.

## Tools of the Mineral Trade

Mineral foundations are usually marketed along with a complex set of brushes. While it's tempting to equip yourself with every possible brush size to ensure a flawless application, in reality you only need two brushes: one for the overall application of the foundation and one for a mineral concealer.

A kabuki brush is by far the best tool to achieve natural, even results when applying a powder foundation. It has a short handle (actually, just a stump of a handle) and a dome-shaped, fluffy, thick head made of goat's hair. Many companies have recently come up with their own version of the original Bare Escentuals kabuki, but often these brushes have either a head too narrow and pointed to produce a really good buffing or they are too stiff and dense so you pick up too much color and end up applying mineral powder so thickly that it looks like fresh plaster. If you decide to buy a foolproof kabuki brush, look for goat hair, not squirrel hair, or at least a blend of both, and a wide, fluffy, flatter, dome-shaped head that looks like a fan, not a furry bullet.

While I do use a Bare Escentuals "minibuki" brush for everyday foundation application, I found that I can achieve even better results with a tapered flat blush brush. You can use the sides of the brush to buff the foundation and the pointed edge to apply touch-ups of concealer. I also found that the use of a good blush brush, coupled with a light-handed application, results in a very fine, almost invisible layer of foundation. Among the better blush brushes are MAC 116 Blush Brush and 227

Large Fluff Brush, and Make Up For Ever 24S Blush Brush.

Make sure you stay away from flat-headed buffing brushes. While they sound like a natural match for powder makeup, the results are horrible: the application is thick, uneven, and all-around messy.

To carefully dot mineral concealer, you will need a special concealer brush. Again, I would recommend straying from traditional options—sleek, flat, stiff nylon brushes. These are good for cream concealer but are worthless with fine mineral powders that simply slide off the brush instead of being buffed into the skin. You simply cannot press and swirl those synthetic Taklon fibers! Your best bet is a tapered, round-edged eye shadow brush made of natural goat or sable hair. Again, head on to MAC for their bestselling 239 Eye Shading Brush, to Sephora for Make Up For Ever Eye Contour Brush 14S made of Russian squirrel fur, or if you're feeling indulgent, splurge on a Natural Brush 13G by Shu Uemura. When in a hurry, don't hesitate to dot the concealer with a clean fingertip: press gently on a blemish or under-eye circle and rub the powder gently.

## Blushers and Highlighters

Choosing a new blush is perhaps the most enjoyable experience after picking a new lip-gloss. Most mineral and other green blush varieties offer pretty, easily blendable, extremely wearable colors that can breathe life and vitality into even the dullest of complexions. There are many types of green blushes available. Loose mineral powder blushes are the most common but can be tricky to apply in a rush. With a loose powder blush, you need to perform a minifoundation application, with swirling, tapping, and buffing, and often you will end up applying more color than you planned. Remember, you can spread foundation across your face, but buffing the blush across your cheeks and close to the nose will result in an overly done, flashy effect. On the plus side, mineral blushes are versatile: you can mix a little bit with your regular foundation to create a subtle glow on your face, or you can custom-mix a perfectly matching lip-gloss color by adding a drop of blusher to any transparent lip-gloss or balm. A good brush is essential in applying mineral blushes evenly and precisely. For a universally flattering, almost foolproof application, try blushes in warm, tawny pinks with a subtle shimmer.

Pressed mineral powder blushers are the easiest to apply. Fine mineral pigments do not sit on the skin's surface like talc-based blushes do; they blend easily and almost disappear into the skin tone. Unfortunately, for some reason, even the makers of perfectly green mineral foundations use paraben preservatives in their blushes. Among the purest pressed blushes, I would recommend Dr. Hauschka Rouge Powder 02 Desert Rose, Jane Iredale PurePressed Blush in Whisper with real 24-carat gold particles, and BeLeeVe Pressed Mineral Blush Sorbet. Pure Minerals makes deep-toned, pressed mineral blushes that are excellent for darker complexions.

Cream and gel blushes are fun to look at but aren't fun to use. The only good thing about them is that you can use them on lips and cheeks. Most gel blushes blend easily into the skin, creating an almost natural, no-makeup look. However, to reap this benefit, you need to eschew foundation and apply blush on bare skin. How many of us can get away with that? Silicone-based, cream-to-powder blushes with a whipped-cream texture are easier to apply, but they usually contain too many chemical additives to be considered green. Among some versatile natural and truly green cream blushes are Kiss My Face 3 Way Color for Lips, Cheeks & Eyes in Dawn Pure Cream Stain by SukiColor in Sandstone. They can double as all-natural lip glosses!

## Green Mascara: Not Just for Ravers

Even if you are a no-makeup type, consider wearing a natural mascara. This amazing makeup product can instantly add definition to your eyes and will pull together any natural makeup look. Finding truly green mascara without alcohol, shellac, preservatives, triethanolamine, phenoxyethanol, and other potential irritants is quite easy. Finding natural mascara that does not run, smudge, sting, bleed, crumble, or dry out after two weeks is mission impossible. After years of testing and tossing, I realized that the following three mascaras are worth considering: Dr. Hauschka Volume Mascara heads the list with a luxurious metal tube and delectable thick lashes after just one sweep; Lavera Volume Organic Mascara is a close second; and Zuzu Luxe Mascara, which is quite basic but water-resistant, is great for summertime use. All of these mascaras do the lengthening and thickening job by using mineral pigments rather than

# MAKEUP APPLICATION TIPS

Here are some application tips I learned from fashion makeup gurus while reporting from backstage at some of the most famous fashion shows in the last ten years.

- Do not try to shape your face with a blush. This is so outdated! To create a prominent cheekbone, makeup artists use shades of light and dark contouring powder. Do not attempt to accentuate cheekbones with a dark blush, applying it in a stripe under your cheekbone, and hoping this will make your cheeks slimmer. Apply the blush to accentuate your healthy glow, starting about an inch from your nose and blending the color just into the cheekbones. Do not paint your entire cheeks with color, either.

- To prop up cheekbones, use a translucent highlighter in skin-friendly, neutral, light warm pink shades. Leave intricate contouring to professional makeup artists, but to instantly add shape and curve to your face, run quickly around your hairline with a large fluffy brush dipped slightly in translucent powder bronzer.

- Most mineral blushers have some glimmer in them. To make this work for you, apply the blush on the apples of your cheeks and keep the color away from the outer corners of your eyes. Do not apply blush in downward motions, and do not rub the brush back and forth. For many mineral blushes, this brings out too much shimmer.

- Don't think that pale colors automatically mean a more natural look. Pale pink or peach blush can look unnatural if you have olive or dark skin. To choose the best color for your complexion, don't pinch your cheeks, but instead, smear some blush on your hand and bring it close to your makeup-free lips. Choose the color that works best with your natural lip tone.

- Do not match your blush to your jewelry, glasses, clothes, or hair color. The only thing that should guide you is the overall undertone of your makeup. If using gray, silver-toned eye shadow, stick to colder tones of blush, such as rose, pink, and berry. If using warm, golden-toned eye shadow and lip-gloss, choose peach, warm pink, or neutral golden beige.

synthetic fibers. Natural beeswax, kaolin, silk powders, and plant extracts keep the mascara in place while nourishing the lashes.

Natural mascaras do not contain preservatives, relying on airtight packaging and your understanding that you should discard any mascara, natural or not, after six months of use. To prolong the life of your natural mascara and help it work well for you for those six months, do not pump the wand into the tube, hoping to squeeze a little bit more color on the brush. All you achieve is pushing more air inside the tube, which makes mascara dry out faster.

You can create exciting effects with your mascara using mineral pigments. If your new natural mascara appears to be too runny, try this trick: lightly dust the mascara wand with just a pinch of very dark brown, purple, or shimmery gray mineral eye shadow. Coat the wand evenly and apply directly onto your lashes. Do not blend the eye shadow and mascara in the palm of your hand! This is messy and possibly contaminates the mascara with germs that are not found on your eyelashes.

## Natural Eyeliners and Eye Shadows

While it's really hard to go overboard and apply clashing, utterly unnatural-looking makeup using mineral and natural-based foundations, blushes, and mascara, mineral eye shadows virtually let you go nuts for color and shimmer. From barely there pastel hues to vivid, strong metallic pigments, myriads of color and texture variations of mineral eye shadows could easily be the one reason you convert into a green makeup junkie. Whether you want to go basic and classic with a single shadow accentuating the shape of your eye, or you are artistically inclined and feel brave enough to combine four shades into a sultry, sexy, smoky eye, you have all the cards.

Mineral eye glimmer and shadows are more intensely pigmented than foundations and blushers, hence there's a higher risk of making a mistake. The technique is basically the same as with the mineral foundation, only the brush is smaller. Tap a pinch of eye shadow powder into the lid or take some on your brush and transfer onto your hand. Don't apply loose powder eye shadows directly from the jar! You need to let the shadow penetrate the brush so that drops of dark eyeshadow do not ruin your foundation.

Mineral eye shadows can be applied wet or dry. With wet applications you can create an intense, long-lasting yet thin layer of color. You can use dark mineral shadows—dark gray, brown, purple, emerald green—as liquid eyeliner by dipping a pointed eyeliner brush into water (not saliva!) and tracing the upper lash line with a strong line of mineral color.

Mineral eye shadows can be applied wet or dry.

Here's a trick of the makeup art trade: before starting an intricate, smoky eye design, apply a heavy layer of translucent loose powder under your eyes. When you are done with the eye makeup, simply whiff off the excess powder with a large brush. Be warned, though: the powder will soak up any moisturizer you have under your eyes, so fine lines may look more prominent. Sometimes, after you are done with the makeup application, you look closely in the mirror and realize that you need some dramatic measures to get rid of wrinkles. Moments like this usually make me run and grab a pair of sunglasses. But there's a better way of hiding the lines around eyes. Simply and carefully dab some hydrating organic mist under the eyes to set the foundation and soften lines. Any floral hydrosol (steam-distilled flower water) will do the trick.

Natural eyeliners were invented long before eye shadows and even other types of makeup. Kohl, a mixture of castor oil, soot, and other ingredients, was used predominantly by Middle Eastern, North African, and Southeastern Asian women. Sometimes called surma or kajal in Southeastern Asia, kohl has been worn traditionally as far back as the Bronze Age.

Traditional kohl is made by burning a white muslin cloth soaked in sandalwood paste in a mud lamp filled with castor oil. The soot is then mixed with cow's milk, butter, or castor oil. All the ingredients are believed to have medicinal properties, and they are still used in ayurvedic therapy. Organic charcoal can be used instead of castor oil soot.

Despite its natural preparation methods, kohl raised a lot of concerns in the 1990s, when commercial kohl preparations from Egypt, Oman, and India were found to contain as much as 84 percent lead, putting its users at risk of lead poisoning. Complications of lead poisoning include anemia, growth retardation, low IQ, convulsions, and in severe cases, death. However, those kohls are completely different from Western cosmetics that only use the term "kohl" to describe the shade and manner of application rather than its actual ingredients. Still, to be safe, purchase traditional kohls only from a reputable manufacturer.

Wearing kohl liner is much easier than you think—if it were otherwise, do you think that Jack Sparrow from the *Pirates of the Caribbean* film trilogy would spend ten minutes every morning on a shaky ship to apply kohl around his eyes? Traditional kohl is applied using a metal or polished wooden stick dipped into the kohl to color the inner rim of the eyelids, darkening lash roots so there's no skin visible. This adds amazing definition and depth to the eye. You can safely experiment with Guerlain Terracotta Loose Powder Kohl in beautiful shades of shimmery black, brown, and teal, packed in a handy tube with a smooth metal applicator. To replicate a powdered kohl application, you can also use a well-sharpened black eyeliner pencil. I highly recommend Dr. Hauschka butter-soft Kajal Eyeliner. Soften the tip by quickly pressing it between your fingertips so it doesn't hurt your eye if your hand slips. Close your eye firmly and quickly run the pencil between the closed lashes. I saw a girl performing this trick on an underground train! Of course, for the first application, you would need to steady your elbow on a table to avoid any injuries. A smudge of organic kohl, a coat of organic mascara, a dab of a natural lip balm, and you are all set for the day!

## Green Lip Balms

Are you a big fan of lip-gloss? I'm sure you are. Millions of women (and thousands of men) claim they are addicted to lip balms and glosses. There's an urban legend that blames a misprint on a little jar of Carmex balm for its widespread use. The original ingredients list put the word "salicylic" on one line and "acid" on the next. I suspect some people thought the wax contained LSD or some other illegal acid! While there are no addictive substances in conventional lip balms, most of them are still loaded with synthetic ingredients that do little to help our lips.

Our lips are protected by the thinnest skin on the body. It has only three to five protective layers of cells, while the rest of our skin has sixteen! This unique structure makes lips very sensitive—and very fragile. Our lips have no sweat or sebum glands, so there's no moisture coming from inside. Technically, a slick of petroleum jelly works just as well to protect our lips as a layer of organic beeswax blended with jojoba oil. The only difference is what ends up inside of us: an average woman eats up to an ounce of lip-gloss a year, and we already know that liquid paraffin has become the main pollutant inside our bodies.

For the everyday protection of lips, natural lip balm is essential. Dry lips can crack and become sore, leaving the skin prone to infection. That's why many natural lip balms are enriched with mild antibacterial and healing ingredients.

## Green Product Guide: Lip Balms

If you don't let nonorganic food pass your lips, why would you wear synthetic goo on them? Here are the top three natural lip balms of choice, as voted by 182 women questioned in July 2006 during a poll on Toronto Fashion Monitor (www.toronto.fashion-monitor.com).

**Burt's Bees Beeswax Lip Balm** is the green beauty's answer to ChapStick. An easy-to-use, skin-friendly stick infuses the lips with plant oils, vitamin E, comfrey root, and rosemary extract. The only drawback is a strong presence of peppermint, which may be bothersome for sensitive skins.

**Unscented Badger Lip Care** has proven itself as the most versatile balm out there. Because it's made of virgin olive and castor oils in a beeswax base, and nothing else, fellow moms reported using it for quick touch-ups of their baby's cheeks in winter and even smearing baby's bottom with it when doing a quick diaper change in a coffeehouse restroom.

**Weleda Everon Lip Balm** is packed to the brim of its happy little orange tube with healing plant oils and extracts, including jojoba oil, shea butter, and rose extract. It is on the heavier side, so you don't need to reapply. It smells like roses in vanilla ice cream—enough to trigger an addiction in me.

# Making Your Own Lip Balms

Finding a good natural lip balm is relatively easy. Preparing your own green balm, surprisingly, is even easier. All you need is a little bit of organic soy wax from your soy candle, an essential oil of your choice, and a bit of mineral blusher or eye shadow to add a delicate shimmery tint.

## Golden Lip Healing Balm

1 tablespoon organic soy wax flakes

1 scoop of coconut butter with a tablespoon

3 drops vanilla extract

1 drop chamomile essential oil

1 drop rose essential oil

1 pinch shimmery pink mineral blush

1 pinch pure golden mineral glimmer

**Yield: 4 ounces**

*I find that beeswax-based lip balms go stiff and dry on my lips faster than those based on other waxes. If formulated incorrectly, when too little beeswax is melted with too much oil, the wax can leave an unpleasant ridge along the lip contour. For this reason, I like to experiment with other waxes, like soy and jojoba, for my lip balms.*

1. Place the soy wax and coconut butter in a metal tin from a cuticle butter or lip balm. Place it in a small enameled pan half-filled with water and double-boil until the wax mixture melts. Do not let mixture boil!

2. Carefully remove the tin and allow the mixture to cool slightly. Add essential oils and extracts and carefully swirl with a wooden toothpick.

3. Carefully spoon in the mineral pigments, adding each color one at a time to allow colorful waves of color to form.

4. Blend well and let the balm cool completely before using.

When combining colors of mineral pigments, be brave! Don't hesitate to mix two or more shades of bright pink, mauve, or bright metallics. When you combine them in a single tin of a lip balm, you can create endless variations of natural-looking shades. If you come up with a particularly interesting color combination, you can make a larger batch of the balm and store it in a half-ounce glass jar, such as a container your eye cream might come in. Many online companies sell inexpensive, small lidded glass jars for lip balm use.

# Basics of Green Lip Colors

Ten years ago, lip coloring was taken rather seriously. You had to use a lip liner, fill it with matching color, blot the lips, and reapply the lipstick. There were tips to make thin lips look fuller or pouty lips appear more modest. There was much emphasis on "correcting flaws" instead of appreciating your unique beauty and highlighting your individual features.

No matter how flattering, invigorating, and chic a red lipstick looks on any complexion, there's a reason why I won't be wearing any: I don't want my brain to hibernate anytime soon. Many conventional lipsticks have been proven to contain considerable amounts of lead, and red lipsticks were especially rich in this toxic metal, according to a CNN report about the findings (full article: http://money.cnn.com/2007/10/12/news/companies/lipstick_lead/index.htm). Lead is a potent neurotoxin that accumulates in soft tissues and bone over time. As we apply lead-containing lipstick several times a day, every day for long periods of time (and aren't we loyal to the perfect color we found once?), it can add up to high exposure levels.

"We tested lipsticks from different stores, different cities, and different price ranges," said Stacy Malkan, the cofounder of Campaign for Safe Cosmetics. "We found lead in all of them. All of the lipsticks were reds, first of all, because red is an iconic lipstick color, and also because we wanted to compare all reds from all the companies. Some reds contained less lead; some contained more." Lead salts in lipstick most often contaminate the pigment, the research found, but lead could also contaminate raw materials used to manufacture lipsticks. Other contaminants in conventional lipsticks include aluminum in the form of color pigments, and glittery particles that are created by aluminum powder and mercury that act as preservative and coloring agents.

### Green Tip

Bright colors on your lips will distract from your eyes and overall complexion. Always accentuate, not hide, your natural beauty.

When it comes to lip color, let the words "green" and "delicate" be your keys. After all, you want the focal point to be your lips, not what's painted on them.

While lip-glosses enjoyed their well-earned fifteen minutes of glory and then shifted to the same style niche where skinny jeans and Hello Kitty handbags belong, lipsticks have made a glorious comeback. Yet finding a pure lippie today is as hard as it was ten years ago. We literally eat lipstick off our lips, yet they often contain potentially toxic components such as petroleum, aluminum, synthetic dyes, and colorings. Even with otherwise perfectly green brands, lipsticks often end up stuffed with silicones, parabens, and FD&C dyes.

Of all the organic beauty products, natural lipsticks feel the most glamorous compared to their synthetic counterparts. Natural brands avoid the use of petrochemicals by using natural ingredients such as carnauba wax, beeswax, jojoba oil, and shea butter. Instead of paraben preservatives, they may use vitamins and citrus oils. Instead of shimmering flakes that may contain lead, aluminum, and even mercury, they use mineral mica. Aveda lipsticks are tinted with organic, plant-derived pigment uruku, while other natural brands use mineral pigments that can deliver a deep, rich color.

Among the safe and pure lipstick brands available, Origins and Aveda (paraben-free versions) have the best selection of colors and textures, while Dr. Hauschka offers the highest moisture and glamour factor. Burt's Bees Lip Shimmers are the most economical option, with pretty, wearable, slender lip products that are a cross between balms and lipsticks. Other perfectly green brands of lipsticks to try include U.S.-based Ecco Bella, German Lavera, and the new Australian organic makeup darling NVEY Eco.

Many natural lipsticks go to great lengths to use sustainable packaging. Aveda uses recycled plastics for lipstick tubes and recycled paper for boxes. They even have refillable lipstick cases! Canadian makeup brand Cargo introduced a line of natural-based lipsticks packed in tubes made entirely from corn. Celebrity-designed shades of Cargo Plant Love Biodegrable Lipstick are sold in boxes that grow wildflowers when planted. Now, that's truly green beauty!

When choosing a lipstick, I recommend subtle, neutral shades, at least for daytime. You can stay neutral and still enjoy a range of options. If you have a yellow-toned complexion, you can use warmer shades, from pale bronze to warm rose. Olive tones can experiment with girly pinks and lilacs for daytime, but save deep berry shades for the night, adding drama to little black dresses. Dark skin tones can try rich chocolate and true reds.

If you have a fair, pink-toned complexion, use subtle colors from light pink to soft plums to enhance your skin tone. For dramatic nighttime use, go for deep plummy (lead-free!) reds for a modern screen siren look. Redheads look gorgeous in apricots and corals, but sheer yet intense raisin tints can really lift up porcelain skin.

If you have a fair, pink-toned complexion, use subtle colors from light pink to soft plums to enhance your skin tone.

As a general rule, lipsticks have more lasting power than lip-glosses, go on more smoothly, and are better for moisturizing your lips. During the summer, or anytime when the sun is shining, try to add some lip protection by rubbing a little bit of mineral foundation on your clean lips before applying the lipstick.

For a quick lip exfoliation, use ripe, juicy papaya. You can use leftovers from a fruit salad or dessert. Mash the papaya flesh into a juicy paste so you get at least a tablespoon of puree. Apply a generous amount of papaya pulp to the lips and skin around the lips. Find a comfortable couch or a recliner to spend a glorious ten or fifteen minutes doing nothing while papaya works on your lips. Rinse off with warm water and enjoy smooth, flake-free lips. For an even quicker exfoliation, rub the inside of papaya skin against your lips for a few minutes.

the green beauty guide

# chapter 15

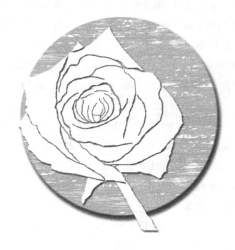

*green*
# fragrances

cannot possibly think of a better introduction to the chapter about natural fragrances than this excerpt from *The Picture of Dorian Gray* by Oscar Wilde:

> And so he would now study perfumes, and the secrets of their manufacture, distilling heavily-scented oils, and burning odorous gums from the East. He saw that there was no mood of the mind that had not its counterpart in the sensuous life, and set himself to discover their true relations, wondering what there was in frankincense that made one mystical, and in ambergris that stirred one's passions, and in violets that woke the memory of dead romances, and in musk that troubled the brain, and in champak that stained the imagination; and seek-ing often to elaborate a real psychology of perfumes, and to estimate the several influences of sweet-smelling roots, and scented pollen-laden flowers, or aromatic balms, and of dark and fragrant woods, of spikenard that sickens, of hovenia that makes men mad, and of aloes that are said to be able to expel melancholy from the soul.

## Ancient Trade Becomes Hottest Trend

The art of making perfumes in the modern sense began in ancient Iran and Egypt. Persian doctor and chemist Avicenna (AD 980–1037) introduced the process of extracting oils from flowers by distillation and began to manufacture musk and rose water. The Persian poet, mathematician, and astronomer Omar Khayyám (1048?–1132) related that Jamshid, one of the first ten mythological kings of ancient Iran, discovered ambergris, myrrh, camphor, and saffron.

The art of distilling and blending aromas was refined by the Romans, but the first modern perfume, made of scented oils blended in an alcohol solution, was made in 1370 for Queen Elizabeth of Hungary and was known throughout Europe as Hungary Water. In the sixteenth century,

France became the center of the perfume art thanks to Catherine de Médicis' personal perfumer, René le Florentin. His laboratory was connected with her apartments by a secret passageway so that no formulas could be stolen on the way. By the eighteenth century, aromatic plants were being grown in Grasse, a town in the southeast of France, to provide the perfume industry with raw materials—rose blossoms, orange flower petals, lavender flowers, and cypress cones.

In early days, perfumes were used primarily by royalty and the wealthy to mask body odors. Scents were applied daily not only to the skin but also to clothing and furniture. Perfume substituted for soap and water. Fragranced gloves became popular, and in the seventeenth century, a French duchess was murdered when poison perfume was rubbed into her gloves and slowly absorbed by her skin. Could this story be the inspiration for Poison perfume by Christian Dior?

> In early days, perfumes were used primarily by royalty and the wealthy to mask body odors.

When Napoleon Bonaparte came to power, the fragrance industry thrived as never before. According to historical documents, no less than two quarts of violet cologne were consumed by Napoleon each month. Same time, he ordered sixty (!) bottles of jasmine extract for his personal use. Venerable French perfume house Creed created a fragrance, Bois du Portugal, for Napoleon, a strong blend of cedar, sandalwood, vetiver, and lavender.

The first completely synthetic perfume wasn't created until the twentieth century. Coco Chanel is to "blame" for the ever-present chemicals in fragrance bottles. Her Chanel No. 5, the first artificial fragrance, relied heavily on synthetic aldehyde, which belongs to the same group of chemicals as the carcinogen formaldehyde and hangover-causing acetaldehyde. It was a novel, avant-garde concept. Coco Chanel opted for synthetic ingredients not for the lack of money: she believed that artificial scents would emphasize the natural beauty of its wearer. However, the phenomenal success of Chanel No. 5 prompted most fragrance labels to swap expensive natural fragrance ingredients for synthetic equivalents.

The U.S. Department of Agriculture, the government agency responsible for overseeing product safety, does not systematically review the safety of fragrances and cannot require that fragrances be tested for safety before they are sold. Instead, the fragrance industry regulates itself, through its trade association, the International Fragrance Association, which funds and conducts safety assessments for fragrance ingredients. This self-regulating scheme has led to the widespread use of chemicals in fragrances that raise concerns when it comes to our health.

What we apply to our skins is our personal choice. What we spray in the air for our kids to breathe is a completely different matter. Pregnant and breast-feeding women who indulge in mainstream fragrances expose their offspring to high levels of toxic chemicals when their endocrine systems aren't mature enough to withstand the damage. As a result, the toxic load accumulates from birth, leading to unknown health consequences that may surface ten or twenty years later.

The wider environmental issue comes into play when you consider what happens to synthetic fragrances when you wash them off your body or launder fragrance-soaked clothes. Most of the synthetic aromatic compounds are discharged into streams, rivers, and other waterways.

Every year the cosmetic industry churns out dozens of designer and celebrity fragrances, not to mention thousands of cosmetic products heavily scented with synthetic chemicals. It's impossible and unreasonable to expect all manufacturers to switch to natural ingredients that are expensive to produce. Natural perfumes are made of rare, precious essences that are considered too costly by the mainstream industry.

Of course, apart from the higher price, natural perfumes are not without limitations. Because there are no chemical fixatives in a natural fragrance formulation, their composition may be unstable or short lasting. And while synthetic perfume makers adhere to strict concentrations of perfume per alcohol and water base, the formulations for natural fragrances can vary from season to season, and ingredients can smell slightly different, depending on the season of harvesting and the weather condition in the particular area. This means that it's close to impossible to create a stable composition that will remain unchanged for years to come. Additionally, the use of some natural materials, like sandalwood and musk, can lead to species endangerment and illegal trafficking.

# The Musky Controversy

Musk, a popular perfume fixative since ancient times, was traditionally obtained from the gland of the male musk deer, *Moschus moschiferus*. The animal was usually killed in the process. Between thirty and fifty deer would die to provide two pounds of musk grains. Due to the high demand of musk, populations of musk deer were severely depleted. Musk deer is now protected by law in China, Mongolia, Afghanistan, Bhutan, India, Nepal, and Pakistan, and international trade of musk from *Moschus moschiferus* is prohibited.

For legal and ethical reasons, many perfume companies use synthetic musk: aromatic nitromusks, polycyclic musk compounds, and macrocyclic musk compounds. Synthetic musk compounds have been found in human fat, breast milk, and in lakes and rivers. Scientists from State University of New York at Albany found synthetic musks in most breast milk samples collected in Massachusetts in 2007 in concentration of "five times greater than the concentrations reported 10 years ago for breast milk samples collected in Germany and Denmark" (Reiner et al. 2007). Synthetic musks, along with bisphenol-A, phthalates, fire retardants, aluminium, and paraben preservatives, are classified as xenoestrogens, synthetic compounds that mimic the action of the hormone beta-estradiol and activating the estrogen receptors (Singleton et al. 2004). Xenoestrogens are linked to reproductive and fertility problems, as well as breast and uterine cancer in women (Donovan et al. 2007) and testicular cancer in men (Irvin 2000).

Today, the European Union has banned the use of some nitromusks in cosmetics and personal care products. In the United States, all musk chemicals are unregulated, and safe levels of exposure have not yet been set.

Some plants, such as garden angelica (*Angelica archangelica*) and ambrette seeds (*Abelmoschus moschatus*), produce musky-smelling aromatic compounds that are widely used in natural perfumery as substitutes for natural musk. Other plant sources of musk include muskflower (*Mimulus moschatus*) and the muskwood (*Olearia argophylla*) of the Guianas and West Indies. So if you are very partial to musk, choose a botanical musk fragrance from a reputable green fragrance brand.

## SHOULD YOU LOVE OR HATE YOUR PERFUME?
### *An Interview with Serge Lutens*

French photographer, stylist, perfumer, and fashion designer Serge Lutens was a creative director for Shiseido and now creates perfumes under his own name sold in Salons du Palais Royal Shiseido in Paris. He uses only natural ingredients and classical techniques in his fragrant masterpieces, such as Sa Majeste la Rose, Santal Blanc, and Douce Amere, which have an extraordinarily devoted following among celebrities and fragrance connoisseurs worldwide. Serge Lutens spoke to us from his home in Morocco:

*On life choices:* "Perfumery was not a conscious choice. It was perfumery that picked me. The powerful desire for making perfumes dates back to my first voyage to Morocco, in 1968, when I smelled aromatic waxes, precious woods. . . . I did not know at that time if I would ever be able to turn this desire into reality."

*On breaking the rules:* "My first perfume was Nombre Noir, created in 1982. At the time, the black-on-black packaging had created a small revolution in the world of perfumery. My idea was to remove gold plating, decorations, and all those lavish ornaments that made me feel that perfumery was becoming fake and more about the embellishment than the scents. Black packaging creates an emotion, and today has become a classic design. The juice in itself—to create a contrast—was based on an aroma of white flowers. At that time, my tastes in perfumes were not well defined. Yet, ten years later, in 1992, a new revolution occurred, this time olfactive, with the launching of Feminite Du Bois, a feminine perfume based on masculine cedar. This perfume became a legend."

*On inspiration:* "I do not know if one can speak about inspiration when it comes to perfume creation. Some of my perfumes were inspired by literature and music; others were inspired by plants. A perfume must always awaken a memorable feeling and reconstitute your personal universe. In Datura Noir I tried to create a violent, dominating atmosphere that would evoke images of decadent

*continued*

nights with the bitter aroma of almonds. The first scent I clearly remember goes back to my childhood years in northern France. It's an overwhelming smell of vanilla and gingerbread cookies from the bakery nearby. The perfume creator makes scents that can stir strong emotions, such as love or hate. He should not have personal preferences in the scents he uses."

*On perfumes and music*: "I do not think, though, that perfumery and music are strongly connected. Perfume is already music by itself. Nevertheless, I like to listen to Johann Sebastian Bach, who is my favorite composer."

*On the allure of perfumes*: "There are two types of people who buy perfumes. The first category determines the perfume like a sociocultural product that helps them create a new identity. This approach helps to market the perfumes, but the success is very short-lived. In this case, you buy an idea, not a juice! Another category of people is attracted by pure smell. They choose more personal scents that relate to them and bring out something new in their characters."

*On personal preferences*: "I do not use perfume often. When I work, it is impossible. I prefer to keep my senses fresh so that nothing interferes with the olfactive tension. However, I wear Ambre Sultan in the evening sometimes . . . and a lot of it!"

*On natural beauty*: "Natural beauty, for me, is to exist as one feels. When something is natural, you feel it instantly."

## Making Your Own Fragrance Blends

To create your own perfume, you only need water, a spirit, and the essential oil blend of your choice. Essential oils can also be diluted by means of neutral-smelling lipids such as jojoba or coconut oil and then blended with wax to create a solid perfume. You'll also need a pipette and small, dark glass bottles for storing your fragrance creations.

The most concentrated perfume extract should contain 20 to 40 percent fragrant oils, the rest being water and spirit mix or neutral oil. Perfume oils should always be diluted because undiluted oils contain high concentrations of volatile components and will likely cause irritation if applied directly to the skin. Please note that many essential oils can adversely interact with drugs. I would not recommend using any fragrances during pregnancy or when breast-feeding.

Nature has provided us with an abundance of beautiful scents—rose, jasmine, ylang-ylang, tea rose, sandalwood, and chamomile, to name a few, all are available as essential oils. Get creative, save money, and make your own earth-friendly perfumes!

You can blend your favorite essential oils to create your signature scent, but don't use more than eight drops of essential oil and fragrant extracts of your choice per ounce beeswax and jojoba oil. Try one or more of the following traditional essential oils that are believed to stimulate the senses and reportedly have aphrodisiac qualities: frankincense, black pepper, myrrh, cinnamon, vetiver, neroli, cardamom, cedarwood, ginger, violet leaf, nutmeg, hyacinth, benzoin, mimosa, and lemon verbena.

## Green Eau de Toilette

1 ounce vodka

4–10 drops essential oil of your choice

2 tablespoons distilled water

**Yield: 4 ounces**

*To practice, start with one or two essential oils and add more as you gain experience. Don't forget to carefully record the amount of each essential oil you use so that you can re-create or refine the formula.*

1. Pour the vodka into a small glass measuring cup (that has a spout) and add the essential oil, stirring slowly until the oil is fully mixed in. Pour mixture into a small, dark, lidded bottle and leave in a dark place (such as a closet) for two days so that the oil can fully blend with the vodka.

2. Slowly add the distilled water, shaking well. Again, let the mixture sit for two days (or more, if you want a more potent mix). Now the perfume is ready! If you like, you can transfer it into a pretty spray bottle.

Here's an even simpler version: add four drops of rosemary and lavender essential oils to two ounces organic grain vodka and two ounces purified water. You may add a few drops of glycerin to prevent the mix from drying your skin.

## Carmelite Water (Eau de Carmes)

3 cups vodka

1 cup dried angelica leaves

1 cup dried lemon balm leaves

1 tablespoon coriander seeds, lightly crushed

1 nutmeg seed, grated

2 teaspoons whole cloves

3 cinnamon sticks, crushed

½ to 1 cup distilled water

Yield: 4 ounces

This unisex plant musk cologne was first made by Carmelite monks in Paris in 1611 and was regarded as a highly effective medicine for nervous headaches and neuralgia. The original recipe includes over a dozen herbs, and the preparation, no doubt, involved Gregorian chants and lengthy fermentation. It is still sold in Germany as Klosterqu Melissen Geise.

1. Place all the spices and herbs in a glass jar, and pour the vodka over them. Seal and shake vigorously. Leave in a warm corner for up to ten days, shaking at least once a day.

2. Strain through unbleached muslin cloth, then siphon through an unbleached coffee filter into a dark glass bottle.

3. Dilute to the strength you want with the distilled water. You may substitute 5 drops citronella oil for the lemon balm leaves, but the fragrance will lack the spicy green scent of dried plants.

## Queen of Hungary Water

2 cups organic grain vodka or grappa (grape spirit)

¼ cup dried rosemary

¼ cup dried lavender flowers

Peel of one unwaxed lemon

Peel of one unwaxed orange

1 tablespoon dried peppermint

4 drops bergamot essential oil

Yield: 5 ounces

This ancient perfume can be used as a facial splash and even as a rubbing alcohol and hand wash. The original recipe published in "Selectiora remedia multiplici usu comprobata, quae inter secreta medica jure recenseas" (a 1656 text by John Prevot) reads: "Take of aqua vitae, four times distilled, three parts, and of the tops and flowers of rosemary two parts; put these together in a close[d] vessel, let them stand in a gentle heat fifty hours, and then distil them. Take one dram of this in the morning once every week, either in your food or drink, and let your face and diseased limb be washed with it every morning." Here's a slightly modernized version of this recipe, which I find more suitable for home preparation.

1. Mix the ingredients well in a glass jar (a mason jar is ideal), stir thoroughly, and allow to blend together in a warm, dark place for up to three days.

2. Strain mixture through a coffee filter and store in a sealed or airtight bottle in a cool, dark place. To use, dilute one part of the mixture with four parts distilled water.

## Summer Garden Splash

4 tablespoons chopped fresh tomato leaves

2 tablespoons chopped fresh geranium leaves

1 teaspoon fresh mint leaves

1 teaspoon grated lemon rind

1 cup vodka or witch hazel

1 teaspoon glycerin

**Yield: 4 ounces**

*This delicious summer scent combines the exquisite fragrance of geranium with the green, tangy aroma of tomato leaves.*

1. Place the leaves and the grated lemon rind in a glass jar with a lid. Pour the vodka or witch hazel and glycerin over the leaves and rind.

2. Cover and let mixture sit in a cool, dark place for at least two weeks.

3. Strain the liquid through a coffee filter to remove the debris. Pour into a spray bottle.

## Aphrodisiac Solid Perfume

1 ounce beeswax

2 tablespoons jojoba oil

2 drops jasmine essential oil

2 drops ylang-ylang essential oil

1 drop sandalwood essential oil

1 drop rose essential oil

2 drops vanilla extract

**Yield: 5 ounces**

*This is a great way to wear perfume because the scent envelopes you, creating subtle differences depending on where you apply the balm. Remember not to exceed the recommended amounts of essential oils, or you risk irritating your skin.*

1. Gently heat the beeswax and jojoba oil in a small enameled saucepan until the wax is melted.

2. Remove from heat and stir in the essential oils and vanilla.

3. Pour the mixture into a clean lip balm container, a vintage silver pillbox, or, if feeling extravagant, an Estée Lauder refillable facial powder container.

4. Let the mixture cool. To use, soften it with your fingers and apply the solid perfume to pulse points.

## Preserving Your Natural Perfumes

You invested in a lavish botanical fragrance or created one of your own. Good for you! Here are some points to help you enjoy your natural fragrance as long as possible.

Keep in mind that fragrance compounds in perfumes will degrade or break down if improperly stored in the presence of heat, light, and oxygen. To prolong the life of your fragrances, keep them away from sources of heat, and store them in dark cabinets where they will not be exposed to light. Perfumes are best preserved in their original packaging and should be stored in a fridge when not in use. An opened full bottle will keep the scent intact for up to a year, but as the level goes down, the oxygen will eventually alter the fragrant composition. Any dust, skin, and debris trapped in a bottle will degrade the quality of the perfume.

> Keep in mind that fragrance compounds in perfumes will degrade or break down if improperly stored in the presence of heat, light, and oxygen.

# All-Natural Deodorants

In the modern world, sweat odor has become unacceptable. While the faint, clean smell of sweat might be considered sexy, nothing is more repulsive than body odor reeking from underarms after a brisk walk in a heavy coat. Pharmacies and drugstores offer a huge selection of sweat-busters loaded with propylene glycol, aluminum, Triclosan, and synthetic fragrances. Fortunately, there are many green alternatives that work against sweat just as well.

First of all, I would not recommend using "rock" deodorants, which are based on aluminum salts. Unlike commercial antiperspirants, rock deodorant does not stop perspiration; it only eliminates odor due to the antibacterial action of potassium alum, a naturally occurring mineral with the chemical name aluminum potassium sulfate. It's still unclear whether rock deodorants load the blood with the same amounts of aluminum as commercial antiperspirants, but if, like me, you prefer to err on the side of caution, you'll want to explore other alternatives.

So, how can we stay fresh-smelling naturally? There are plenty of reliable odor-busters in natural food stores. Unlike antiperspirants, they do not block sweat glands, causing toxin buildup under the skin. Instead, they sanitize the underarm area and kill the odor-causing bacteria. Weleda, Desert Essence, Dr. Hauschka, Aubrey Organics, Neal's Yard, and Origins make excellent green deodorants that can also double as room sprays, if the emergency arises.

Need a quick refresher on the run? According to natural health guru Dr. Andrew Weil, you could just rub alcohol under your arms because it acts as an antibacterial agent. A light dusting of baking soda deodorizes and keeps underarms dry. You can also prepare a deodorant at home. Try this easy recipe.

## Green Spice Deodorant

1 cup vodka
2 tablespoons witch hazel
3 drops tea tree essential oil
1 drop juniper essential oil
1 drop lemon essential oil

Combine all the ingredients in a sterilized pump bottle. Shake before each use. This unisex blend can be used as an aftershave splash as well.

**Yield:**
4 ounces

## Green Bug Repellants

Organic living means avoiding pesticides in your food. So why would you want to spray them on your skin? Millions of people do just that in an attempt to keep mosquitoes and other bugs at bay. Ironically, the result of this spraying is that the pests themselves are becoming more resistant, and we are required to cover ourselves in ever-stronger chemicals to counteract them.

There are dozens of natural mosquito and bug repellant recipes. Some recommend boiling garlic in mineral oil and diluting it with dishwasher liquid—hardly green and hardly pleasant to use! Some people prefer to use plain rubbing alcohol or pure lavender oil, but I would not recommend indulging in lavender due to its potential hormone-disrupting effects. Neem (*Azadirachta indica*) oil blended with coconut or jojoba oil in equal proportions makes a traditional Indian insect repellant. Catnip, thyme, and amyris essential oils have been reported to be more effective in warding off mosquitoes and other nasties than DEET, the widely used chemical insect repellent (Zhu et al. 2006).

I have found that citronella, also known as lemongrass, naturally keeps the mosquitoes away when planted in the backyard. The U.S. Environmental Protection Agency considers citronella oil a safe and natural insect repellent, a "biopesticide with a nontoxic mode of action." What else can you wish for? You can rub citronella leaves and stalks directly on skin, and the effect lasts for about five hours.

## Green Chai Mosquito Guard

2 cups grain alcohol

20 drops eucalyptus essential oil

20 drops citronella essential oil

10 drops thyme essential oil

10 drops catnip essential oil

**Yield: 4 ounces**

*The following recipe repels even the most fanatical bugs.*

Blend all the ingredients in a spray bottle, shake well, and spray on exposed skin and clothing frequently, avoiding the eye area.

If you substitute grain alcohol for 1 ounce of grape seed or any other unscented oil, you can also use this blend in aroma lamps and burners when enjoying a quiet summer night on the patio.

## Green Air Fresheners

Let's be honest: do you really enjoy the smell of violets, or maybe you need that little synthetic plug-in to cover up the smell of not-so-clean curtains, the dog's lack of toilet manners, another burned dinner, or even worse, stale tobacco smoke? There are many reasons you reach for that aerosol spray or scented candle. But the surprising fact is that most air fresheners may be making you ill. They work by emitting heavily scented chemicals that mask unwanted odors, using synthetic perfumes such as musk and other aromatic hydrocarbons to provide fragrance.

The toxic chemicals released by air fresheners—particularly those with pine, orange, and lemon scents—are known as volatile organic compounds (VOCs). These are well-proven toxins, many of which have been linked to a range of diseases and conditions when inhaled even in low concentrations over a long period of time. Some of these chemicals include benzene, a petroleum-derived chemical that causes cancer in animals and has been linked to leukemia; xylene, which has been linked to nausea and "sick building syndrome," as well as liver and kidney damage; phenol, which can cause kidney, respiratory, neurological, and skin problems; naphthalene, a suspected carcinogen that has been linked to blood, kidney, and liver problems; and formaldehyde, a colorless, unstable gas. Inhaling formaldehyde fumes in even small amounts can cause coughing, a sore throat, and respiratory and eye problems. Formaldehyde has been linked to cancer, particularly in the nasal cavity.

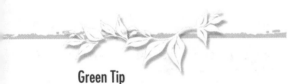

**Green Tip**

Try filling your home with plants. Plants can effectively detoxify the air by absorbing toxic vapors and releasing oxygen back into the atmosphere, which also improves air quality. The spider plant *(Chlorophytum comosum)* and rubber tree *(Ficus elastic)* are especially good. Research by NASA found that a single spider plant could reduce dangerous levels of toxins in a room by 96 percent in 24 hours.

So what should we do to keep our homes smelling like vanilla cookies if we aren't in the mood to bake? Try green air fresheners. Look for nonaerosol canisters and words such as "biodegradable," "plant-based," "formulated without synthetic fragrance," and "contains no formaldehyde/phthalates." Green, nontoxic air freshener sprays are made by Seventh Generation, Miessence, and Rainforest Organic, while California Scents now makes organic gel fresheners that are practical and spill-proof. Of course, you can use an all-natural body deodorant (Weleda, for example) in citrus or wild rose scent and generously spray it around the house whenever you need to. Most natural nonaerosol air fresheners are quite concentrated, and a little squirt will last a long time.

You may also try some of Grandma's recipes. Put some whole cloves in a pan of water and simmer it on the stove. Another way to fill your

  **the green beauty guide**

home with a natural fragrance is to simmer four lemons cut into quarters or bake them in the oven for about forty-five minutes. The citric acid can also destroy airborne toxic particles. For bathroom odors, a simple lit match often does the trick.

Soy candles are fun and easy to make from loose soy wax chips and premade wicks using essential oils such as lavender, vanilla, and lemon. (These are also safe to use if you're pregnant.) If you are not in the DIY mood, try a lush candle by the Organic Pharmacy, Diptyque, or an ultra-luxurious candle with essential oils by Costes. For the baby's room, try a candle by California Baby with scents of lavender, lemon, or orange—these scents quickly eliminate a soiled diaper odor.

Potpourri is another good replacement for toxic air fresheners. Browse your local thrift stores or take a walk at an antique market and pick up a lovely "shabby chic" shallow and wide china or crystal vase. Fill it with dried rose petals, pinecones, or lavender florets. Add five to six drops of an essential oil blend of your choice and place the vase in your bathroom or kitchen. To create an uplifting aromatherapy potpourri, mix orange, lemon, and clove essential oils in equal proportions. For an air-purifying concoction, blend tea tree, eucalyptus, and lemon essential oils.

**Green Tip**

Potpourri is another good replacement for toxic air fresheners.

Now that you have learned how to prepare some of the world's most exquisite fragrance blends, it's highly unlikely you'll ever choose conventional aerosol sprays to scent your home.

chapter **16**

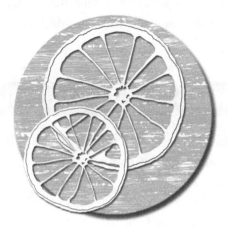

*green*
*beauty* detox

Who doesn't like shortcuts and magic fixes? We all do, even though most of the quick fixes don't work in the long run. This three-day detox, however, is different from your usual fad diet. Instead of burning calories and fighting hunger pangs, you will be burning bad beauty habits and cleaning up your act—while losing a few pounds and a handful of zits in the process! The ultimate three-day green makeover, the Green Beauty Detox, will help you start your skin-friendly and ecoconscious living from a clean page.

## Is Your Food Making You Old?

The connection between our skin's health and the toxic burden in our bodies is so important I cannot help but stress it again: the more toxins we accumulate in our system, the faster our skin ages. No matter how many antiwrinkle serums you rub into your face, your body is crippling under the weight of the industrial toxins that have entered our food, air, and personal care products in the last fifty years—and it is these toxins, not the sun or gravity, that are aging our skin. Let's take a look at how this happens.

You buy a lean chicken breast and plan to prepare a healthy low-fat chicken Caesar salad. As you eat it, you ingest the hormone-laden chicken that was fed with antibiotics and drugs to help it gain weight unnaturally fast. If you decide to barbecue the chicken, keep in mind that carcinogenic compounds form in char-grilled meats. Your hormones are further disrupted by pesticides and chemical fertilizers found in lettuce leaves. Your "healthy" dessert of strawberries comes with a spoonful of pesticides and fertilizers, and the mercury-laden fish you ate earlier adds to a lifetime load of toxic metals accumulated in the bones and fat tissue. All of these toxins come from homemade, "wholesome" food. What about salads prepared at a fast-food counter? The average person in North America each year consumes up to 12 pounds of food additives and 1 gallon of pesticides and herbicides sprayed on fruit, vegetables, and animal feed.

Add the synthetic chemicals creeping into our bodies from household cleaning products, cigarette smoke, hair dyes, cosmetics and antiperspirants, chlorinated water, office supplies, and beauty and personal care products—and the picture starts to look frightening, to say the least. Traces of Agent Orange and other pesticides, petroleum-based fertilizers, preservatives, antibiotics, mercury, lead, heavy metals, and paraffin are found in everybody, no matter what their age, location, or occupation. This body burden causes a host of diseases—and most visibly, it makes us age at a faster rate.

Environmental toxins speed up premature aging by mimicking estrogen hormones in our bodies. The feed that nonorganic farmers give to their cows, chickens, pigs, and lambs is loaded with hormones that make animals gain weight at an incredibly high rate, unseen in nature. When we eat meat and dairy products from these farms, we consume these hormones, too. Even if you are vegetarian, you are still eating your load of estrogen-mimicking chemicals. Pesticides used to protect crops from bugs or fungus and fertilizers that speed up crop growth have an estrogenic effect on humans.

Xenoestrogens, or man-made, artificial hormones, are different from natural estrogens present in plants and human bodies. Xenoestrogens were introduced into the environment only seventy years ago, and they have a cumulative effect on the human body. First of all, they damage the reproductive system, causing problems with fertility in women and low sperm count in men. Xenoestrogens are directly linked to hormone-induced cancers, most importantly to breast cancer. While estrogen regulates such vital female processes as menstruation, pregnancy, and menopause, excess estrogen overstimulates cell growth in breasts, uteruses, or ovaries. Symptoms of excess estrogen include hair loss, allergies, thyroid dysfunction, cysts in breasts and ovaries, irregular periods, and premenstrual syndrome.

Here is the list of most common sources of xenoestrogens entering our bodies on a daily basis:

*Cosmetics:* paraben preservatives, butylated hydroxyanisole, aluminum
*Makeup:* FD&C Red No. 3 (erythrosine), phenosulfothiazine
*Sunscreen lotions:* 4-methylbenzylidene camphor
*Plastics:* bisphenol-A
*Insecticides:* atrazine, dieldrin, DDT, endosulfan, heptachlor, lindane, nonylphenol

*Furniture:* polychlorinated biphenyls (PCBs), plasticizer for PVC

*Water:* chlorine

When synthetic chemicals enter our body, they face an encounter with the liver, our living filter that destroys toxins and releases the leftovers into the bloodstream. Many synthetic chemicals, including xenoestrogens, petrochemicals, nitrates from processed meats, secondhand smoke, antibiotics, and alcohol, disrupt the vital processes in the liver. Toxins slow up bile production, making it thick and viscous. As we keep the liver busy by throwing more toxins in its direction, it becomes sluggish and overtired. It begins to convert toxins into other toxic compounds that create free radicals, causing damage to cells in various body parts, including the skin, which is prone to free radical damage and irritation. Tired livers and thick bile cannot break down food properly, which results in a clogged, toxic colon—meaning more acne outbreaks, allergic dermatitis, and wrinkles on our faces.

## Eating Organic for Healthy Skin

Now that you understand what the lifetime of toxic living has done to your skin and overall health, you are no doubt feeling a bit overwhelmed. The bad news: your health has already been damaged. The good news is that you can still do much to improve the situation. By following the guidelines of the Green Beauty Detox, you will help your body eliminate the toxic load accumulated for decades and defend against future attacks.

*Start with food.* Conventional produce is often contaminated with chemical fertilizers, pesticides, sewage sludge residue, polluted underground water, lead from cans, phthalates from plastic lids and containers, and aluminum from foil and packaging. Fish is often polluted with mercury, while imported fruits and vegetables may carry a load of DDT (banned in the United States, but still used in many countries) and airplane fuel emissions from being flown across the globe. You can even find radioactive materials in some foods, since radioactive municipal and medical waste make a cheap commercial fertilizer. The use of municipal sewage sludge is not regulated in the United States, meaning that industrial refuse ends up in livestock and on our plates.

*Go organic.* What's the point of avoiding chemical toxins in your cosmetics if you load your plate with pesticides, herbicides, artificial sweeteners, antibiotics, petrochemicals, and preservatives? Nothing will save your skin and hair if you continue eating conventionally produced food. Fortunately, organic produce is easy to find, and you can replace every single food item in your menu with organic versions. Organic foods taste better and contain more nutrients. Organic farming considers the health of the planet by preserving soil and waterways. Yes, organic produce can cost 5 to 20 percent more than conventionally farmed food. Consider these extra costs as monthly payments for the most effective health insurance you'll ever find.

## Foods That Cure Your Skin

Here are the foods that form the foundation of Green Beauty Detox eating. If possible, everything you eat should be organic or locally grown by responsible farmers. Many grocery stores are now stocking organic produce and other food items, so look for these sections when you're shopping.

### Protein

Protein is vital for your skin, nails, and hair. Without an adequate supply of protein, your skin ages prematurely and loses collagen and elastin, becoming dull and pale, while facial muscles lose strength, and hair and nails weaken.

During the Green Beauty Detox, you should avoid all kinds of animal proteins. This includes meat, poultry, fish, whey, and dairy. In his groundbreaking book *The China Study,* Dr. Colin Campbell found that a typical Western diet, high in fat and animal protein, resulted in increased levels of estrogen hormones that play a role in breast cancer and premature aging. "Women who consume a diet rich in animal-based foods . . . reach puberty earlier and menopause later, thus extending their reproductive lives," writes Dr. Campbell. "They also have higher levels of female hormones throughout their life span." According to *The China Study,* a lifetime's exposure to estrogen among Western women is three times higher than in Chinese women. Other studies consistently prove the destructive role of animal fats and protein in the hormonal balance. Recent studies show that animal fat can also boost the risk for breast cancer (Wu et al. 1999) and endometrial cancer (Bandera et al. 2007). Animal protein appears to boost estrogen levels no matter where it comes from.

So what should you eat instead? I am not asking you to go vegan, since strict elimination diets have never worked for everyone. Instead, let plant-based foods take the center stage—or the center of your plate. Let meat and dairy play supporting roles while you indulge in fruits, vegetables, mushrooms, beans and peas, nuts, and seeds. Plant foods have more antioxidants, minerals, and vitamins than animal foods, and plant proteins, cholesterol, and fats are healthier than those of animal origin, especially if they are grown in organic soil. Experimental studies on laboratory animals show that diets with reduced calories, fat, and protein can even prevent breast, prostate, and possibly other types of cancer (Hede et al. 2008).

**Green Tip**

Eliminate sugar, hydrogenated fat, and starches, which are known to increase the risk of cancer.

Eat smaller amounts of plant protein throughout the day. That way, your energy levels remain stable, and you can avoid late afternoon fatigue. Eat plant protein, such as rice, tofu, soy milk, nuts, and seeds for breakfast, lunch, and dinner. Of course, three days of vegetarian eating will not lower your estrogen levels, but you will hopefully develop a taste for plant-based foods and understand that eating vegetarian is not as hard as it seems.

## Essential Fatty Acids (EFAs)

Essential fatty acids are your skin's best friends. Essential fatty acids serve lots of important functions: they reduce inflammation, improve cell signaling, ease mood disorders, and protect DNA from damage. Last but not least, they can literally save your face, nourishing the skin, keeping it glowing, and even improving eczema and psoriasis. Omega-6 fatty acids are particularly helpful in restoring the barrier function of the epidermis, and omega-3 fatty acids preserve collagen and elastin.

You can add essential fatty acids to your salads and stews. You can drink them undiluted (as in the Green Liver Flush, described later in this chapter) or take them as a food supplement. Fish oil capsules should be the only source of animal-derived fat in your diet during the detox. Plant sources of EFAs include flaxseed (linseed), hemp oil, soya oil, canola (rapeseed) oil, chia seeds, pumpkin seeds, sunflower seeds, leafy vegetables, and walnuts.

> Omega-6 fatty acids are particularly helpful in restoring the barrier function of the epidermis, and omega-3 fatty acids preserve collagen and elastin.

## Fruits and Vegetables

Fresh, organic fruits and vegetables are the key ingredients of your Green Beauty Detox. Every piece of fruit, every bunch of salad, should be organic or locally grown without fertilizers, pesticides, or herbicides. Some stores do not carry as many organic varieties as we would like. If you're buying nonorganic produce, stay away from the most contaminated fruits and vegetables, which include apples, apricots, bananas, cabbage, cantaloupe, celery, cherries, lettuce, pears, peppers, potatoes, raspberries, spinach, strawberries, and watermelon. Whenever you want one of these delicious creations of nature, buy only organic. However, the following fruits and vegetables are found to be lower in chemical additives and can be eaten in limited quantities even when grown conventionally: asparagus, avocados, beans, broccoli, carrots, cauliflower, onions, peas, tomatoes, and zucchini.

## What to Avoid

By all means avoid the following during the Green Beauty Detox: alcohol, artificial sweeteners, hydrogenated fats, butter, refined sugar (other than in body rubs and facial scrubs), and refined carbohydrates (white bread, white rice, cereal or pasta made from white flour, etc.).

# Water: The Essential Skin Remedy

There's so much water in our bodies, one may wonder why we don't drown in all the water in our brain, blood, and lungs! Water regulates body temperature; carries glucose, oxygen, and nutrients; cushions joints; and removes waste from the body. Drinking water is a well-known health and beauty tool, but how many of us actually drink the recommended eight glasses a day?

Keep water flowing. Dehydration is the surefire way to increase the toxic burden in your body. It has been estimated that when we feel thirsty, approximately 28 percent of blood plasma is lost. Even mild dehydration slows cell metabolism by 5 percent, which speeds up the accumulation of toxic metabolites in your blood. Skin cell turnover slows down and bowel movements become scarce, which leads to clogging your body's "plumbing system" with waste. Not drinking enough water has been linked to colon and bladder cancer as well as fatigue and worsening memory (Altieri et al. 2003; Manz, Wentz 2005). Dehydration can intensify the symptoms of diabetes and has been shown to raise blood pressure (Manz 2007).

Some rural communities, especially when located on organically certified soil, can safely drink tap water, but most of us don't have this luxury anymore. Fertilizers, pesticides, and herbicides constantly seep into waterways, while the dumping of sewage and industrial wastes and toxins pollutes rivers and lakes, disrupting delicate ecosystems. From 1971 to 2002, there were 764 documented waterborne outbreaks associated with drinking water in the United States, resulting in more than half a million cases of illness and 79 deaths, according to a report by the University of Arizona (Reynolds et al. 2008). Scientists noted that, according to epidemiological studies, people who drank filtered water had 20–35 percent less gastrointestinal illnesses than those consuming regular tap water.

Fortunately, there are so many sources of pure water available, you don't need to quench your thirst from the tap or water fountains. You can drink bottled water made by a reputable company, ideally from a certified organic source, or you can filter your tap water using carbon or reverse osmosis filters. Store your filtered water in glass or stainless steel bottles.

Not all bottled water is created equal. Glacial water comes from melted ice caps, which is then purified using reverse osmosis or deionization, so it becomes indistinguishable from distilled water. Spring and well water is bottled from natural sources or holes drilled in the ground, and then treated to remove any possible contaminants. Then there's plain purified water, which is basically tap water that has been filtered and deionized. Another name for purified water is "demineralized." Some types of bottled water are labeled as "ozonated," which means that water has been purified with ozone and contains a higher amount of oxygen. Studies show that ozonation helps kill bacteria and degrade antibiotics and other toxins in tap water. There's also mineral water, which contains minerals and trace elements from geologically and physically protected underground water sources.

Which type of bottled water is best? It's mineral water certified by a dependable source and bottled in glass, not plastic. Bottled water in plastic containers is bad for two reasons: first, plastic is known to leach phthalates and other toxins into the water, especially when heated during storage or transportation or when you leave the bottle in a warm place. Have you ever noticed that plastic-y smell your water emits after it has spent a whole day in your beach bag? This is a sign that the volatile compounds of the plastic are migrating into your water. PETE or #1 PET (polyethylene terephthalate) plastic water bottles have been shown to leach antimony into water, while the xenoestrogen bisphenol-A has been routinely added to polycarbonate (#7) plastic water and baby bottles.

The second reason to give plastic bottles the boot is ecological. The processing and manufacturing of petroleum-based plastic water bottles is energy consuming. And since plastics are made of petroleum, they deplete the world's most valuable resource and increase our dependence on oil. The plastic industry contributes more than 15 percent of the most carcinogenic industrial releases, including styrene, benzene, trichloroethane, sulfur oxides, nitrous oxides, methanol, ethylene oxide, and volatile organic compounds (VOCs). Then there's the problem of waste: #1 PET plastic bottles generate 100 times more waste than glass bottles, and plastic polymers never fully biodegrade.

If you must buy bottled water on the run, choose glass bottles of Perrier or San Pellegrino, to name a few. Reuse your glass bottles by filling them with filtered water, and always, always recycle glass bottles. When eating out, ask the waiter which water comes in a glass bottle before ordering, and request that he or she bring you an unopened bottle so you know it hasn't been opened and refilled with tap water. (Unfortunately, this happens sometimes.) Some people think that plain water is blunt and adds nothing to the flavors of food. To make plain water more palatable, add a squeeze of lemon or orange to it.

The most ecoconscious and economical way to have unlimited access to pure drinking water is to install a tap water filter. Jug filters, such as Brita made of nonpolycarbonate plastic certified by U.S. National Sanitation Foundation, are a good, inexpensive option, but a tap water filter gives you more water for your buck.

During the Green Beauty Detox, drink more water than you think you need. These three days you will be eliminating lots of toxins, so you will need extra water to keep fibrous food moving smoothly in your bowels and toxins flushing away.

## Three-Day Green Beauty Detox

When you are ready to start your three-day cleansing ritual, closely follow the detailed protocol given here. Begin the routine upon rising every morning. You don't have to perform all the procedures at the exact same time, but be sure to have all three meals and two snacks plus all servings of the Green Detox Drink and at least six cups of water. You'll need to prepare a fresh batch of the Green Detox Drink (recipe follows) on each of the three days.

### Day One: Body Detox

This day you focus on the whole-body rejuvenation. This is the most taxing day, as you will be doing your deep Green Liver Flush.

*Upon rising:* Drink one glass (8 ounces) of mineral/filtered water.

*Before shower:* Brush your dry skin with a natural bristle brush. Starting at your feet, brush in circular motions toward your heart. Spend at least one minute on each leg. Now move on to your arms. Brush from your fingertips, again toward your heart. Spend at least one minute on each arm. Now brush from your back toward your stomach. Do not dry brush your neck, breasts, or face. When you are done brushing, shower using plain olive, grape seed, or jojoba oil as a body cleanser. Gently pat dry, not rub, your body with a clean towel.

*Throughout the day:* Drink one glass of the Green Detox Drink every two hours. The recipe provides enough drink for the whole day. Spend your day doing relaxing and thoughtful things such as reading, tending to your garden, playing with children, walking or shopping for ecofriendly things. Your breakfast, lunch, and snacks should be vegetarian, without any dairy, refined wheat, or sugar.

*After dinner:* Prepare for the Green Liver Flush.

## The Green Detox Drink

1 organic lemon

1 organic orange

1 tablespoon maple syrup

½-inch piece fresh ginger root, chopped

2 tablespoons virgin olive oil

1 clove organic garlic, chopped

¼ teaspoon cayenne pepper

¼ teaspoon ground cloves

¼ teaspoon chopped organic or local parsley

Yield: 1 quart

*The Green Detox Drink is thick, nourishing, and loaded with vitamins, but it is not a meal replacement. However, you might feel quite full after a glass. It tastes like a thick orange juice with a bit of a kick. The drink is very easy to prepare (five to six minutes total, including peeling and chopping), and the ingredients are quite affordable, too. Note: The Green Detox Drink is not compatible with dairy of any kind.*

1. Peel the lemon and orange and cut them into chunks. Place all the remaining ingredients into a blender with the lemon and orange. Blend for 10 minutes. The mixture should be quite thick.

2. Dilute mixture with the water of your choice to make 1 quart and store it in the refrigerator.

## Green Liver Flush

This is a traditional East European technique now making news among holistic healers. It is effective in removing fat-soluble toxins, such as pesticide residues, from the body. The effectiveness and safety of conducting a home liver flush has been debated among medical professionals. If you have any liver or gallbladder problems or other health concerns, you should consult your doctor before doing this procedure.

Here's what you need: the juice from five medium-sized lemons, a slightly heated bottle of virgin olive oil, a hot water bottle, and a shot glass for measuring. Arrange everything, including this book and the TV remote if desired, on a coffee table so you won't have to jump up and down too often. It's important not to perform the liver cleansing when you are home alone, in case you feel dizzy or weak in the bathroom. Folk medicine recommends starting the flush at 7 PM.

Make sure you follow these steps precisely:

1. Fill the water bottle with hot water, place it on your upper right abdomen, and relax for thirty minutes.
2. Drink one shot (2 tablespoons) of lemon juice.
3. Wait fifteen minutes, then drink one shot (2 tablespoons) of olive oil.
4. Alternate shots of lemon juice and olive oil every fifteen minutes until you are out of lemon juice. Keep the hot water bottle on your right-hand side!

Be ready for a massive bowel movement in an hour or two. Don't be afraid to see some extraordinary things coming out of you! You may even pass small gallstones and tar-colored goo, which signals that your liver was crippling under the weight of toxins.

As you finish in the bathroom, take a quick shower, massaging your body and hair with grape seed oil, then washing it off with your regular shampoo. Go to bed.

The classic liver flush routine prescribes an enema next morning to complete the cleansing process, but this is truly optional.

## Day Two: Hair Detox

This day you'll take really good care of your hair. Relax and enjoy the newfound sense of lightness and purity in your right side!

*Upon rising:* Drink one 8-ounce glass of mineral/filtered water.

*In the shower:* Give yourself a head massage with almond or jojoba oil. Stand on a clean towel to minimize the risk of slipping on oil drops! Pour some oil into your palms and rub them to warm the oil. Rub the oil into your scalp in circular motions. When you have saturated your whole scalp and all your hair with oil, apply stronger pressure to stimulate circulation and help the oil penetrate deeper into the hair follicles. Spend not less than five minutes massaging your head. Shower and wash your hair as usual.

*Breakfast:* Have one 8-ounce glass of Green Detox Drink, a cup of instant miso soup (available from health food stores), twenty almonds, and an organic apple.

*One hour after breakfast:* Drink one 8-ounce glass of mineral/filtered water.

*Two hours after breakfast:* Drink one 8-ounce glass of Green Detox Drink.

*Lunch:* Have a Warm Avocado Reuben sandwich (recipe follows) with green tea. For dessert, drink one glass of Green Detox Drink.

*One hour after lunch:* Drink one 8-ounce glass of mineral/filtered water.

*Two hours after lunch:* Drink one 8-ounce glass of Green Detox Drink and eat a light snack of five strawberries, a half cup of blueberries, and one sliced banana topped with nondairy whipped cream such as Natural by Nature Organic Whipped Cream.

This is a great day to spend time doing what you really like to do. Meditate, read, walk, tidy up your garden, write in your journal, practice some yoga—please yourself anyway possible to direct thoughts away from possible caffeine or sugar cravings.

*Three hours after lunch:* Drink one 8-ounce glass of mineral/filtered water.

*Dinner:* Prepare and eat Vegetarian Chili (recipe follows). Finish the dinner with one 8-ounce glass of Green Detox Drink.

*One hour after dinner:* Drink one 8-ounce glass of mineral/filtered water.

*Three hours after dinner:* Drink one 8-ounce glass of mineral/filtered water.

*Before sleep:* Take a purifying hot bath. Fill the bath with hot water, add 1 pound of Epsom salts and 1 pound of baking soda. Let the salt and soda dissolve completely. Apply a homemade hair treatment from the assortment of green recipes in Chapter 12 and place a glass of cool water

## Warm Avocado Reuben

2 slices whole-wheat, rye, or pumpernickel bread

1 avocado, peeled and sliced

¼ cup sauerkraut

1 tablespoon virgin olive oil

Splash of balsamic vinegar

A dash of black pepper

1. Place the bread slices in a lightly oiled skillet. Place avocado on one slice and sauerkraut on the other.
2. Over medium heat, warm the sandwich until lightly browned and hot.
3. Drizzle olive oil and vinegar over the avocado and add black pepper to taste.

**Yield: 1 sandwich**

## Vegetarian Chili

3 to 4 tablespoons vegetable oil

1 medium-sized white onion, diced

3 medium-sized carrots, peeled and finely chopped

3 cloves garlic, finely chopped

1 yellow and 1 red bell pepper, chopped

¾ cup celery, chopped

2 teaspoons chipotle puree or ½ teaspoon chili powder

1 lb. white mushrooms, cut in half

14 oz (400 g) can organic diced tomatoes in own juice

14 oz (400 g) can organic kidney beans, drained

2 cups sweet corn or 6 to 8 baby corns, broken in half

3 tablespoons coarsely chopped cilantro

2 tablespoons chopped fresh mint

¼ teaspoon salt

2 tablespoons toasted cumin seed

*Drink lots of sparkling mineral water with this chili—it's hot! This recipe feeds two.*

1. Sauté the onions, carrots, and garlic in olive oil in a large stainless steel or cast iron saucepan until tender.
2. Stir in the yellow and red peppers, celery, and chipotle puree or chili powder. Cook until the vegetables are tender, about six minutes.
3. Stir in the mushrooms, and cook for an additional four minutes. Stir in the tomatoes, kidney beans, and corn. Add cilantro, mint, and salt, and stir thoroughly. Bring to a boil, then reduce the heat to medium.
4. Cover and simmer for 20 minutes, stirring occasionally.

**Yield: 2 servings**

nearby. Soak in the bath until the water cools down. Do not shower! Dry off, wrap yourself in cotton pajamas, and get ready to sleep.

*Bedtime snack:* A medium apple or a medium-sized orange or two tangerines, plus 10–15 almonds. Keep a glass of water on your bedside table.

## Day Three: Face Detox

Today you are going to reward yourself for all your efforts of the previous two days. Most likely, you have already noticed that under-eye circles have diminished greatly and many skin problems are now less visible. Seal the deal with facial pampering!

*Upon rising:* Drink one 8-ounce glass mineral/filtered water.

*In the shower:* Wash your face with Sugar Mommy Scrub (Chapter 8).

*After showering:* Apply a deep cleansing Kinky Oatmeal mask. Relax until the mask is dry. Wash it off with tepid water and give yourself a light facial massage with ten drops of jojoba or almond oil. Do not wear makeup today.

*Breakfast:* Banana French Toast (recipe follows) with green tea and one 8-ounce glass of Green Detox Drink.

*One hour after breakfast:* Drink one 8-ounce glass of mineral/filtered water.

*Two hours after breakfast:* Drink one 8-ounce glass of Green Detox Drink.

*Lunch:* Green Fettuccine Alfredo (recipe follows). For dessert, drink one 8-ounce glass of Green Detox Drink.

*One hour after lunch:* Drink one 8-ounce glass of mineral/filtered water.

*Two hours after lunch:* Drink one 8-ounce glass of Green Detox Drink and eat a light snack of sliced apple on top of one slice of whole-wheat toast covered with a generous amount of almond butter.

*Three hours after lunch:* Drink one 8-ounce glass of mineral/filtered water.

*Dinner:* Green Chow Mein (recipe follows) followed by one 8-ounce glass of Green Detox Drink.

*One hour after dinner:* Drink one 8-ounce glass of mineral/filtered water.

*Three hours after dinner:* Drink one 8-ounce glass of mineral/filtered water.

*Before sleep:* Treat yourself to a spa-style facial. Start with an herbal steam bath. Boil a kettle of water and pour it into a shallow basin. Throw in a handful of dried chamomile flowers and three tea bags of green tea. Lean over the basin and steam your face for ten to fifteen minutes. When the water cools down, pat your face with a towel.

Apply a White for Sake Scrub (Chapter 8) and massage your face with circular movements for at least three minutes. Rinse off the scrub with warm water and pat your face dry.

Apply a nourishing, rich homemade facial mask of your choice. Relax for twenty minutes while reading or meditating. Rinse off the mask with warm water, pat your face dry, and perform a calming facial massage with Soothing Face Oil (Chapter 9). Let the oil soak in completely.

*Bedtime snack:* Eat a cup of strawberries, a small packet of rice crackers with hummus, or one apple. Keep a glass of water on your bedside table.

This program is a simple and completely green way to detoxify your life and adopt new skin care and hair care methods. Hopefully you learned that you can survive without animal fats and protein and still feel great. Try this detox twice a year, and enjoy any part of it whenever you feel like your life needs a little bit of cleaning up.

## Green Fettuccine Alfredo

4 ounces fettuccine pasta

1 cup sweet corn

1 cup soy or almond milk

2 tablespoons hummus

14 oz (400 g) can green beans, drained

Salt and black pepper

**Yield: 2 servings**

1. Cook the fettuccine in a large pot of boiling water until tender.

2. While the fettuccine is cooking, blend the corn, milk, hummus, and black pepper with a stick blender until smooth.

3. Heat the mixture in a small saucepan and stir in the beans. Continue heating and stir often until beans have warmed through. Season with a pinch of salt.

4. Drain the fettuccine well and return to the pot. Pour in the hot sauce mixture and toss. Serve immediately. Add freshly ground black pepper to taste.

## Banana French Toast

2 medium bananas

1 cup soy milk

2 tablespoons maple syrup

⅛ teaspoon vanilla extract

4 slices whole-wheat bread

Yield:
2 servings

1. Blend bananas, soy milk, maple syrup, and vanilla with a stick blender until smooth. Pour into a shallow dish and soak the bread slices for two minutes until all liquid disappears into the bread.

2. Carefully transfer the bread to a lightly oiled skillet. Cook each side for two minutes or until browned.

3. Serve with organic whipped cream, berries, and almonds.

## Green Chow Mein

4 ounces fresh egg noodles

1 tablespoon virgin olive oil

1 tablespoon finely chopped garlic

½ red bell pepper

¼ cup snow peas, trimmed

1-inch piece of ginger root, sliced

3 tablespoons dark soy sauce

1 tablespoon rice wine or dry sherry

3 tablespoons finely chopped shallots

1 cup soybean sprouts

1 cup mung bean sprouts

1 teaspoon sesame seed oil

Black pepper

Yield:
2 servings

1. Cook the noodles three to five minutes in a pan of boiling water. Drain and plunge into cold water; drain and toss with a little sesame oil. Set aside.

2. Heat a wok until it is very hot. Add one tablespoon olive oil. You can add a few drops of chili oil for an extra sparkle. When the oil is very hot and slightly smoking, add the garlic and stir-fry for 10 seconds.

3. Add the bell pepper and snow peas and stir-fry for one minute; transfer to a plate.

4. Return noodles to wok and add soy sauce, rice wine, and shallots, and stir-fry for two minutes. Add snow peas and peppers to the noodle mixture.

5. Add the sprouts and continue to stir-fry for three to four minutes until the sprouts are soft. Stir in the sesame oil, and add black pepper to taste.

# Gorgeous Green Finale

If there is one lesson you learn from this book, make it this: scientists have yet to discover exactly what kind of damage paraben preservatives, phthalates, triethanolamine, and DMAE do to us, and we probably won't find out in the next twenty or thirty years. Well, many of us have already celebrated our thirtieth birthday (or as I prefer to call it, twenty-tenth), and we are still alive after fifteen to twenty years of rubbing esters of para-hydroxybenzoic acid and formaldehyde into our faces. Luckily, today we have everything we need to adopt a healthier attitude toward our looks. We exercise and make efforts to eat less junk food, so why would we put up with "junk beauty"? Remember, skincare is the food for our skin. Just like junk food is loaded with refined wheat and sugar, hydrogenated fat, and artificial additives, so is junk beauty loaded with synthetic chemicals, petroleum-derived fats, and artificial flavors. Do your health a favor, and don't eat junk food. Do your skin a favor, and ditch junk beauty. It's bad for you; it's bad for our planet.

You are your only hope. Science does not have all the answers to everything. Neither do government regulators. If you want proof, ask your dermatologist when you go for a yearly checkup of your moles and freckles what she thinks of mercury whitening cream. Watch her face go pale and ashen, and her voice turn reproachful. Only fifteen years ago, mercury bleaching creams were widely recommended. Today, mercury in cosmetics is banned. What will be the next mercury? Phthalates? Lead? Formaldehyde? Parabens? Do you really want to wait to find out?

Set yourself apart from the rest by going green. Learn to spot the dangerous chemicals that undermine your health and put your family and children, now and tomorrow, at a higher risk for allergies, autism, or cancer. Pass on buying anything proven to be carcinogenic, even in animal studies. That's right, humans are not rodents—but then again, DNA is DNA. If a substance is damaging a living creature's DNA and causing it to mutate, there's a very high chance it will mess up human cells, too.

Your common sense is your best guide to sorting through the organic hype. Remember that the cosmetics industry spends billions of dollars each year to sell you one myth or another. Many of the so-called organic products give you a false sense of safety. Spend a second or two scanning ingredients lists and refuse to buy anything that doesn't comply with your understanding of truly pure and natural cosmetics.

You can influence the industry by making smart buying choices. You may think that one bottle of conventional shampoo won't really change the world, but stop right there and think for a moment. If a drugstore sells ten fewer bottles of shampoo in one week, the store manager will become curious. If a drugstore chain sells a thousand fewer bottles of shampoo, the supplier will take notice. If ten thousand bottles of chemical goo are left unsold, then the manufacturer gets the message. Every bottle counts.

You can make your point every time you open your wallet to buy a toxic cosmetic product. You can buy the chemical, fruity-smelling goop and support the current twisted state of the cosmetic industry. Manufacturers will get more proof that the public buys their products, as is, without batting an irritated, swollen eye. And they will keep churning out shampoos that make our hair fall out, toners that burn and sting our faces, and baby powders with ingredients that cause lung cancer. So the next time you reach for that pretty bottle, stop for a second, read the list of ingredients, and ask yourself: would I eat any of it? Think about it for a moment. Then close your wallet, head on to that humble health food store, and grab an unpretentious bottle of herbal body and hair wash. Your hair will be just as clean. The only difference is that you may sleep a little bit better.

I have seen the future of beauty, and it looks rosy and green.

# appendix a
# recommended resources

## Online Green Beauty Shopping

Online shopping is the most time-efficient and money-saving way to shop for organic beauty products or ingredients to make DIY green cosmetics. Here are some of my favorite online shopping destinations:

### Saffron Rouge (www.saffronrouge.com)

What started as a humble yet stylish online store with Dr. Hauschka and Jurlique in stock evolved into a comprehensive information portal on all things pretty, green, and eco-friendly. Kirstien Binder handpicks organic brands to represent, and her roster now includes Pangea, Dr. Hauschka, Jo Wood, Weleda, Primavera, Erbaviva, Balm Balm, Dr. Alkaitis, John Masters Organics, Jurlique, Nvey Eco, Santaverde, Suzanne Aux Bains, and Florascent. Everything you buy here is guaranteed organic or biodynamic. The website offers tons of samples, a no-hassle return policy, and reasonable shipping charges.

### Drugstore.com/Beauty.com

For organic bathroom staples, head to the largest online pharmacy, which is Drugstore.com. It has a cute "Green&Natural" tab with a green leaf on the home page, with green offerings including Burt's Bees, Juice Organics, Seventh Generation, Avalon Organics, Weleda, Desert Essence, Earth Science, Kiss My Face, Nature's Gate Organics, Annemarie Borlind, Ecco Bella, Zia Natural Skincare, Frownies, JASON Organic Products, Rachel Perry, Alba Botanica, and Moom Organic Hair Removal. Other natural products to note include Natracare (organic feminine hygiene products), Chicken Poop lip balms, Baby's Only organic baby formulas, and nontoxic house cleaning products by Method.

Beauty.com specializes in more upscale brands, and its natural section includes Inara Organics, Astara, Caudalie, Lavanila, Juice Beauty, John Masters Organics, BORBA, Malie Kauai, and Crabtree & Evelyn. All ingredients are clearly listed, so you see what you are buying. Both sites have decent shipping charges and convenient return policies.

## Amazon.com

This online shopping empire features such brands as Pangea Organics, Juice Beauty, Crabtree & Evelyn, John Masters Organics, Dr. Hauschka, BORBA, Nvey Eco, Organic Bath Company, Davie's Gate, Erbaviva, Bare Escentuals, Jo Wood Organics, Suki, Weleda, and Eminence. Shipping charges and delivery time vary from retailer to retailer, but the overall experience is pleasant, and you can spread the word about organic beauty by leaving reviews.

## Sephora.com

Sephora earns extra kudos for consistent listing of ingredients and clear, accurate color swatches. Sometimes the online shopping experience is far more pleasant than dawdling around the store and bickering with sales associates who cannot always grasp why you want a humble Dr. Hauschka's lotion if there's such a gorgeous, shimmering, luxuriously smelling and fast-absorbing dermatologist-tested cream that "contains natural ingredients." Green brands handpicked by Sephora experts include CARE by Stella McCartney, Juice Beauty, Bare Escentuals, CARGO, Lavanila, Nvey Eco, and Caudalie.

## eBay.com

This is the route to take when you want to save up to 50 percent on organic beauty products, create your own green cosmetic products from scratch, or try a new, niche brand. Many stores sell organic beauty products with a substantial discount, although shipping charges may be on the high end, and be prepared to receive a Dr. Hauschka lotion from Germany with instructions in German, or even to spend up to a month waiting for your purchase or not receive it at all.

A word of online shopping wisdom: be ruthless and file the claim with PayPal after ten days of waiting. But the savings make it all worth the trouble. I head to eBay for plant hydrosols for toners and masks, rare and discontinued Black Phoenix Alchemy Lab perfume oils, powdered plant extracts for creams and hair treatments, pure henna, inexpensive antioxidants, organic soy wax chips for homemade candles, organic essential oils from all over the world, and, of course, for vintage perfume bottles or cobalt glass jars that will contain my homemade beauty creations.

## Skin Actives Scientific (www.SkinActives.com)

If you are a cosmetic DIY enthusiast, make this online store your source of continual inspiration. All Skin Actives products are synthesized in an Arizona lab by acclaimed chemist and research scientist Dr. Hannah Sivak and her team.

 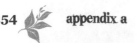

Be prepared to frantically jump from one active to another, pretty much like a kid in a candy store: active ingredients include potent antioxidants idebenone, kinetin, resveratrol, and green tea extracts; collagen boosters matrixyl and epidermal growth factor; antiwrinkle *Boswellia serrata* and hyaluronic acid; anti-inflammatory bisabolol and copper peptide, and the bestselling fermented sea kelp that will allow you to prepare your Creme De La Mer duplicate without petrochemicals or parabens. All active ingredients are shipped in sterile containers, complete with detailed instructions, pipettes, and spatulas.

## MountainRoseHerbs.com

If you prefer to blend your masks and toners from scratch, head over to this online store that has been selling certified organic plant extracts, essential oils, and hydrosols since 1987. Aloe vera gel, almond meal, borax powder, castile soap, witch hazel, vegetable glycerine, and all other basic cosmetic ingredients are sold in various amounts, depending on your needs. You will find bulk organic herbs and spices, butters, waxes, carrier oils, clays, natural flavors, boxes and bottles, as well as seaweeds, sprouting seeds, and herbal teas to complete your green journey. The store has a no-hassle return policy and reasonable shipping fees.

## There Must Be a Better Way Ltd. (theremustbeabetterway.co.uk)

This humble Brit store sells rare, hard-to-find organic labels, such as Mother Earth, Living Nature, Eselle, Miessense, and Logona. You can also find Britain's own organic creations here, including Spiezia, Green People, and Trevarno, alongside bestselling Weleda, Aubrey Organics, and Dr. Bronner's Magic Soaps. Try this store if you are looking for products that are not available in North America, including hidden treasures such as rare (and probably discontinued) Burt's Bees Vitamin E Body and Bath Oil, Weleda Aloe Body Lotion, and the ingenuous mineral shampoo Logona Ghassoul Clay Powder. The store ships worldwide, but shipping charges are on the higher side, especially if you buy more than 5 pounds of green goodies.

## Additional Online Green Resources

*The Campaign for Safe Cosmetics* (www.safecosmetics.org) is a coalition of public health, educational, religious, labor, women's, environmental, and consumer groups that aims to protect our health by requiring the health and beauty industry to phase out chemicals linked to cancer, birth defects, and other health problems, and replace them with safer alternatives.

*Department of Health and Human Services' Agency for Toxic Substances & Disease Registry (ATSDR) ToxFAQs* (www.atsdr.cdc.gov/toxfaq.html) is a series of summaries about hazardous substances developed by the ATSDR Division of Toxicology. Information for this series is excerpted from the ATSDR Toxicological Profiles and Public Health Statements. Each fact sheet serves as a quick and easy-to-understand guide.

*Environmental Working Group's Body Burden Studies* (ewg.org/reports/bodyburden2/execsumm.php) provides information on EWG's Human Toxome Project and its various body burden studies of more than five hundred chemicals in babies, children, and adults.

*Environmental Working Group's National Tap Water Quality Database* (www.ewg.org/tapwater) contains data on drinking water contamination for more than 39,751 water utilities in forty-two states through contact with state environmental and health agencies. For the first time ever, you will see how your tap water measures up against other cities and towns throughout the United States.

*Environmental Working Group's Shopper's Food Guide* (www.food news.org) teaches about the "best and worst" food products, and explains how to buy and eat healthier from EWG's analysis of forty thousand government tests of pesticides in popular fruits and vegetables.

*Environmental Working Group's Skin Deep Database on Safe Personal Care Products* (www.cosmeticdatabase.com) is the most complete, interactive guide to personal care product safety. It checks the safety of ingredients in nearly twenty-five thousand cosmetic products by looking into fifty toxicity and regulatory databases, making it the largest data resource of its kind. You can search by cosmetic product, brand, or an ingredient.

*Healthy Child, Healthy World* (www.healthychild.org) is dedicated to protecting the health and well-being of children from harmful environmental exposures. It educates parents, supports protective policies, and engages communities to make responsible decisions, simple everyday choices, and well-informed lifestyle improvements to create healthy environments where children and families can flourish.

*Our Stolen Future* (www.ourstolenfuture.org) provides a host of information about a new category of toxic chemicals called endocrine disruptors. Many man-made chemicals fall into this category—chemicals that in some way block, trigger, or change our normal endocrine function.

*Scorecard* (www.scorecard.org) provides an in-depth pollution report for your state or town, covering air, water, chemicals, and more.

 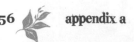

*Toxicology Data Network* (TOXNET) (www.toxnet.nlm.nih.gov) is another great way to check the toxic potential of chemical ingredients in your cosmetic products.

To report adverse side effects in cosmetics, contact these organizations:

**CFSAN Adverse Event Reporting System (CAERS)**
Phone: 301-436-2405
E-mail: CAERS@cfsan.fda.gov

**British Association of Dermatologists**
Willan House, 4 Fitzroy Square, London W1T 5HQ
Phone: 0207-383-0266
E-mail: admin@bad.org.uk

## Green Reading

So, you are almost done. Where do you go next? Try these books if you have more questions about living a healthy, ecoconscious lifestyle.

Ausubel, Kenny, ed. *Ecological Medicine: Healing the Earth, Healing Ourselves*. San Francisco: Sierra Club, 2004.

Campbell, T. Colin, with Thomas M. Campbell II. *The China Study: The Most Comprehensive Study of Nutrition Ever Conducted*. Dallas, TX: BenBella Books, 2006.

Colborn, Theo, Dianne Dumanoski, and John Peterson Myers. *Our Stolen Future: Are We Threatening Our Fertility, Intelligence, and Survival? A Scientific Detective Story*. New York: Plume, 1997.

Cox, Jeff. *The Organic Cook's Bible*. Hoboken, NJ: Wiley, 2006.

Dadd, Debra Lynn. *Home Safe Home: Creating a Healthy Home Environment by Reducing Exposure to Toxic Household Products*. New York: Tarcher/Putnam, 2007.

Fagin, Dan, Marianne Lavelle, and the Center for Public Integrity. *Toxic Deception: How the Chemical Industry Manipulates Science, Bends the Law, and Endangers Your Health*. Monroe, ME: Common Courage, 1999.

Goodall, Jane. *Harvest for Hope: A Guide to Mindful Eating*. New York: Wellness Central, 2006.

Gore, Al. *Earth in the Balance: Ecology and the Human Spirit*. New York: Rodale, 2006.

———. *An Inconvenient Truth*. New York: Rodale, 2006.

Hicks, India. *Island Beauty*. London: Stewart, Tabori & Chang, 2006.

Krimsky, Sheldon. *Science in the Private Interest: Has the Lure of Profits Corrupted Biomedical Research?* Lanham, MD: Rowman & Littlefield, 2004.

Kurz, Susan West. *Awakening Beauty, the Dr. Hauschka Way*. New York: Clarkson Potter, 2006.

Malkan, Stacy. *Not Just a Pretty Face: The Ugly Side of the Beauty Industry*. Gabriola Island, Canada: New Society, 2007.

Markowitz, Gerald, and David Rosner. *Deceit and Denial: The Deadly Politics of Industrial Pollution*. Berkeley and Los Angeles: University of California Press, 2003.

Nestle, Marion. *Food Politics: How the Food Industry Influences Nutrition and Health*. Berkeley and Los Angeles: University of California Press, 2007.

Pollan, Michael. *The Omnivore's Dilemma: A Natural History of Four Meals*. New York: Penguin, 2007.

Schlosser, Eric. *Fast Food Nation*. New York: Harper Perennial, 2005.

# appendix b
# 100 toxic cosmetic ingredients you don't want in your beauty products

Here's the most comprehensive list of harmful chemicals currently used in skincare, hair care, makeup, and fragrances. Use this list anytime you buy a beauty product. Don't keep it secret: photocopy it and give it to your family and friends. Minimize your exposure to these chemicals. Ideally, eliminate them from your beauty routine. They are the worst enemies of your skin and hair.

1. **Acrylic Acid**: respiratory toxin for humans; causes asthma, severe skin burns, and allergic reaction in the skin or lungs; causes renal and kidney damage in animals; causes blood tumors and skin tumors in animals

2. **Aluminum (Pure Aluminum Powder)**: strong human neurotoxicant; causes irritation of eyes, skin, and lungs; endocrine disruptor; linked to Alzheimer's disease and breast cancer; causes birth disorders in animals

3. **Aluminium Chloride**: nose and lung irritant; causes liver and bladder abnormalities in animals; causes brain disorders in animals; human endocrine disruptor linked to breast cancer and Alzheimer's disease; aluminum compounds are neurotoxic to humans

4. **Aluminium Hydrochloride**: endocrine disruptor linked to breast cancer and Alzheimer's disease; aluminum compounds are neurotoxic to humans

5. **Aluminium Oxide**: strong nose and lung irritant; causes skin cancer in animals; endocrine disruptor linked to breast cancer and Alzheimer's disease; aluminum compounds are neurotoxic to humans

6. **Ammonium Laureth Sulfate**: causes skin irritation; water contaminant; may be contaminated with carcinogen 1,4-Dioxane

7. **Ammonium Persulfate**: strong eye, respiratory system, and skin irritant; can trigger asthma; restricted in cosmetics

8. **Amyl Acetate**: neurotoxin; eye and lung irritant; lung allergen

9. **Benzalkonium Chloride**: immune system, lung, and skin toxicant; can trigger asthma; restricted in Canada and Japan

10. **Benzyl Alcohol**: strong neurotoxicant; can cause allergic reaction in lungs; causes itching, burning, scaling, hives, and blistering of skin; causes liver damage, coma, and death in animals

11. **Boric Acid**: strong reproductive toxin; potent endocrine disruptor; unsafe for use on infants and injured or damaged skin; causes death and birth defects in animals; banned in Canada and Japan

12. **Bronopol (2-bromo-2-nitropropane-1,3-diol)**: one of the strongest lung and skin toxicants; endocrine disruptor; forms carcinogenic nitrosamine; causes allergic contact dermatitis; environmental contaminant; poisonous to wildlife

13. **Butylated Hydroxyanisole (BHA)**: human carcinogen; causes brain and liver tumors in animals at low doses; endocrine disruptor; causes allergic contact dermatitis and skin depigmentation; banned in European Union; persistent environmental toxin

14. **Butylated Hydroxytoluene (BHT)**: endocrine disruptor, skin and lung toxicant at low doses; causes death, liver and stomach cancers, thrombosis, fibrosis, and liver and brain damage in animals; strong skin and eye irritant

15. **Butylene Glycol**: skin, lung, and eye irritant; environmental toxin

16. **Butylparaben**: skin and eye irritant; endocrine disruptor linked to breast and ovarian cancer; environmental contaminant

17. **Calcium Fluoride**: neurotoxic to humans; leads to bone weakness; causes birth abnormalities and depression in animals

18. **Ceteareth (with any numeral following it)**: unsafe for use on broken skin; eye and lung irritant; may be contaminated with 1,4-Dioxane

19. **Cetrimonium Chloride**: skin and eye sensitizer that can include itching, burning, scaling, hives, and blistering; causes cell mutations and lung cancer in animal studies

20. **Cetyl Alcohol**: skin and eye irritant in humans

21. **Chloroacetamide**: strong skin, eye, and lung irritant; toxic if inhaled; causes paralysis, goiter, and birth defects in animals; banned in Canada

22. **Coal Tar**: known human carcinogen; causes lung and urinary tract cancer; potent skin irritant; causes multiple cancers in animals; banned in most countries including Canada and European Union; still used in anti-dandruff shampoos in the US

23. **Cocamide DEA (Ethanolamide of Coconut Acid)**: strong human skin toxicant and suspected carcinogen; causes irritation of skin, eyes, and lungs in humans; causes liver and bladder cancer in animals

24. **D&C Red 30 Lake**: strong nervous system toxicant; as an aluminum compound, disrupts endocrine system and linked to breast and ovarian cancer; persistent wildlife contaminant

 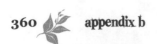

25. **D&C Violet 2**: coal tar dye; skin and eye irritant; long-time use of coal tar hair dye is linked to bladder cancer

26. **Dibutyl Phthalate**: neurotoxicant; linked to impaired fertility and urinary abnormalities; linked to breast and ovarian cancers; contaminates wildlife

27. **Diethanolamine (DEA)**: linked to brain abnormalities in animals; may be contaminated with carcinogen 1,4-Dioxane

28. **Dimeticone (Dimethicone)**: petroleum derivative; environmental toxicant

29. **Direct Black 38**: diethanolamine-containing dye that is a confirmed human carcinogen; strong evidence of causing bladder cancer; may harm unborn child; causes liver and kidney cancer in animals; banned in European Union

30. **DMDM Hydantoin**: contains carcinogenic formaldehyde; skin, eye, and lung irritant; environmental toxicant

31. **EDTA (Disodium EDTA)**: this penetration enhancer is a neurotoxin linked to brain damage in animals; caused liver changes and endocrine damage in animals; caused fetal death and birth abnormalities in animals; made from formaldehyde; approved for use in cosmetics and baby food

32. **Ethylparaben**: skin and eye irritant; endocrine disruptor linked to breast and ovarian cancer; environmental contaminant

33. **Eugenol**: endocrine disruptor; skin, eye, and lung irritant; well-recognized consumer allergen; causes death, coma, insomnia, convulsions, hematuria, pulmonary edema, and liver cancer in animals

34. **Ext. D&C Violet 2**: this coal tar dye is a strong skin irritant; long-time use of coal tar dyes is linked to increased risk of bladder cancer; restricted in cosmetics

35. **FD&C Blue 1**: derived from coal tar; linked to allergies and hyperactivity disorders

36. **FD&C Green 3**: causes sarcomas and bone marrow hyperplasia in animals; not studied for safety in humans; prohibited in European Union

37. **FD&C Yellow 5 (E104, Tartrazine)**: causes severe allergic and intolerance reactions, especially among asthmatics and those with an aspirin intolerance; linked to thyroid tumors, chromosomal damage, hives, and hyperactivity in humans

38. **FD&C Yellow 5 Aluminum Lake**: aluminum compounds are neurotoxic to humans

39. **FD&C Yellow 6**: human skin and eye irritant; causes coma, convulsions, testicular damage, and changes in leucocytes in animals; cannot be used in eye cosmetics

40. **Fig *(Ficus Carica)* Extract**: immune system toxin; cannot be used as

fragrance ingredient due to potential carcinogenicity; banned in European Union; allowed in the US as fragrance ingredient in shampoos and body washes

41. **Formaldehyde**: known human carcinogen linked to leukemia, pancreatic, skin, liver, and lung cancer; strong skin, eye, and lung irritant; irritates human liver (causes cirrhosis), stomach, kidneys, and bladder; can cause skin burns; triggers asthma; hazardous air pollutant; environmental toxin; banned in Canada and Japan; determined as safe for use in cosmetics in the US

42. **Formaldehyde Resin**: contains formaldehyde and carries same risks; can trigger allergic reaction in the skin or lungs

43. **Formaldehyde Solution (Formalin)**: neurotoxin in humans and animals; restricted in Canada and European Union; known human carcinogen linked to leukemia, nasal and nasopharyngeal, pancreatic, skin, liver, bladder, and lung cancer; strong skin, eye, and lung irritant; irritates human liver (causes cirrhosis), stomach, kidneys, and bladder; can cause skin burns; triggers asthma; hazardous air pollutant; environmental toxin; banned in Canada and Japan; determined as safe for use in cosmetics in the US

44. **Glyceryl Stearate**: weak skin, eye, and lung irritant

45. **Hydroquinone**: eye, lung, and nervous system toxin; can cause itching, burning, scaling, hives, and blistering of skin; suspected liver and stomach carcinogen; causes liver cancer, and DNA and ovary mutations in animals; restricted in Canada

46. **Iodopropynyl Butylcarbamate**: contains Diethanolamine; can affect thyroid function; gastrointestinal and liver toxicant; cannot be used in aerosols; causes allergic contact dermatitis; restricted in Japan

47. **Imidazolidinyl Urea (Uric Acid)**: can cause itching, burning, scaling, hives, and blistering of skin

48. **Isobutylparaben**: skin and eye irritant; endocrine disruptor linked to breast and ovarian cancer; environmental contaminant

49. **Isoparaffin**: petroleum derivative; environmental toxin; mildly irritating; produces kidney damage in animals; not carcinogenic in humans

50. **Isopropyl Alcohol (SD-40)**: human neurotoxin; skin, eye, and lung irritant; vapors cause drowsiness and dizziness; causes skin dehydration; may promote brown spots and premature aging of skin; petroleum derivative

51. **Lactic acid**: strong skin and eye irritant; can cause skin burns; causes changes in liver, brain, and blood in animals; causes mutations and birth defects in animals; restricted in Canada

52. **Lanolin**: strong skin irritant and toxicant; can cause allergic reaction in the lungs

 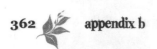

53. **Laureth-7 (Polyethylene Glycol Ether of Lauryl Alcohol)**: may be contaminated with carcinogen 1,4-Dioxane

54. **Lead Acetate**: possible human carcinogen and neurotoxin; skin and eye irritant; environmental toxin; banned in the European Union

55. **Lecithin**: can irritate lungs in aerosol form; a potent asthma trigger; forms carcinogenic nitrosamine compounds if mixed with nitrosating agents

56. **Manganese Sulfate**: strong human neurotoxin; harmful during prolonged exposure or inhalation; causes convulsions, DNA mutations, and protein loss in animals; toxic to wildlife

57. **Methamine**: strong skin, eye, nose, and lung irritant; can cause itching, burning, scaling, hives, and blistering of skin; may be contaminated with carcinogenic 1,4-Dioxane; cannot be used in aerosol cosmetics

58. **Methyl Methacrylate**: strong neurotoxin; strong eye and lung irritant; causes asthma and skin burns; causes cancer and stomach bleeding in animals; hazardous air pollutant; banned in Canada and recently in the US

59. **Methylparaben**: skin and eye irritant; endocrine disruptor linked to breast and ovarian cancer; environmental contaminant

60. **Mineral Oil (Liquid Petrolatum)**: causes blood and skin cancer formations in animals; eye and skin irritant; derived from petroleum; non-biodegradable environmental toxin

61. **Monoethanolamine (MEA)**: skin and eye irritant at low doses; can be irritating to the respiratory tract

62. **Nonoxynol (ethoxylated alkyl phenol)**: endocrine disruptor; skin and lung irritant; causes liver damage in animals; may be contaminated with 1,4-Dioxane

63. **Octoxynol (10, 11, 13, 40)**: strong skin and eye toxin that can cause itching, burning, scaling, hives, and blistering of skin; may contain carcinogen 1,4-Dioxane; causes cancer of reproductive organs in animals

64. **Oxybenzone (Benzophenone–4)**: strong photoallergen; endocrine disruptor; produces free radicals that can increase skin aging; environmental toxicant

65. **Padimate O (Octyl Dimethyl PABA/PABA Ester)**: has estrogenic activity; releases free radicals that damage DNA when exposed to sunlight; causes allergic reactions and photoallegenic dermatitis; restricted in Japan

66. **Para Amino Benzonic Acid (PABA)**: causes allergic dermatitis and photosensitivity; produces free radicals that cause mutations, lead to cell death, and may be implicated in cardiovascular disease; causes changes in blood components and muscle weakness in animals; banned in Canada

67. **Paraffin (Paraffinum Liquidum, Paraffin Petrolatum)**: petrochemical

bleached with carcinogen acrolyn; releases carcinogens benzene and toluene upon heating; causes kidney or renal system tumor in animals; environmental toxin

68. **PEG-100 Stearate**: polyethylene glycols are often contaminated with 1,4-Dioxane; suspected endocrine disruptor; linked to cancer in animals; skin and eye irritant

69. **Petrolatum (Soft Paraffin, White Petrolatum, Petroleum Jelly)**: lung irritant upon inhalation; derived from petroleum; non-biodegradable environmental toxin

70. **Phenol**: strong respiratory irritant; toxic by skin contact; causes skin burns; causes kidney damage and cyanosis in humans; causes skin cancer, birth defects, and brain and nervous system damage in animals at very low doses; environmental contaminant; banned in Canada, restricted in Japan, permitted in the US

71. **Phenoxyethanol**: endocrine disruptor and carcinogen in animals; linked to allergic contact uritica and dermatitis

72. **Picric Acid**: human immune system toxicant; toxic by inhalation, skin contact, and ingestion; causes allergic reaction in the skin or lungs; causes coma, convulsions, and body temperature increase in animals; banned in Canada and European Union

73. **Placental Extract**: endocrine disruptor containing estradiol and progesteron; banned in Canada

74. **Polyethylene Glycol (PEG)**: often contaminated with carcinogenic 1,4-Dioxane; suspected endocrine disruptor; linked to cancer in animals; skin and eye irritant

75. **Polyethylene Terephthalate**: causes cancer in animals; not studied for safety in humans

76. **Polysorbate 80**: may be contaminated with 1,4-Dioxane; suspected endocrine disruptor; linked to cancer in animals; skin and eye irritant

77. **Potassium Persulfate**: strong irritant to eyes, lungs, respiratory system, and skin; restricted for use in cosmetics

78. **P-phenylenediamine**: linked to bladder and prostate cancer; human neurotoxin; skin and lung irritant; causes liver cancer and birth defects in animals; very strong environmental toxin

79. **Propyl Acetate**: skin, eye, nose, and lung irritant

80. **Propylene Glycol (PG)**: can cause eye irritation and conjunctivitis, as well as upper respiratory tract irritation

81. **Propylparaben**: skin and eye irritant; endocrine disruptor linked to breast and ovarian cancer; environmental contaminant

82. **Quaternium–7, 15, 31, 60**: formaldehyde releasing; can cause skin and eye irritation; linked to several cancers (see **Formaldehyde**)

 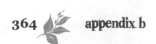

83. **Resorcinol (m-Hydroquinone, Euresol, 1,3-Benzenediol)**: strong skin irritant; linked to adenomas in animals; suspected to trigger skin cancer in humans; environmental toxin

84. **Saccharin**: suspected human carcinogen; causes liver, kidney, and bladder damage in animals, as well as reproductive damage and birth abnormalities

85. **Silica**: linked to esophageal cancer, renal disease, pulmonary fibrosis, mesothelioma, sarcoma, rheumatoid arthritis, and bronchitis; strong nasal and lung irritant; wildlife toxicant; accumulates in human body.

86. **Sodium Laureth Sulfate**: skin irritant; water contaminant; may be contaminated with carcinogen 1,4-Dioxane

87. **Sodium Lauryl Sulfate**: skin and eye irritant; in toothpaste may cause canker sores

88. **Sodium Metabisulfite**: immune system toxicant; eye and skin irritant; emits toxic gas when in contact with acids; dangerous for asthmatics; causes stillbirth, muscle weakness, and brain degeneration in animals

89. **Sodium Methylparaben**: endocrine disruptor; causes mild brain damage in animals; skin irritant causing itching, burning, scaling, hives, and blistering; causes depigmentation of skin; banned for use in European Union

90. **Sodium Monofluorophosphate**: nervous system toxin; harmful if swallowed during teeth bleaching; causes convulsions, proteinuria, osteoporosis, and changes in DNA in animals; restricted in Canada

91. **Talc**: even when it contains no asbestos, was proven fibrogenic (causes tissue injury and fibrosis); skin and lung irritation

92. **Teflon**: causes toxic pneumonitis and skin cancer in animals; not studied for safety in humans

93. **Tetrasodium EDTA**: contains formaldehyde; cytotoxic and genotoxic in animals; strong skin and lung irritant in humans; most widespread poison to waterways

94. **Thimerosal (Thiomersal, Merthiolate)**: strong toxin to skin, nervous, and immune system; mercury is linked to autism; causes cancer in animals; environmental toxin

95. **Thioglycolic Acid**: strong human skin irritant; causes itching, burning, scaling, hives, and blistering of skin; lung allergen; restricted in cosmetics; banned in Canada

96. **Toluene (Methylbenzene)**: skin and lung toxicant; accumulates in fat tissue; soil contaminant

97. **Triclosan**: endocrine disruptor, affects thyroid hormone–associated gene expression, caused fetal death in animals; strong skin irritant; environmental toxicant

98. **Triethanolamine (TEA)**: causes lymphoid, kidney; and renal tumors in animals; may be contaminated with carcinogen 1,4-Dioxane; skin and eye irritant even when used in low doses

99. **Triphenyl Phosphate**: human neurotoxin; skin, eye, and lung irritant; causes tremors, depression, and diarrhea in animals

100. **Xanthene (AKA106, CI 45100)**: found unsafe for use in cosmetics in the US; causes cancer and various organ mutations in animals

And the list can go on and on. This is not a complete list of all harmful and toxic chemicals found in beauty products. Last time I counted, a popular hair highlighting kit contained forty chemicals that are linked to various health disorders even at low doses. However, these are some of the most common staples of junk beauty products. Try to avoid them at all costs.

Sources: Cosmetic Ingredient Review (CIR); Environmental Protection Agency (EPA); European Union: Classification & Labelling; Health Canada: List of Prohibited and Restricted Cosmetic Ingredients; EPA Water Quality Standards Database; EPA Hazardous Air Pollutants; National Library of Medicine; CHE Toxicant and Disease Database; Scorecard.org Toxicity Information; U.S. Association of Occupational and Environmental Clinics; International Agency for Research on Cancer (IARC)

# references

## Introduction

Hildenbrand GL, Hildenbrand LC, Bradford K, Cavin SW. "Five-year survival rates of melanoma patients treated by diet therapy after the manner of Gerson: a retrospective review." *Alternative Therapies in Health and Medicine.* 1995 Sep; 1(4):29–37.

## Chapter 1. The Nature of Skin

HAE Benson. "Transdermal drug delivery: penetration enhancement techniques." *Current Drug Delivery.* 2005 (2): 223–33.

Niculescu MD, Wu R, Guo Z, da Costa KA, Zeisel SH. "Diethanolamine alters proliferation and choline metabolism in mouse neural precursor cells." *Toxicological Sciences.* 2007 Apr; 96(2):321–6.

Williams, AC, Barry, BW. "Penetration enhancers." *Advanced Drug Delivery Reviews.* 2004 Vol. 56, No. 5: 603–618.

## Chapter 2. Beauty and the Toxic Beast

Adibi JJ, Whyatt RM, Williams PL, Calafat AM, Camann D, Herrick R, Nelson H, Bhat HK, Perera FP, Silva MJ, Hauser R. "Characterization of phthalate exposure among pregnant women assessed by repeat air and urine samples." *Environmental Health Perspectives.* 2008 Apr; 116(4):467–73.

Alijotas-Reig J, Garcia-Gimenez V. "Delayed immune-mediated adverse effects related to hyaluronic acid and acrylic hydrogel dermal fillers: clinical findings, long-term follow-up and review of the literature." *Journal of European Academy of Dermatology and Venereology.* 2008 Feb; 22(2):150–61.

Andersen A. "Final report on the safety assessment of benzaldehyde." *International Journal of Toxicology.* 2006; 25 Suppl 1:11–27.

Anderson D, Brinkworth MH, Jenkinson PC, Clode SA, Creasy DM, Gangolli SD. "Effect of ethylene glycol monomethyl ether on spermatogenesis, dominant lethality, and F1 abnormalities in the rat and the mouse after treatment of F0 males." *Teratogenicity, Carcinogenicity, and Mutagenicity.* 1987; 7(2):141–58.

Baxter KF, Wilkinson SM, Kirk SJ. "Hydroxymethyl pentylcyclohexene- carboxaldehyde (Lyral) as a fragrance allergen in the UK." *Contact Dermatitis.* 2003 Feb; 48(2):117–8.

BCC Research. "Chemicals for Cosmetics and Toiletries." May 1, 2006. http://www.market research.com/product/display.asp?productid=1507343&SID=45507473-415408409-443859592 (accessed May 19, 2008).

Begoun, Paula. *The Beauty Bible.* The Beginning Press, 2002 (2nd Edition): 13–14.

Bisaccia E, Lugo A, Torres O, Johnson B, Scarborough D. "Persistent inflammatory reaction to hyaluronic acid gel: a case report." *Cutis.* 2007 May; 79(5):388–9.

Blackwell M, Kang H, Thomas A, Infante P. "Formaldehyde: evidence of carcinogenicity." *American Industrial Hygiene Association Journal.* 1981 Jul; 42(7):A34, A36, A38, passim.

Bosetti C, McLaughlin JK, Tarone RE, Pira E, La Vecchia C. "Formaldehyde and cancer risk: a quantitative review of cohort studies through 2006." *Annals of Oncology.* 2007 Sep 25.

Buckley DA. "Fragrance ingredient labelling in products on sale in the U.K." *British Journal of Dermatology.* 2007 Aug; 157(2):295–300.

Centers for Disease Control and Prevention (CDC). "CDC reports higher levels of other phthalates than of DEHP in humans, despite greater environmental exposure." *American Journal of Health-System Pharmacy.* 2001 May 15; 58(10):857–8.

Colón I, Caro D, Bourdony CJ, Rosario O. "Identification of phthalate esters in the serum of young Puerto Rican girls with premature breast development." *Environmental Health Perspectives.* 2000 Sep; 108(9):895–900.

Cosmetic Ingredient Review Expert Panel. "Final report on the safety assessment of Triethylene Glycol and PEG–4." *International Journal of Toxicology.* 2006; 25(2):121–38.

Cosmetic, Toiletry, and Fragrance Association. "Cosmetic, Toiletry, and Fragrance Association 2005 Annual Report." http://www.ctfa.org/Content/NavigationMenu/About_CTFA/Annual_Report/48661a_CTFA_Lowres.pdf (accessed May 18, 2008).

Curtis L. "Toxicity of fragrances." *Environmental Health Perspectives.* 2004 Jun; 112(8):A461.

Daniells S. "UK women spend big to look better." *Cosmetics Design Europe.* http://www.cosmeticsdesign-europe.com/news/ng.asp?id=66942 (accessed May 19, 2008).

Darbre PD, Aljarrah A, Miller WR, Coldham NG, Sauer MJ, Pope GS. "Concentrations of parabens in human breast tumours." *Journal of Applied Toxicology.* 2004 Jan-Feb; 24(1):5–13.

Darbre PD. *"Environmental oestrogens, cosmetics and breast cancer."* Best Practices and Research: Clinical Endocrinology and Metabolism. 2006 Mar; 20(1):121–43.

Darbre PD, Byford JR, Shaw LE, Horton RA, Pope GS, Sauer MJ. "Oestrogenic activity of isobutylparaben in vitro and in vivo." *Journal of Applied Toxicology.* 2002 Jul-Aug; 22(4):219–26.

de Groot AC, Bruynzeel DP, Jagtman BA, Weyland JW. "Contact allergy to diazolidinyl urea (Germall II)." *Contact Dermatitis.* 1988 Apr; 18(4):202–5.

Diepgen TL, Weisshaar E. "Contact dermatitis: epidemiology and frequent sensitizers to cosmetics." *Journal of European Academy of Dermatology and Venereology.* 2007 Sep; 21 Suppl 2:9–13.

DiGangi J, Norin H. "Pretty Nasty—Phthalates in European Cosmetic Products." *Health Care Without Harm.* http://www.wen.org.uk/health/Reports/Prettynasty.pdf (accessed May 17, 2008).

Euromonitor International. "Fragrance Markets: Reinvigorating Fragrances." *Global Cosmetic Industry.* Oct 2007. http://www.gcimagazine.com/marketdata/10488727.html (accessed May 19, 2008).

Exley C, Charles LM, Barr L, Martin C, Polwart A, Darbre PD. "Aluminum in human breast tissue." *Journal of Inorganic Biochemistry.* 2007 Sep; 101(9):1344–6.

Frosch PJ, Johansen JD, Menné T, et al. "Further important sensitizers in patients sensitive to fragrances." *Contact Dermatitis.* 2002 Aug; 47(2):78–85.

Gee RH, Charles A, Taylor N, Darbre PD. "Oestrogenic and androgenic activity of triclosan in breast cancer cells." *Journal of Applied Toxicology.* 2008 Jan; 28(1):78–91.

Gonzalo MA, et al. "Allergic contact dermatitis to propylene glycol." *Allergy.* 1999; 54:82–3.

Gwinn MR, Whipkey DL, Tennant LB, Weston A. "Gene expression profiling of di-n-butyl phthalate in normal human mammary epithelial cells." *Journal of Environmental Pathology, Toxicology and Oncology.* 2007; 26(1):51–61.

Hannuksela M, Pirila V, Salo OP. "Skin reactions to propylene glycol." *Contact Dermatitis.* 1975; 1:112–6.

Harris CA, Henttu P, Parker MG, Sumpter JP. "The estrogenic activity of phthalate esters in vitro." *Environmental Health Perspectives.* 1997 Aug; 105(8):802–11.

Hauser R. "The environment and male fertility: recent research on emerging chemicals and semen quality." *Seminars in Reproductive Medicine.* 2006 Jul; 24(3):156–67.

Held E, Johansen JD, Agner T, Menné T. "Contact allergy to cosmetics: testing with patients' own products." *Contact Dermatitis.* 1999 Jun; 40(6):310–5.

Högberg J, Hanberg A, Berglund M, Skerfving S, Remberger M, Calafat AM, Filipsson AF, Jansson B, Johansson N, Appelgren M, Håkansson H. "Phthalate diesters and their metabolites in human breast milk, blood or serum, and urine as biomarkers of exposure in vulnerable populations." *Environmental Health Perspectives.* 2008 Mar; 116(3):334–9.

Johnson W Jr. "Final report on the safety assessment of PEG–25 propylene glycol stearate, PEG–75 propylene glycol stearate, PEG–120 propylene glycol stearate, PEG–10 propylene glycol, PEG–8 propylene glycol cocoate, and PEG–55 propylene glycol oleate." *International Journal of Toxicology.* 2001; 20 Suppl 4:13–26.

Jørgensen PH, Jensen CD, Rastogi S, et al. "Experimental elicitation with hydroxyisohexyl-3-cyclohexene carboxaldehyde-containing deodorants." *Contact Dermatitis.* 2007 Mar; 56(3):146–50.

Kim IY, Han SY, Moon A. "Phthalates inhibit tamoxifen-induced apoptosis in MCF–7 human breast cancer cells." *Journal of Toxicology and Environmental Health A.* 2004 Dec; 67(23–24):2025–35.

Kleinsasser NH, Weissacher H, Kastenbauer ER, Dirschedl P, Wallner BC, Harréus UA. "Altered genotoxicity in mucosal cells of head and neck cancer patients due to environmental pollutants." *European Archives of Otorhinolaryngology.* 2000; 257(6):337–42.

Kuykendall JR, Jarvi EJ, Finley BL, Paustenbach DJ. "DNA-protein cross-link formation in Burkitt lymphoma cells cultured with benzaldehyde and the sedative paraldehyde." *Drug and Chemical Toxicology.* 2007; 30(1):1–16.

Larsen WG. "Allergic contact dermatitis to the fragrance material lilial." *Contact Dermatitis.* 1983 Mar; 9(2):158–9.

Lotery H, Kirk S, Beck M, et al. "Dicaprylyl maleate—an emerging cosmetic allergen." *Contact Dermatitis.* 2007 Sep; 57(3):169–72.

Madslien J. "Jewellery and Perfume Sales Rise." *BBC News Online.* http://news.bbc.co.uk/1/hi/business/1753472.stm (accessed May 19, 2008).

National Toxicology Program. "NTP-CERHR Monograph on the Potential Human Reproductive and Developmental Effects of Di-n-Butyl Phthalate (DBP)." *NTP CERHR MON.* 2003 Apr; (4):i–III90.

Neppelberg E, Costea DE, Vintermyr OK, Johannessen AC. "Dual effects of sodium lauryl sulphate on human oral epithelial structure." *Experimental Dermatology.* 2007 Jul; 16(7):574–9.

Nguema PN, Matsiegui PB, Nsafu DN. "Severely burned patients: epidemiology and treatment (a study of 104 Gabonese cases)." *Sante.* 2000 Jan-Feb; 10(1):37–42.

Organic Consumers Association. "Carcinogenic 1,4–Dioxane Found in Leading 'Organic' Brand Personal Care Products." http://www.organicconsumers.org/bodycare/Dioxane Release08.cfm (accessed May 19, 2008).

Reid FR, Wood TO. "Pseudomonas corneal ulcer. The causative role of contaminated eye cosmetics." *Archives of Ophthalmology.* 1979 Sep; 97(9):1640–1.

Reiner JL, Wong CM, Arcaro KF, Kannan K. "Synthetic musk fragrances in human milk from the United States." *Environmental Science and Technology.* 2007 Jun 1; 41(11):3815–20.

Ross G. "A perspective on the safety of cosmetic products: a position paper of the American Council on Science and Health." *International Journal of Toxicology.* 2006 Jul-Aug; 25(4):269–77.

Sathyanarayana S, Karr CJ, et al. "Baby care products: possible sources of infant phthalate exposure." *Pediatrics.* 2008 Feb; 121(2):260–268.

Scaife MC. "An in vitro cytotoxicity test to predict the ocular irritation potential of detergents and detergent products." *Food and Chemical Toxicology.* 1985 Feb; 23(2):253–8.

Shcherbatykh I, Carpenter DO. "The role of metals in the etiology of Alzheimer's disease." *Journal of Alzheimer's Disease.* 2007 May; 11(2):191–205.

Singh AR, Lawrence WH, Autian J. "Maternal-fetal transfer of 14C–di-2-ethylhexyl phthalate and 14C-diethyl phthalate in rats." *Journal of Pharmaceutical Sciences.* 1975 Aug; 64(8):1347–50.

Stahlhut RW, van Wijngaarden E, Dye TD, Cook S, Swan SH. "Concentrations of urinary phthalate metabolites are associated with increased waist circumference and insulin resistance in adult U.S. males." *Environmental Health Perspectives.* 2007 Jun; 115(6):876–82.

Stickney JA, Sager SL, Clarkson JR, Smith LA, Locey BJ, Bock MJ, Hartung R, Olp SF. "An updated evaluation of the carcinogenic potential of 1,4–dioxane." *Regulatory Toxicology and Pharmacology.* 2003 Oct; 38(2):183–95.

United States Environmental Protection Agency. "OPPT Chemical Fact Sheets 1,4–Dioxane (CAS No. 123–91–1)." *United States Environmental Protection Agency: Pollution Prevention and Toxics.* http://www.epa.gov/chemfact/dioxa-sd.pdf (accessed on June 10, 2008).

United States Environmental Protection Agency. "1,4–Dioxane (1,4–Diethyleneoxide). Hazard Summary—Created in April 1992; Revised in January 2000." *Technology Transfer Network Air Toxics Web Site.* www.epa.gov/ttn/atw/hlthef/dioxane.html (accessed on June 10, 2008).

Waddell WJ. "Thresholds of carcinogenicity of flavors." *Toxicological Sciences.* 2002 Aug; 68(2):275–9.

Williams RM. "Cosmetic chemicals and safer alternatives—Health Risks and Environmental Issues." *Townsend Letter for Doctors and Patients.* Feb–March 2004. http://findarticles.com/p/articles/mi_m0ISW/is_247-248/ai_113807003 (accessed May 19, 2008).

Women's Environmental Network. "Chemicals and Cosmetics: What's the Problem?" www.wen.org.uk/general_pages/Newsitems/pr_cosmeticscoverup.htm (accessed May 18, 2008).

Wojnarowska F, Calnan CD. "Contact and photocontact allergy to musk ambrette." *British Journal of Dermatology.* 1986 Jun; 114(6):667–75.

Zhang Y, Sanjose SD, Bracci PM, Morton LM, Wang R, Brennan P, Hartge P, Boffetta P, Becker N, Maynadie M, Foretova L, Cocco P, Staines A, Holford T, Holly EA, Nieters A, Benavente Y, Bernstein L, Zahm SH, Zheng T. "Personal use of hair dye and the risk of certain subtypes of non-hodgkin lymphoma." *American Journal of Epidemiology.* 2008 Apr 11:1321–31.

 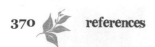

## Chapter 3. Become an Ingredients List Expert

Sepp DT. "DEA: Setting the Record Straight." *Laboratory Shelf.* http://labshelf.com/dea.html (accessed April 21, 2008).

## Chapter 4. Understanding Green Beauty

Animal Liberation. "Cosmetic testing: What are some alternatives?" http://www.animal liberation.org.au/costest.php (accessed June 10, 2008).

Jha A. "RSPCA outrage as experiments on animals rise to 2.85 m." *The Guardian.* December 9, 2005. http://education.guardian.co.uk/higher/news/story/0,,1663421,00.html (accessed June 10, 2008).

Organic Consumers Association. "Industry Creates New Bogus OASIS Organic Standard for Personal Care Products." http://www.organicconsumers.org/articles/article_10886.cfm (accessed May 19, 2008).

Organic Consumers Association. *"Italian Law Calls for All Organic Foods in Nation's Schools."* http://www.organicconsumers.org/organic/italy062804.cfm (accessed June 10, 2008).

Osborn A, Gentleman A. *"Secret French move to block animal-testing ban." The Guardian.* August 19, 2003. http://www.guardian.co.uk/world/2003/aug/19/eu.businessofresearch (accessed June 10, 2008).

## Chapter 5. Do-It-Yourself Green Beauty

Agarwal A, Malhotra HS. "Camphor ingestion: an unusual cause of seizure." *The Journal of the Association of Physicians of India.* 2008 Feb; 56:123–4.

Ashour HM. "Antibacterial, antifungal, and anticancer activities of volatile oils and extracts from stems, leaves, and flowers of Eucalyptus sideroxylon and Eucalyptus torquata." *Cancer Biology & Therapy.* 2007 Dec 2; 7(3).

Atsumi T, Tonosaki K. "Smelling lavender and rosemary increases free radical scavenging activity and decreases cortisol level in saliva." *Psychiatry Research.* 2007 Feb 28; 150(1):89–96.

Beaumont DM, Mark TM Jr, Hills R, Dixon P, Veit B, Garrett N. "The effects of chrysin, a Passiflora incarnata extract, on natural killer cell activity in male Sprague-Dawley rats undergoing abdominal surgery." *AANA Journal.* 2008 Apr; 76(2):113–7.

Bell SG. "The therapeutic use of honey." *Neonatal Network.* 2007 Jul–Aug; 26(4):247–51.

Blaut M, Braune A, Wunderlich S, Sauer P, Schneider H, Glatt H. "Mutagenicity of arbutin in mammalian cells after activation by human intestinal bacteria." *Food and Chemical Toxicology.* 2006 Nov; 44(11):1940–7.

Burke KE. "Interaction of vitamins C and E as better cosmeceuticals." *Dermatological Therapy.* 2007 Sep–Oct; 20(5):314–21.

Conney AH, Kramata P, Lou YR, Lu YP. "Effect of caffeine on UVB-induced carcinogenesis, apoptosis, and the elimination of UVB-induced patches of p53 mutant epidermal cells in SKH-1 mice." *Carcinogenesis.* 2008 26(8):1465–1472.

Cosgrove MC, Franco OH, Granger SP, Murray PG, Mayes AE. "Dietary nutrient intakes and skin-aging appearance among middle-aged American women." *American Journal of Clinical Nutrition.* 2007 Oct; 86(4):1225–31.

Cosmetic Ingredient Review Expert Panel. "Final report on the safety assessment of Ricinus Communis (Castor) Seed Oil, Hydrogenated Castor Oil, Glyceryl Ricinoleate, Glyceryl Ricinoleate SE, Ricinoleic Acid, Potassium Ricinoleate, Sodium Ricinoleate,

Zinc Ricinoleate, Cetyl Ricinoleate, Ethyl Ricinoleate, Glycol Ricinoleate, Isopropyl Ricinoleate, Methyl Ricinoleate, and Octyldodecyl Ricinoleate." *International Journal of Toxicology.* 2007; 26 Suppl 3:31–77.

Elmore AR, Cosmetic Ingredient Review Expert Panel. "Final report on the safety assessment of aluminum silicate, calcium silicate, magnesium aluminum silicate, magnesium silicate, magnesium trisilicate, sodium magnesium silicate, zirconium silicate, attapulgite, bentonite, Fuller's earth, hectorite, kaolin, lithium magnesium silicate, lithium magnesium sodium silicate, montmorillonite, pyrophyllite, and zeolite." *International Journal of Toxicology.* 2003; 22 Suppl 1:37–102.

Facino RM, Carini M, Aldini G, Saibene L, Pietta P, Mauri P. "Echinacoside and caffeoyl conjugates protect collagen from free radical-induced degradation: a potential use of Echinacea extracts in the prevention of skin photodamage." *Planta Medica.* 1995 Dec; 61(6):510–4.

Foitzik K, Hoting E, Förster T, Pertile P, Paus R. "L-carnitine-L-tartrate promotes human hair growth in vitro." *Experimental Dermatology.* 2007 Nov; 16(11):936–45.

Frosch PJ, Peiler D, Grunert V, Grunenberg B. "Efficacy of barrier creams in comparison to skin care products in dental laboratory technicians—a controlled trial." *Journal der Deutschen Dermatologischen Gesellschaft.* 2003 Jul; 1(7):547–57.

Habashy RR, Abdel-Naim AB, Khalifa AE, Al-Azizi MM. "Anti-inflammatory effects of jojoba liquid wax in experimental models." *Pharmacological Research.* 2005 Feb; 51(2):95–105.

Heber GK, Markovic B, Hayes A. "An immunohistological study of anhydrous topical ascorbic acid compositions on ex vivo human skin." *Journal of Cosmetic Dermatology.* 2006 Jun; 5(2):150–6.

Henley DV, Lipson N, Korach KS, Bloch CA. "Prepubertal gynecomastia linked to lavender and tea tree oils." *New England Journal of Medicine.* 2007 Feb 1; 356(5):479–85.

Higa Y, Kawabe M, Nabae K, Toda Y, Kitamoto S, Hara T, Tanaka N, Kariya K, Takahashi M. "Kojic acid—absence of tumor-initiating activity in rat liver, and of carcinogenic and photogenotoxic potential in mouse skin." *The Journal of Toxicological Sciences.* 2007 May; 32(2):143–59.

Ho YS, Lai CS, Liu HI, Ho SY, Tai C, Pan MH, Wang YJ. "Dihydrolipoic acid inhibits skin tumor promotion through anti-inflammation and anti-oxidation." *Biochemical Pharmacology.* 2007 Jun 1; 73(11):1786–95.

Jacobson EL, Kim H, Kim M, Williams JD, Coyle DL, Coyle WR, Grove G, Rizer RL, Stratton MS, Jacobson MK. "A topical lipophilic niacin derivative increases NAD, epidermal differentiation and barrier function in photodamaged skin." *Experimental Dermatology.* 2007 Jun; 16(6):490–9.

Janson M. "Orthomolecular medicine: the therapeutic use of dietary supplements for anti-aging." *Clinical Interventions in Aging.* 2006; 1(3):261–5.

Jarrahi M. "An experimental study of the effects of Matricaria chamomilla extract on cutaneous burn wound healing in albino rats." *Natural Product Research.* 2008 Mar 20; 22(5): 423–8.

Jun SY, Park KM, Choi KW, Jang MK, Kang HY, Lee SH, Park KH, Cha J. "Inhibitory effects of arbutin-beta-glycosides synthesized from enzymatic transglycosylation for melanogenesis." *Biotechnology Letter.* 2008 Apr 1; 30(4):743–8.

Katiyar SK. "Grape seed proanthocyanidines and skin cancer prevention: inhibition of oxidative stress and protection of immune system." *Molecular Nutrition & Food Research.* 2008 Apr 2. http://www.ncbi.nlm.nih.gov/pubmed/18384090 (accessed June 10, 2008).

Katiyar S, Elmets CA, Katiyar SK. "Green tea and skin cancer: photoimmunology, angiogenesis and DNA repair." *Journal of Nutritional Biochemistry.* 2007 May; 18(5):287–96.

Kwakman PH, Van den Akker JP, Güçlü A, Aslami H, Binnekade JM, de Boer L, Boszhard L, Paulus F, Middelhoek P, te Velde AA, Vandenbroucke-Grauls CM, Schultz MJ, Zaat SA. "Medical-grade honey kills antibiotic-resistant bacteria in vitro and eradicates skin colonization." *Clinical Infection Diseases.* 2008 Jun 1; 46(11):1677–82.

Lotfy M, Badra G, Burham W, Alenzi FQ. "Combined use of honey, bee propolis and myrrh in healing a deep, infected wound in a patient with diabetes mellitus." *British Journal of Biomedical Sciences.* 2006; 63(4):171–3.

Marel AK, Lizard G, Izard JC, Latruffe N, Delmas D. "Inhibitory effects of trans-resveratrol analogs molecules on the proliferation and the cell cycle progression of human colon tumoral cells." *Molecular Nutrition and Food Research.* 2008 May; 52(5):538–48.

McDaniel DH, Neudecker BA, Dinardo JC, Lewis JA 2nd, Maibach HI. "Idebenone: a new antioxidant—Part I. Relative assessment of oxidative stress protection capacity compared to commonly known antioxidants." *Journal of Cosmetic Dermatology.* 2005 Jan; 4(1):10–7.

Monroe KR, Murphy SP, Kolonel LN, Pike MC. "Prospective study of grapefruit intake and risk of breast cancer in postmenopausal women: the Multiethnic Cohort Study." *British Journal of Cancer.* 2007 Aug 6; 97(3):440–5.

Morissette G, Germain L, Marceau F. "The antiwrinkle effect of topical concentrated 2-dimethylaminoethanol involves a vacuolar cytopathology." *The British Journal of Dermatology.* 2007 Mar; 156(3):433–9.

Nandakumar V, Singh T, Katiyar SK. "Multi-targeted prevention and therapy of cancer by proanthocyanidins." *Cancer Letters.* 2008 May 3. http://www.cancerletters.info/article/S0304–3835(08)00253-X/pdf (accessed June 10, 2008).

Schuhmacher A, Reichling J, Schnitzler P. "Virucidal effect of peppermint oil on the enveloped viruses herpes simplex virus type 1 and type 2 in vitro." *Phytomedicine.* 2003; 10(6–7):504–10.

Schwarz A, Maeda A, Gan D, Mammone T, Matsui MS, Schwarz T. "Green tea phenol extracts reduce UVB-induced DNA damage in human cells via interleukin-12." *Photochemistry and Photobiology.* 2008 Mar–Apr; 84(2):350–5.

Segaert S, Duvold LB. "Calcipotriol cream: a review of its use in the management of psoriasis." *Journal of Dermatological Treatment.* 2006; 17(6):327–37.

Spasov AA, Orobinskaia TA, Mazanova LS, Motov AA, Sysuev BB. "Antiinflammatory effect of bischofit ointment." *Eksperimentalnaya i Klinicheskaya Farmakologia.* 2007 Nov–Dec; 70(6):32–5.

Steerenberg PA, Garssen J, Dortant P, Hollman PC, Alink GM, Dekker M, Bueno-de-Mesquita HB, Van Loveren H. "Protection of UV-induced suppression of skin contact hypersensitivity: a common feature of flavonoids after oral administration?" *Photochemical Photobiology.* 1998 Apr; 67(4):456–61.

Thiboutot D. "Versatility of azelaic acid 15% gel in treatment of inflammatory acne vulgaris." *Journal of Drugs in Dermatology.* 2008 Jan; 7(1):13–6.

Tournas JA, Lin FH, Burch JA, Selim MA, Monteiro-Riviere NA, Zielinski JE, Pinnell SR. "Ubiquinone, idebenone, and kinetin provide ineffective photoprotection to skin when compared to a topical antioxidant combination of vitamins C and E with ferulic acid." *Journal of Investigative Dermatology.* 2006 May; 126(5):1185–7.

Villaseñor IM, Simon MK, Villanueva AM. "Comparative potencies of nutraceuticals in chemically induced skin tumor prevention." *Nutrition and Cancer.* 2002; 44(1):66–70.

Walle UK, Walle T. "Induction of human UDP-glucuronosyltransferase UGT1A1 by flavonoids-structural requirements." *Drug Metabolism and Disposition.* 2002 May; 30(5):564–9.

Yusuf N, Irby C, Katiyar SK, Elmets CA. "Photoprotective effects of green tea polyphenols." *Photodermatology, Photoimmunology and Photomedicine.* 2007 Feb; 23(1):48–56.

## Chapter 9. Green Moisturizers

Johnson W Jr, Cosmetic Ingredient Review Expert Panel. "Final report on the safety assessment of PEG–25 propylene glycol stearate, PEG–75 propylene glycol stearate, PEG–120 propylene glycol stearate, PEG–10 propylene glycol, PEG–8 propylene glycol cocoate, and PEG–55 propylene glycol oleate." *International Journal of Toxicology.* 2001; 20 Suppl 4:13–26.

## Chapter 10. Green Sun Protection

Alpert PT, Shaikh U. "The effects of vitamin D deficiency and insufficiency on the endocrine and paracrine systems." *Biological Research for Nursing.* 2007 Oct; 9(2):117–29.

Armas LA, Dowell S, Akhter M, Duthuluru S, Huerter C, Hollis BW, Lund R, Heaney RP. "Ultraviolet-B radiation increases serum 25-hydroxyvitamin D levels: the effect of UVB dose and skin color." *Journal of American Academy of Dermatology.* 2007 Oct; 57(4): 588–93.

Armstrong BK, Kricker A. "Sun exposure and non-Hodgkin lymphoma." *Cancer Epidemiology, Biomarkers and Prevention.* 2007 Mar; 16(3):396–400.

Azizi E, Iscovich J, Pavlotsky F, Shafir R, Luria I, Federenko L, Fuchs Z, Milman V, Gur E, Farbstein H, Tal O. "Use of sunscreen is linked with elevated naevi counts in Israeli school children and adolescents." *Melanoma Research.* 2000 Oct; 10(5):491–8.

Beissert S, Loser K. "Molecular and cellular mechanisms of photocarcinogenesis." *Photochemistry and Photobiology.* 2008 Jan–Feb; 84(1):29–34.

Blount AM. "Amphibole content of cosmetic and pharmaceutical talcs." *Environmental Health Perspectives.* 1991 Aug; 94:225–30.

Chatelain E, Gabard B, Surber C. "Skin penetration and sun protection factor of five UV filters: effect of the vehicle." *Skin Pharmacology and Applied Skin Physiology.* 2003 Jan–Feb; 16(1):28–35.

Cook N, Freeman S. "Report of 19 cases of photoallergic contact dermatitis to sunscreens seen at the Skin and Cancer Foundation." *The Australasian Journal of Dermatology.* 2001 Nov; 42(4):257–9.

Gorham ED, Mohr SB, Garland CF, Chaplin G, Garland FC. "Do sunscreens increase risk of melanoma in populations residing at higher latitudes?" *Annals of Epidemology.* 2007 Dec; 17(12):956–63.

Heller, Eklund SP, Bartels LE, Agnholt J, Glerup H, Nielsen SL, Hvas CL, Dahlerup JF. "Vitamin D insufficiency—possible etiologic factor of autoimmune diseases." *Ugeskrift for Laeger.* 2007 Oct 22; 169(43):3655–60.

Institute of Food Technologists (IFT) (press release). "Difference Between Some Organic, Conventional Produce." Newswise.com. http://www.newswise.com/articles/view/506144 (accessed June 06, 2008).

 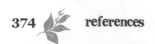

Jung K, Seifert M, Herrling T, Fuchs J. "UV-generated free radicals (FR) in skin: Their prevention by sunscreens and their induction by self-tanning agents." *Spectrochim Acta A Mol Biomol Spectrosc.* 2007 Oct 10.

Langseth H, Hankinson SE, Siemiatycki J, Weiderpass E. "Perineal use of talc and risk of ovarian cancer." *Journal of Epidemiology and Community Health.* 2008 Apr; 62(4):358–60.

Lin FH, Lin JY, Gupta RD, Tournas JA, Burch JA, Selim MA, Monteiro-Riviere NA, Grichnik JM, Zielinski J, Pinnell SR. "Ferulic acid stabilizes a solution of vitamins C and E and doubles its photoprotection of skin." *Journal of Investigative Dermatology.* 2005 Oct; 125(4):826–32.

Lin JY, Selim MA, Shea CR, Grichnik JM, Omar MM, Monteiro-Riviere NA, Pinnell SR. "UV photoprotection by combination topical antioxidants vitamin C and vitamin E." *Journal of American Academy of Dermatology.* 2003 Jun; 48(6):866–74.

Litonjua AA, Weiss ST. "Is vitamin D deficiency to blame for the asthma epidemic?" *Journal of Allergy and Clinical Immunology.* 2007 Nov; 120(5):1031–5.

Miniño AM, Heron MP, Murphy SL, Kochanek, KD. "Deaths: Final Data for 2004." *National Vital Statistics Reports. National Center for Health Statistics.* 2007; Vol. 55 (19):30–37.

Morley N, Clifford T, Salter L, Campbell S, Gould D, Curnow A. "The green tea polyphenol (-)-epigallocatechin gallate and green tea can protect human cellular DNA from ultraviolet and visible radiation-induced damage." *Photodermatology, Photoimmunology and Photomedicine.* 2005 Feb; 21(1):15–22.

Rass K, Reichrath J. "UV damage and DNA repair in malignant melanoma and nonmelanoma skin cancer." *Advances in Experimental Medicine and Biology.* 2008; 624:162–78.

Reichrath J. "Vitamin D and the skin: an ancient friend, revisited." *Experimental Dermatology.* 2007 Jul; 16(7):618–25.

Schlumpf M, Cotton B, Conscience M, Haller V, Steinmann B, Lichtensteiger W. "In vitro and in vivo estrogenicity of UV screens." *Environmental Health Perspectives.* 2001 Mar; 109(3):239–44.

Shaheen SO. "Vitamin D deficiency and the asthma epidemic." *Thorax.* 2008 Mar; 63(3):293.

Sies H, Stahl W. "Carotenoids and UV protection." *Photochemical and Photobiological Sciences.* 2004 Aug; 3(8):749–52.

Stahl W, Sies H. "Bioactivity and protective effects of natural carotenoids." *Biochimica et Biophysica Acta.* 2005 May 30; 1740(2):101–7.Tuohimaa P, Pukkala E, Scélo G, Olsen JH, Brewster DH, Hemminki K, Tracey E, Weiderpass E, Kliewer EV, Pompe-Kirn V, McBride ML, Martos C, Chia KS, Tonita JM, Jonasson JG, Boffetta P, Brennan P. "Does solar exposure, as indicated by the non-melanoma skin cancers, protect from solid cancers? vitamin D as a possible explanation." *European Journal of Cancer.* 2007 Jul; 43(11):1701–12.

Weinstock MA. "Do sunscreens increase or decrease melanoma risk: an epidemiologic evaluation." *Journal of Investigative Dermatology.* 1999 Sep; 4(1):97–100.

## Chapter 11. Green Body Care

Bassin EB, Wypij D, Davis RB, Mittleman MA. "Age-specific fluoride exposure in drinking water and osteosarcoma (United States)." *Cancer Causes and Controls.* 2006 May; 17(4):421–8.

Blaszczyk I, Grucka-Mamczar E, Kasperczyk S, Birkner E. "Influence of fluoride on rat kidney antioxidant system: effects of methionine and vitamin E." *Biological Trace Elements Research.* 2008 Jan; 121(1):51–9.

Bosetti C, McLaughlin JK, Tarone RE, Pira E, La Vecchia C. "Formaldehyde and cancer risk:

a quantitative review of cohort studies through 2006." *Annals of Oncology.* 2008 Jan; 19(1):29–43.

Bryan GT, Ertürk E, Yoshida O. "Production of urinary bladder carcinomas in mice by sodium saccharin." *Science.* 1970 Jun 5; 168(936):1238–40.

Chen GR, Dong L, Ge RS, Hardy MP. "Relationship between phthalates and testicular dysgenesis syndrome." *Zhonghua Nan Ke Xue (National Journal of Andrology).* 2007 Mar; 13(3):195–200.

Coplan MJ, Patch SC, Masters RD, Bachman MS. "Confirmation of and explanations for elevated blood lead and other disorders in children exposed to water disinfection and fluoridation chemicals." *Neurotoxicology.* 2007 Sep; 28(5):1032–42.

Edgar WM. "Sugar substitutes, chewing gum and dental caries—a review." *British Dental Journal.* 1998 Jan 10; 184(1):29–32.

Energy Information Administration. The Official Statistics of the U.S. Government. "Carbon Dioxide Emissions from the Consumption of Energy (Consumption of Petroleum, Natural Gas, and Coal and Flaring of Natural Gas), Selected Countries, Most Recent Annual Estimates, 1980-2006." The Energy Information Administration (EIA). http://www.eia.doe.gov/emeu/international/carbondioxide.html (accessed June 10, 2008).

Freni SC. "Exposure to high fluoride concentrations in drinking water is associated with decreased birth rates." *Journal of Toxicology and Environmental Health.* 1994 May; 42(1):109–21.

Heller KE, Eklund SA, Burt BA. "Dental caries and dental fluorosis at varying water fluoride concentrations." *Journal of Public Health and Dentistry.* 1997 Summer; 57(3):136–43.

Huang XH, Ip HS, Yu JZ. "Determination of trace amounts of formaldehyde in acetone." *Analytica Chimica Acta.* 2007 Dec 5; 604(2):134–8.

Lee DE, Pai J, Mullapudui U, Alexoff DL, Ferrieri R, Dewey SL. "The effects of inhaled acetone on place conditioning in adolescent rats." *Pharmacology and Biochemistry Behavior.* 2008 Mar; 89(1):101–5.

Lottrup G, Andersson AM, Leffers H, Mortensen GK, Toppari J, Skakkebaek NE, Main KM. "Possible impact of phthalates on infant reproductive health." *International Journal of Andrology.* 2006 Feb; 29(1):172–80; discussion 181–5.

Main KM, Mortensen GK, Kaleva MM, Boisen KA, Damgaard IN, Chellakooty M, Schmidt IM, Suomi AM, Virtanen HE, Petersen DV, Andersson AM, Toppari J, Skakkebaek NE. "Human breast milk contamination with phthalates and alterations of endogenous reproductive hormones in infants three months of age." *Environmental Health Perspectives.* 2006 Feb; 114(2):270–6.

National Toxicology Program. "NTP Toxicology and Carcinogenesis Studies of Sodium Fluoride (CAS No. 7681–49–4) in F344/N Rats and B6C3F1 Mice (Drinking Water Studies)." *National Toxicology Program Technical Report Series.* 1990 Dec; 393:1–448.

Park KK, Sohn Y, Liem A, Kim HJ, Stewart BC, Miller JA. "The electrophilic, mutagenic and tumorigenic activities of phenyl and 4-nitrophenyl vinyl ethers and their epoxide metabolites." *Carcinogenesis.* 1997 Feb; 18(2):431–7.

Redmond AF, Cherry DV, Bowers DE Jr. "Acute illness and recovery in adult female rats following ingestion of a tooth whitener containing 6% hydrogen peroxide." *American Journal of Dentistry.* 1997 Dec; 10(6):268–71.

Ribeiro DA, Marques ME, Salvadori DM. "Study of DNA damage induced by dental bleaching agents in vitro." *Brazilian Oral Research.* 2006 Jan-Mar; 20(1):47–51.

Sainio EL, Engström K, Henriks-Eckerman ML, Kanerva L. "Allergenic ingredients in nail polishes." *Contact Dermatitis.* 1997 Oct; 37(4):155–62.

Tripathi M, Khanna SK, Das M. "Usage of saccharin in food products and its intake by the population of Lucknow, India." *Food Additives and Contaminants.* 2006 Dec; 23(12):1265–75.

Watt BE, Proudfoot AT, Vale JA. "Hydrogen peroxide poisoning." *Toxicological Reviews.* 2004; 23(1):51–7.

Wurtz T, Houari S, Mauro N, Macdougall M, Peters H, Berdal A. "Fluoride at non-toxic dose affects odontoblast gene expression in vitro." *Toxicology.* 2008 July 10; 249(1):26–34.

## Chapter 12. Green Hair Care

Ambrosone CB, Abrams SM, Gorlewska-Roberts K, Kadlubar FF. "Hair dye use, meat intake, and tobacco exposure and presence of carcinogen-DNA adducts in exfoliated breast ductal epithelial cells." *Archives of Biochemistry and Biophysics.* 2007 Aug 15; 464(2):169–75.

Bolt HM, Golka K. "The debate on carcinogenicity of permanent hair dyes: new insights." *Critical Reviews in Toxicology.* 2007; 37(6):521–36.

de Sanjosé S, Benavente Y, Nieters A, Foretova L, Maynadié M, Cocco PL, Staines A, Vornanen M, Boffetta P, Becker N, Alvaro T, Brennan P. "Association between personal use of hair dyes and lymphoid neoplasms in Europe." *American Journal of Epidemiology.* 2006 Jul 1; 164(1):47–55.

Heineman EF, Ward MH, McComb RD, Weisenburger DD, Zahm SH. "Hair dyes and risk of glioma among Nebraska women." *Cancer Causes and Control.* 2005 Sep; 16(7):857–64.

Kelsh MA, Alexander DD, Kalmes RM, Buffler PA. "Personal use of hair dyes and risk of bladder cancer: a meta-analysis of epidemiologic data." *Cancer Causes and Controls.* 2008 Feb 20. [Epub ahead of print] Accessed on June 07, 2008 via Pubmed.com.

La Vecchia C, Tavani A. "Epidemiological evidence on hair dyes and the risk of cancer in humans." *European Journal of Cancer Prevention.* 1995 Feb; 4(1):31–43.

McCall EE, Olshan AF, Daniels JL. "Maternal hair dye use and risk of neuroblastoma in offspring." *Cancer Causes and Control.* 2005 Aug; 16(6):743–8.

Miligi L, Costantini AS, Benvenuti A, Veraldi A, Tumino R, Ramazzotti V, Vindigni C, Amadori D, Fontana A, Rodella S, Stagnaro E, Crosignani P, Vineis P. "Personal use of hair dyes and hematolymphopoietic malignancies." *Archives of Environmental Occupational Health.* 2005 Sep-Oct; 60(5):249–56.

Park KK, Sohn Y, Liem A, Kim HJ, Stewart BC, Miller JA. "The electrophilic, mutagenic and tumorigenic activities of phenyl and 4-nitrophenyl vinyl ethers and their epoxide metabolites." *Carcinogenesis.* 1997 Feb; 18(2):431–7.

Zhang Y, Sanjose SD, Bracci PM, Morton LM, Wang R, Brennan P, Hartge P, Boffetta P, Becker N, Maynadie M, Foretova L, Cocco P, Staines A, Holford T, Holly EA, Nieters A, Benavente Y, Bernstein L, Zahm SH, Zheng T. "Personal use of hair dye and the risk of certain subtypes of non-Hodgkin lymphoma." *American Journal Epidemiology.* 2008 Jun 1; 167(11):1321–31.

## Chapter 13. Green Baby Care

Al-Saleh I, Arif J, El-Doush I, Al-Sanea N, Jabbar AA, Billedo G, Shinwari N, Mashhour A, Mohamed G. "Carcinogen DNA adducts and the risk of colon cancer: case-control study." *Biomarkers.* 2008 Mar-Apr; 13(2):201–16.

Concin N, Hofstetter G, Plattner B, Tomovski C, Fiselier K, Gerritzen K, Fessler S, Windbichler G, Zeimet A, Ulmer H, Siegl H, Rieger K, Concin H, Grob K. "Mineral oil paraffins in human body fat and milk." *Food and Chemical Toxicology.* 2008 Feb; 46(2):544–52.

Huhtala V, Lehtonen L, Heinonen R, Korvenranta H. "Infant massage compared with crib vibrator in the treatment of colicky infants." *Pediatrics.* 2000 Jun; 105(6):E84.

Lahat S, Mimouni FB, Ashbel G, Dollberg S. "Energy expenditure in growing preterm infants receiving massage therapy." *Journal of American College of Nutritionists.* 2007 Aug; 26(4):356–9.

Macioszek VK, Kononowicz AK. "The evaluation of the genotoxicity of two commonly used food colors: Quinoline Yellow (E 104) and Brilliant Black BN (E 151)." *Cellular and Molecular Biology Letter.* 2004; 9(1):107–22.

O Higgins M, St James Roberts I, Glover V. "Postnatal depression and mother and infant outcomes after infant massage." *Journal of Affective Disorders.* 2008 Jul; 109(1–2):189–92.

Peleg O, Bar-Oz B, Arad I. "Coma in a premature infant associated with the transdermal absorption of propylene glycol." *Acta Paediatrica.* 1998 Nov; 87(11):1195–6.

Rundle A, Tang D, Zhou J, Cho S, Perera F. "The association between glutathione S-transferase M1 genotype and polycyclic aromatic hydrocarbon-DNA adducts in breast tissue." *Cancer Epidemiology, Biomarkers and Prevention.* 2000 Oct; 9(10):1079–85.

Sankaranarayanan K, Mondkar JA, Chauhan MM, Mascarenhas BM, Mainkar AR, Salvi RY. "Oil massage in neonates: an open randomized controlled study of coconut versus mineral oil." *Indian Pediatrics.* 2005 Sep; 42(9):877–84.

Underdown A, Barlow J, Chung V, Stewart-Brown S. "Massage intervention for promoting mental and physical health in infants aged under six months." *Cochrane Database of Systemic Reviews.* 2006 Oct 18; (4): CD005038.

Wang S, Chanock S, Tang D, Li Z, Jedrychowski W, Perera FP. "Assessment of interactions between PAH exposure and genetic polymorphisms on PAH-DNA adducts in African American, Dominican, and Caucasian mothers and newborns." *Cancer Epidemiology, Biomarkers and Prevention.* 2008 Feb; 17(2):405–413.

## Chapter 14. Organic and Mineral Makeup

Jones N, Ray B, Ranjit KT, Manna AC. "Antibacterial activity of ZnO nanoparticle suspensions on a broad spectrum of microorganisms." *FEMS Microbiology Letters.* 2008 Feb; 279(1):71–6.

Preussmann R, Ivankovic S. "Absence of carcinogenic activity in BD rats after oral administration of high doses of bismuth oxychloride." *Food and Cosmetic Toxicology.* 1975 Oct; 13(5):543–4.

Reddy KM, Feris K, Bell J, Wingett DG, Hanley C, Punnoose A. "Selective toxicity of zinc oxide nanoparticles to prokaryotic and eukaryotic systems." *Applied Physics Letter.* 2007 May 24; 90(213902):2139021–2139023.

Wilson MR, Foucaud L, Barlow PG, Hutchison GR, Sales J, Simpson RJ, Stone V. "Nanoparticle interactions with zinc and iron: implications for toxicology and inflammation." *Toxicology and Applied Pharmacology.* 2007 Nov 15; 225(1):80–9.

## Chapter 15. Green Fragrances

Chen GR, Dong L, Ge RS, Hardy MP. "Relationship between phthalates and testicular dysgenesis syndrome." *Zhonghua Nan Ke Xue (National Journal of Andrology).* 2007 Mar; 13(3):195–200.

Donovan M, Tiwary CM, Axelrod D, Sasco AJ, Jones L, Hajek R, Sauber E, Kuo J, Davis DL. "Personal care products that contain estrogens or xenoestrogens may increase breast cancer risk." *Medical Hypotheses.* 2007; 68(4):756–66.

Irvine DS. "Male reproductive health: cause for concern?" *Andrologia.* 2000 Sep; 32(4–5):195–208.

Reiner JL, Wong CM, Arcaro KF, Kannan K. "Synthetic musk fragrances in human milk from the United States." *Environ Science and Technology.* 2007 Jun 1; 41(11):3815–20.

Singleton DW, Feng Y, Chen Y, Busch SJ, Lee AV, Puga A, Khan SA. "Bisphenol-A and estradiol exert novel gene regulation in human MCF-7 derived breast cancer cells." *Molecular and Cellular Endocrinology.* 2004 Jun 30; 221(1–2):47–55.

Zhu J, Zeng X, Liu T, Qian K, Han Y, Xue S, Tucker B, Schultz G, Coats J, Rowley W, Zhang A. "Adult repellency and larvicidal activity of five plant essential oils against mosquitoes." *Journal of American Mosquito Control Association.* 2006 Sep; 22(3):515–22.

## Chapter 16. Green Beauty Detox

Altieri A, La Vecchia C, Negri E. "Fluid intake and risk of bladder and other cancers." *European Journal of Clinical Nutrition.* 2003 Dec; 57 Supplement 2:S59–68.

Bandera EV, Kushi LH, Moore DF, Gifkins DM, McCullough ML. "Dietary lipids and endometrial cancer: the current epidemiologic evidence." *Cancer Causes and Control.* 2007 Sep; 18(7):687–703.

Bissonauth V, Shatenstein B, Ghadirian P. "Nutrition and breast cancer among sporadic cases and gene mutation carriers: an overview." *Cancer Detection and Prevention.* 2008; 32(1):52–64.

Campbell T. Colin. *The China Study: The Most Comprehensive Study of Nutrition Ever Conducted and the Startling Implications for Diet, Weight Loss and Long-Term Health.* (BenBella Books, 2006): 161–162.

Hede K. "Fat may fuel breast cancer growth." *Journal of National Cancer Institute.* 2008 Mar 5; 100(5):298–9.

Kobayashi N, Barnard RJ, Said J, Hong-Gonzalez J, Corman DM, Ku M, Doan NB, Gui D, Elashoff D, Cohen P, Aronson WJ. "Effect of low-fat diet on development of prostate cancer and Akt phosphorylation in the Hi-Myc transgenic mouse model." *Cancer Research.* 2008 Apr 15; 68(8):3066–73.

Manz F. "Hydration and disease." *Journal of American College of Nutrition.* 2007 Oct; 26(5 Suppl):535S–541S.

Manz F, Wentz A. "The importance of good hydration for the prevention of chronic diseases." *Nutritional Reviews.* 2005 Jun; 63(6 Pt 2):S2–5.

Reynolds KA, Mena KD, Gerba CP. "Risk of waterborne illness via drinking water in the United States." *Reviews of Environmental Contamination and Toxicology.* 2008; 192:117–58.

Wu AH, Pike MC, Stram DO. "Meta-analysis: dietary fat intake, serum estrogen levels, and the risk of breast cancer." *Journal of the National Cancer Institute.* 1999 Mar 17; 91(6): 529–34.

# index

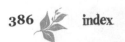

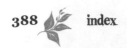

LSD, 310
L-Theanine, 120
lubricants, propylene glycol and, 24
Lucretius, 34
Lumene, 259
Lutens, Serge, 322–23
LVMH. *See* Moet-Hennessy Louis Vuitton
lycophene, 119, 124
lymph, 6, 201, 249
lymph ducts, toxins and, 6
lymphoma, 14, 278
Lyral, 36, 39

**M**
MAC, 21, 304–5
macadamia oil, 56
macrocyclic musk compounds, 321
Madonna, 57–58
magnesium, 118, 126, 145
magnesium salts, 4
Make Up For Ever brushes, 305
makeup. *See* cosmetics; mineral makeup
makeup remover, 153, 157
Malkan, Stacy, 18, 313
mandarin, 146, 155, 241, 247
manganese sulfate, 363
manufacturers, contacting, 47, 70
maple syrup, 343, 349
Marceau, Francois, 117
marigold, 290
marketing, 41, 42, 55, 139–41
marshmallow, 281
Mary Kay, 260
mascara, 306–8
masks, 173–75, 179–81. *See also* exfoliants
massage
    baby, 292–94
    hair care and, 345
Masters, John, 264, 274
*Matricaria recutita. See* chamomile
Max Factor, 21
mayblossom, 149
mayonnaise, 151
McCartney, Stella, 67
McLuhan, Martin, 294–96
MEA. *See* monoethanolamine
measuring glasses, 101–2
meats, 334, 336
medical waste, 337
medications
    eye circles and, 201
    skin and, 5
medicine droppers, 102
medulla, 262
melanocytes, 3
melanoma. *See* skin cancer
melissa oil, 168
*Mentha piperita. See* peppermint
menthol, 163

mercury, 314
merthiolate, 365
metalloestrogen, 23
methamine, 363
methoxycinnamate, 219, 220
methyl eugenol, 39
methyl methacrylate, 363
methylbenzene, 365
methylbenzylidene, 219
methylparaben, 28, 363. *See also* parabens
mica, 74, 224, 314
microdermabrasion, 172–73. *See also* exfoliants
microwaves, 101–2
migraines, 38–39
Milani, 259
milk, 125, 150, 151, 152, 155, 156–57, 177, 181,
    192, 239, 240, 241, 245, 291, 349
milk of magnesia, 151, 157
mimosa, 324
*Mimulus moschatus. See* muskflower
mineral makeup
    application tips for, 307
    blushers/highlighters and, 305–6
    eyeliners/eye shadows and, 308–10
    foundations and, 300–305
    homemade, 312
    lip balms and, 310–11
    lip colors and, 313–15
    mascara and, 306–8
    overview of, 298–300
mineral oil, 52, 97, 146, 267, 272, 287, 363
mineral shimmer, 247
minerals
    in aloe vera, 109
    in cosmetics (*see* mineral makeup)
    cosmetics and, 5
    as element in green beauty products, 74
    in sunscreens, 225
mint, 147, 326, 346
mixing bowls, 102
Moet-Hennessy Louis Vuitton, 21
moisturizers
    acne and, 207
    cleansers and, 143
    costs of, 94
    eye creams and (*see* eye creams)
    homemade, 194–96
    necessity of, 186–87
    need for separate, 46–47, 191–92
    as part of daily routine, 10, 136
    skin and, 3–4
    types of, 187–92
    wrinkles and, 204
Moisturizers by Dr. Hauschka, 193
moles, 216
monoethanolamine, 85, 146, 233, 363
morning cleansing, 142
mortars, 101–2
*Moschus moschiferus. See* musks

index ❦ 391

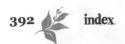

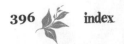

# about the website

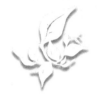

## www.thegreenbeautyguide.com

**W**ant to know more about going green when it comes to beauty? Head on to *The Green Beauty Guide's* homepage www.thegreenbeauty guide.com. Here you will find in-depth information and up-to-date research, as well as some of the most amazing facts about the cosmetic industry and chemicals that won't ever appear in print in glossy magazines. There are tons of useful tips and checklists, as well as reviews of latest offerings in the organic beauty trade. The website also holds great contests with green beauty prizes from both well-known organic and all-natural brands, including Julie Garbriel's skincare line Petite Marie Organics, as well as autographed copies of this book.

When you register as a Green Beauty Guide blog user, you are entitled to receive a monthly *Green Beauty Bulletin* newsletter. That's your mini-guide to the latest organic offerings in skin care, makeup, hair care, and baby care. From the latest facts in health-conscious beauty to environmentally friendly beauty finds, it's all here, at your fingertips.

Green living is, of course, much more than shunning toxic cosmetic ingredients and switching to organic olive oil as a beauty cure-all. Still, it's an important step in diminishing the toxic load that has accumulated over years. Going green in your beauty routine may become your first and probably most enjoyable step toward good health and good looks. So visit www.thegreenbeautyguide.com.

Buy less, waste less, worry less, and enjoy life even more!

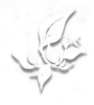

# about the author

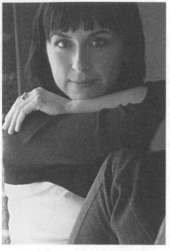

**Julie Gabriel** is a registered holistic nutritionist, writer, and editor of beauty and fashion. In the early 1990s, she worked in production at *CNN's Style with Elsa Klensch*. Gabriel was the associate beauty editor for *Harper's Bazaar* (Eastern European editions) and beauty editor for *Atmospheres*. She has written more than five hundred articles and features on fashion, beauty, and lifestyle.

Since 2002 Julie Gabriel has worked as a founding editor of *Toronto Daily News* (www.torontodailynews. com), *Fashion Monitor* (www.toronto.fashion-monitor. com), and *Organic Life&Style* (www.organiclifeand style.com), promoting an organic lifestyle and environmental awareness.

Gabriel's first book, *Clear Skin: Organic Action Plan for Acne*, was published in January 2007. She created an organic skin care line called Petite Marie Organics to help women and men easily jumpstart a green beauty routine. This organic line includes zero synthetic preservatives, detergents, or artificial fragrances. Julie Gabriel lives in England with her husband and their daughter.